Praise for

Chronic

"This book shines an alarming light on emerging infections that cause chronic illnesses. Brimming with bulletproof science, *Chronic* is an insightful clarion call for more attention to this plague of the twenty-first century."
— **Sanjay Gupta, MD**

"History will reflect back upon this book as a revelation for millions living with chronic illness. It's a fascinating, superbly researched dive into the mysteries of autoimmune diseases and provides critical insights to patients and clinicians. *Chronic* is bold, iconoclastic, and addresses one of the most important and challenging problems facing modern medicine with compassion, love, and hope."
— **Ying Zhang, MD, PhD,** professor of molecular microbiology and immunology, Johns Hopkins University

"This trailblazing book should serve to galvanize efforts to solve the autoimmune crisis in the same way *And the Band Played On* did for HIV."
— **George Church, PhD,** professor of genetics, Harvard Medical School and Harvard–MIT Health Sciences and Technology

"Phillips and Parish take us on a personal, illuminating journey of scientific discovery. Their brilliant work could not have come at a more urgent time. *Chronic* is both thoughtful and thought-provoking, but perhaps most of all, it's intellectually and emotionally honest. A must-read for everyone, but even more so for physicians of all specialties."
— **Haideh Hirmand, MD, MPA, FACS,** clinical assistant professor of surgery, Weill Cornell Medical College

"Speaking truth to power is hard. Speaking truth to established medical and scientific institutions is nearly impossible . . . and extraordinarily rare. But this book does exactly that — it is an act of bravery in its purest form, and it's for all of us, as none of us are immune."

— **Kristen T. Honey, PhD, PMP,** policy advisor, White House Office of Science and Technology Policy (2015–17); senior research scholar, Stanford University

"A powerfully informative guide for patient and practitioner from a misinformed past toward a future of recovery and health."

— **David Perlmutter, MD,** #1 *New York Times* best-selling author of *Grain Brain* and *Brain Wash*

"A clarion call to start reversing the enormous human cost of autoimmune and chronic disease by finally addressing actual root causes."

— **Michael VanElzakker, PhD,** neuroscientist, Massachusetts General Hospital/Harvard Medical School

"With fascinating case studies and the latest science, *Chronic* offers hope for achieving a better future for the millions suffering with complex and severe symptoms."

— **Terry Wahls, MD,** author of *The Wahls Protocol*

"Phillips and Parish show us where and how the medical paradigm for chronic illness has failed us all and exposes the truth. It's a modern-day version of *The Emperor's New Clothes.*"

— **Holly Ahern,** associate professor of microbiology, SUNY

"An informative guide to 'the pandemic in plain sight,' urgent without undue alarmism." — *Kirkus Reviews*

Chronic

Chronic

The Hidden Cause of the
Autoimmune Pandemic and
How to Get Healthy Again

Steven Phillips, MD, and Dana Parish

with Kristin Loberg

MARINER BOOKS
An Imprint of HarperCollins*Publishers*
Boston ▪ New York

The information contained in this book is intended to provide helpful and informative material on the subject addressed. It is not intended to serve as a replacement for professional medical advice. Any use of the information in this book is at the reader's discretion. The authors and publisher disclaim any and all liability arising directly and indirectly from the use or application of any information contained in this book.

First Mariner Books edition 2022
marinerbooks.com

Designed by Chrissy Kurpeski

Library of Congress Cataloging-in-Publication Data has been applied for.
ISBN 9780358561903 (trade paper)
ISBN 9780358066699 (e-book)
ISBN 9780358311256 (audio)

1 2021
4500844314

To the broken ones.
May this book empower you to feel whole again.

"Out of suffering have emerged the strongest souls;
the most massive characters are seared with scars."
—*Edwin Hubbell Chapin*

"Education is the most powerful weapon
which you can use to change the world."
—*Nelson Mandela*

Contents

Foreword

Imagine a pandemic that has affected 50 million Americans. The underlying cause is unknown and therefore there's no cure. No one is immune and there is nowhere to hide. It has already spread throughout all 50 states and across the globe. This could easily be the storyline for a Michael Crichton or Stephen King novel. Unfortunately, this is not fiction.

In *Chronic: The Hidden Cause of the Autoimmune Pandemic and How to Get Healthy Again*, Dr. Steven Phillips and Dana Parish issue a clarion call that an autoimmune pandemic is ravaging America and other parts of the world. The estimated 50 million Americans diagnosed with an autoimmune disease is not a number concocted by someone on social media but rather statistics from the American Autoimmune Related Diseases Association. You would expect that government agencies and scientists would be feverishly working to determine the cause of this steadily growing scourge. Sadly, that doesn't appear to be the case.

Contrast this rather anemic effort to that of the mysterious disease that was killing its victims by suppressing their immune systems in the 1980s and 1990s. The fear that no one was immune triggered an all-out race to find its cause and a cure. Without that intensive research effort in AIDS/HIV, we would not have developed the combination HAART therapy, which has effectively controlled the disease. This begs the question raised in *Chronic*: Why is the medical community complacently treating patients with inflammatory autoimmune diseases with immunosuppressives when these drugs only treat symptoms — not root cause — and put patients at greater risk for developing potentially life-threatening opportunistic infections and cancers?

To do this is contradictory to the principles of precision medicine, which is based upon the notion that development of effective therapeutic interventions requires an understanding of the processes underlying the pathogenesis of the disease. How can we expect to cure autoimmune diseases when we don't even know what we are treating?

In *Chronic*, Phillips and Parish provide compelling evidence that infections play a prominent role in the cause of autoimmune diseases. They illustrate how MS, RA, lupus, fibromyalgia, and others are simply names given to a set of symptoms rather than identifying the underlying cause.

This book also reveals the fact that the rise of these infections mirrors the spreading pandemic of autoimmune diseases. The sad reality is that patients with unrecognized infections are being labeled as having autoimmune diseases and sentenced to lifelong treatment with powerful immunosuppressive drugs, while their physicians won't consider the possibility that pathogens play a causative role in chronic inflammatory illness. And some of these doctors, to whom patients entrust their lives, are ridiculing them for even suggesting they be tested.

Blind allegiance to what you are spoon-fed by a professional medical society is the antithesis of being intellectually curious and scientific. *Chronic* looks at the field of autoimmunity with new eyes. It's filled with useful information for readers at all levels of medical and scientific background. It is extensively researched, thoroughly vetted, and contains information you can use to educate your doctor, family, and friends.

As a survivor of a chronic infection that nearly claimed my life, and a physician for nearly 30 years, I can't help but mourn the dying practice of the Art of Medicine. Here, we see it on full display in Dr. Steven Phillips, who still relies on his clinical skills and judgment as a practitioner of the healing art of medicine. I know Steven personally and can attest to the fact that he spends hours with his patients, learning through observation and being an attentive listener.

Dr. Phillips adapts his treatment to the needs of the individual patient. That is personalized medicine in its purest form. There is a detailed description of the rationale for the antibiotics he uses and his approach to administering them, and an equally informative section on non-antibiotic antimicrobials and medicinal herbs. Perhaps most importantly, *Chronic* describes a therapeutic approach that considers the patient as a human being, and addresses emotional healing using a variety of techniques that have proven effective. As reinforced in this book, healing the mind and body are equally important.

Chronic is a beautiful blend of the perspectives of two highly respected professionals who come from different backgrounds but share a common journey. Anyone who knows Dana Parish can see her influence in this book, a humanistic approach articulated through the lens of a prolific singer/songwriter whose life was derailed by chronic infections. That's how she met Steven, and the two have since been on a singular mission to educate others through the press, public lectures, and social media. Dana's song, "I See You," which she wrote for Idina Menzel, has become somewhat of an anthem for those suffering in silence, alienated by family and friends, and shunned by much of the medical field. Dana, perhaps as much as any individual, has elevated the conversation and visibility of these patients in the public eye.

I've been involved in biomedical research at prestigious academic cancer centers where we have published our work in top-tier journals, and was fortunate to have led translational research programs for two cancer therapies that were approved by the FDA. I've seen excellent science, and conversely, lots of people who talk a good game but have nothing to support their claims. *Chronic* is extensively backed by published scientific research. If you are looking for a book that provides facts that you can use to counter naysayers point by point, want to understand how pathogens can play a causative role in autoimmune, neurodegenerative, and psychiatric illnesses, and catch a glimpse of how this pre-eminent physician treats his patients with complex chronic infections, mind and body, look no further than this book.

Neil Spector, MD,
Medical Oncologist / Cancer Biologist,
Duke University School of Medicine

Introduction

Three things cannot long be hidden:
the sun, the moon, and the truth.

—*Buddha*

It was the 3:00 am request that would stop any mother's heart: "Mommy, you need to take the knives out of my room . . . and the scissors . . . because I'm going to hurt myself."

Dr. Marna Erikson's son was only sixteen years old at the time, and the keeper of those long-forgotten but dangerously sharp family heirlooms. His symptoms had started two years earlier — joint pain, anxiety, insomnia, headaches, an intolerance to light, and sensitivity to sound. This was all due to a devastating but wily infection that doctors had failed to recognize. That night, Marna realized just how bad things had gotten and rushed her son to the local hospital, where he would spend the following week in the psych ward. By then he'd already seen fifty doctors, including at one of the world's most prestigious medical clinics, who turned him away because they could not diagnose his infection using their methods. Three positive tests from North Carolina State University, a leader in infectious disease research, had already come in. But it didn't matter. They still refused to treat him.

Marna is not just a warrior mom but a PhD senior research scientist in the department of dermatology at the University of Minnesota Medical School. There, she uses advanced imaging techniques to study how certain infections manifest in skin conditions. The struggle for her son's life was ferocious and desperate, but after taking matters into her own hands, she was ultimately victorious. Marna found a proper diagnosis and treatment for her son, with a near cure that you'll read about later. It's a chilling story of many lost years, due to the perfect storm of mysterious microbes and medical arrogance, but, ultimately, one of hope.

We like to think of ourselves as truth-tellers in an area of medicine where the truth is hard-won and difficult to find: the field of autoimmune and chronic illness. We teamed up to help people understand the staggering reach of common infections and offer a roadmap to healing. In particular, we're referring to a group of ancient and highly evolved vector-borne diseases, meaning they are transmitted by a biting arthropod. "Arthropod" is just a fancy word for bug, such as a tick, flea, louse, mosquito, fly, or even a spider. These infections are some of the most misunderstood in all of medicine, causing chronic illnesses that are tough to diagnose and even tougher to treat. The result is that most patients never even get an accurate diagnosis, and instead end up being labeled with an autoimmune disease or illness of unknown origin.

We first met in 2015 as doctor and patient. Throughout the book, you'll read about our individual health crises, alongside vignettes from others who've also suffered greatly, but, more importantly, *survived and flourished*. Between the two of us, we've got the medical credentials, the access to leading-edge science, and the personal experience of having survived these wrenching infections ourselves. The fact that a medical expert — who has been studying and lecturing to healthcare professionals about these very germs for more than twenty years — can himself become a victim of the system and come close to death speaks volumes. If it happened to him, then what chance does the average person have of a swift, accurate diagnosis and proper treatment? Millions around the world suffer needlessly from these undiagnosed infections, never living the lives they deserve. In recent years we've seen lots of celebrities speak out about their own plight; they are a voice for those who do not have such platforms. But those voices often don't provide solutions. We've come together to write this book and provide all patients — famous or not — a way back to their lives. The costs of not doing so are enormous. These infections are the plague of our time. They can appear in so many varied ways, able to cause a huge array of diseases, from fibromyalgia and multiple sclerosis to rheumatoid arthritis and severe psychiatric disorders.

Nothing is more agonizing than feeling inexplicably sick. Whether it's constant, or you're experiencing periodic bouts of illness, when attempts to find permanent relief through both conventional and alternative medicine fail, it's soul-crushing. Perhaps you yourself are among those who have struggled with chronic illness, or strange, migrating symptoms that no one seems to take seriously. And if you're not being taken seriously, no one is looking for the cause of your symptoms. You may have been told "it's all in your head." Maybe you asked your doctor (or multiple doctors) whether an underlying infection could be triggering your symptoms that were carelessly labeled as "autoimmune." And it might be that they dismissed your questions and prescribed drugs to treat your symptoms without addressing the underlying cause. Maybe you were referred to a psychiatrist or prescribed an antidepressant by your general practitioner.

You are not alone. We've heard and seen an untold number of patients treating their chronic pain and autoimmune disorders with everything *but* what they truly need to get better, and we've been there ourselves. Between the two of us, we saw thirty-seven doctors before we got real answers. And in my case (Dr. Phillips), sadly, the only real answers came from my own detective work and experience. (Note: Although this book is written from a collective "we," there will be times when we will need to break into our respective individual voices. It will be clear who is talking — Parish or Dr. Phillips — and whose perspective is driving the narrative.) Looking back, we think it's so obvious — 20/20 hindsight is crystal clear, but it was sure mysterious when we were in its midst. Think back to your childhood. Most of us lived outside, especially during the summer, whether at camp, in our suburban backyards, or in a park within a big city. Getting sick from a bug bite was the furthest thing from our minds. We all coped with the temporary itch of mosquito bites, but never thought about bites that would lead to long-term, disabling disease.

As much as we love nature, it's become a veritable hazard zone throughout the world. Though dangerous microbes are far from new, their potential to infect millions has never been more apparent. Bugs of the twenty-first century have not only gone rogue with the long list of diseases they can carry, but they have also physically gone viral, spreading to places where they could not previously survive, due in part to global warming, and finding new, unwitting hosts. And don't be lulled into a false sense of security just because you live in a colder climate; illness-causing microbes have even been found to infect colonies of king penguins off the coast of Antarctica. In many parts of the world, 50 percent of ticks carry pathogens, which are germs that cause disease. Pathogens include viruses, bacteria, fungi, and parasites, such as worms and protozoa. To counter our 24/7 lives with its attendant "nature deficit disorder," we're urged to take in some sunshine, with little thought that the outdoors could bring life-changing, even lethal, health consequences.

There's a reason we haven't used the word "Lyme" yet, several pages into this book. Although it's one vector-borne infection to crawl its way into the public consciousness, the term has been grossly abused and wholly misunderstood, with little consensus on something even as basic as its meaning. Lyme is an ever-exploding landmine on a seedy political battlefield. We feel confident in calling it the most contentious disease in the history of medicine. But we want to get one thing straight from the get-go: this book is about so much more than Lyme disease. For starters, most patients diagnosed with Lyme likely harbor a mixture of infections, most of which get eclipsed by Lyme in the eyes of physicians who lack the knowledge to differentiate them. So when we're referring to *only* Lyme disease, we'll refer to it simply as Lyme. But when we're referring to the collective of these infections, we'll be using the term "Lyme+." And that "plus," as you're about to learn, is dizzyingly comprehensive.

We make strong claims in this book, backed up by equally strong scientific data, with access to insider knowledge and perspective, including jaw-dropping interviews. We'll change the way you look at chronic illness. There's an old saying that you can't fill a cup that's already full. Along those lines, we hope you can empty your cup of any preconceptions you may have about Lyme+. Our goal is to empower those coping with the label of chronic or autoimmune illness, to lead them to its root, and to put them on the path to wellness. It's also our hope that this book will open the minds of doctors who were not looking for infections as a cause of autoimmune diseases. You'll come to understand why we take issue with the term "autoimmune"; we certainly know that these symptoms and disease manifestations are excruciatingly real, but the term puts people in a box. Once that label is assigned, the investigation into *cause* evaporates—and with it, any hope of a cure. And so the origins of these illnesses remain missed by mainstream medicine despite the blaring truth that's long been documented in the medical literature.

We spoke with dozens of authorities on this topic while writing this book, and we'll be featuring their insights. These include infectious disease doctors at our finest institutions, psychiatrists, ophthalmologists, pathologists, rheumatologists, pediatricians, veterinarians, ecologists, medical ethicists, and even top brass in the military. They bring clarity and context to this difficult and infinitely complex subject. Many have gone on the record with us for the first time ever, bringing perspective and information that everyone needs to know. Some of what they share is so sensitive, however, that a few could only speak candidly to us off the record and we've had to remove identifying details to protect them. They would only talk to us under the condition of total anonymity, avoiding any reference to their titles and jobs for fear that they'd be demoted, fired, stripped of credentials, or shunned by colleagues. Some of these conversations were deeply troubling and heartbreaking. And some led to tears. There were long, silent pauses and whispered responses—gasps for air after getting choked up and losing composure. The fear, shame, and anger were palpable. At times we felt like investigative journalists or spies listening to conversations that could only be heard by a select few. The experience reminded us of what Jeffrey Wigand must have felt like when he blew the whistle on the tobacco industry. Wigand, you may recall, was a biochemist for a big tobacco company. He became an informant for the media in the mid-1990s, exposing how Big Tobacco made their products so addictive and doggedly promoted them knowing they were addictive and carcinogenic. Wigand was famously played by Russell Crowe in 1999's *The Insider*. With this book, we — the insiders of Lyme+ — bring you to the truth exposed.

LYME+

Lyme disease is the fastest growing vector-borne infectious disease in the United States today, and among the most common vector-borne diseases worldwide.[1] The confluence of climate change, deforestation, changes in land use, and population growth has paved the way for a proliferation of disease-causing ticks and increased human exposure. Questions do remain, and we don't necessarily know how this infectious stew is evolving, but one thing is certain: infections are on the rise. And they don't discriminate: anyone can get infected regardless of age, gender, affluence, political affiliation, and even geography. The number of new Lyme cases reported annually has increased nearly 25-fold since national surveillance began in 1982.[2] The Centers for Disease Control and Prevention (CDC) report that there are nearly 427,000 new cases of Lyme disease a year in this country; this is almost twice as many as the number of women diagnosed with breast cancer each year in the U.S. and greater than eight times more than the number diagnosed with HIV/AIDS annually in the U.S.[3] Many researchers believe that the true number of Lyme cases is at least twice what the CDC estimates if you account for those who are undiagnosed or misdiagnosed.[4]

When we think about the panic that's erupted throughout history when epidemics have struck, we marvel at how quickly awareness and research for life-saving treatments have often emerged. Yet the current Lyme+ pandemic has raged for the past forty-five years and counting, with no cure in sight, due to divisive chaos within the medical community. Some people have gone so far as to compare the denialism and scandal around Lyme to the HIV/AIDS epidemic of the 1980s and 1990s.[5] It took time for HIV/AIDS to be taken seriously, but once it was, research and treatments came fast and furiously. Lyme+ continues to be a silenced epidemic and its victims are marginalized. One of the biggest Lyme researchers, Russell Johnson of the University of Minnesota, famously said in the *Los Angeles Times* in 1987: "Were it not for AIDS, Lyme disease would be what we are all worrying about."[6] Today, the same could probably be said if other health scares didn't routinely steal the media's attention: Zika, measles, and Ebola. But with Lyme+, there are so many more victims compared to these other relatively rare infections.

It has been estimated that by 2050, 55.7 million people in the United States (12 percent of the U.S. population) will be affected.[7] Many of these infections will become chronic, yet patients are being told that there's "no such thing" as "chronic Lyme." This massive scourge is costing us billions annually by conservative estimates, with lives ruined, careers crushed, savings depleted, and marriages ended. Still, bizarrely, some claim that it doesn't exist.

The U.S. government is finally awakening to this growing epidemic. In 2016 it established the Twenty-first Century Cures Act to address emerging public health problems, especially tick-borne diseases, for which there's now a Tick-Borne Disease Working Group under the Act. In the Group's report published in late 2018, the committee writes: "As tick populations continue to grow and infected ticks expand geographically, the threat to human health intensifies."[8] The report includes poignant stories from patients, like the following from one unlucky gentleman and veteran: "Untreated patients can lose everything, as I did, and become part of the unemployed, underemployed, disabled, and homeless populations."

At least twenty known diseases can result from tick bites—from Rocky Mountain spotted fever to tularemia—and innumerable more from the bites of other bugs. Researchers also continue to find new germs that were previously unknown and undocumented, and which continue to shock even experts in the field.

When we mention Lyme+, virtually everyone has a story. While each has its nuance, they all share something in common: These infections have altered daily life for many, often terrifyingly and unpredictably so. The most heartbreaking stories are the ones in which there are no definitive diagnoses for months, years, sometimes decades, while the effects from these infections have caused untold pain and irreversible damage. Some people are fortunate to experience the early stages of fever, joint pain, and general malaise, which can lead to a timely diagnosis and a chance at more successful treatment. Others are not so lucky and either suffer from a failed treatment or end up disabled, in heart failure, or dead. Between these two extremes are myriad other symptoms—from memory loss, headaches, depression, anxiety, and insomnia, to arthritis, numbness, and immense, unshakable fatigue.

Many unfortunate Lyme+ sufferers whose infections evade a cure with the current recommendations set by the Infectious Disease Society of America (IDSA)—a few weeks of antibiotics—become saddled with an autoimmune diagnosis. Think about it like this: If you are not feeling all better by day 21 of antibiotics, you'll likely be given an entirely different diagnosis on day 22. And by day 23, you might be sentenced to dangerous and exorbitantly expensive immunosuppressants, which cure nothing but may suppress symptoms. You could be dependent on these drugs for the rest of your life. The result is that many children and adults are never fully treated for Lyme+. Worse, most Lyme+ cases are likely never treated at all. They go undiagnosed, their diagnosis defaulted to autoimmune or rheumatic conditions (e.g., multiple sclerosis, arthritis, fibromyalgia, lupus, chronic fatigue syndrome, and so on), and the investigation for cause abruptly stops. How do we know this? It's based on volumes of published medical research demonstrating a causal link between infection and autoimmune disease, as well as my (Dr. Phillips') professional experience after more than twenty-three years of treating thousands of patients, including myself. I have witnessed countless chronic mystery illnesses resolve once an underlying infectious cause was found and appropriately treated.

Lyme is known as The Great Imitator. But we consider Lyme, or more accurately Lyme+, "The Great Cause." To call it an imitator is to misrepresent the truth: These infections cause a range of chronic and autoimmune diseases. They're deceiving. The wording matters, because it guides patients' care.

The diagnosis of Lyme is elusive, given that a tick bite is rarely seen, there is no telltale bull's-eye rash history in most cases of late Lyme, and symptoms are so variable that they're often chalked up to an autoimmune or psychiatric condition (again, patients are often told it's "all in their head" or "psychosomatic"). Additionally, the diagnosis can be missed because testing is flawed, with high rates of false-negative results. And even more frustrating, lab results on the very same blood specimen, if split up and sent to different labs, will vary enormously among those labs. Or another vector-borne infection in the Lyme+ group, like *Bartonella* or *F. tularensis* (which causes tularemia), is actually causing the illness but not considered or tested for properly. Those who have persistent (or chronic) Lyme+ face rejection and belittlement by the medical community. Chronic Lyme+ is often dismissed by mainstream medicine, including the CDC and IDSA. We know what it's like to have an illness that's minimized and underestimated because we, too, have chronic Lyme+ that we beat into submission.

This will be the first time that I (Dr. Phillips) disclose my own near-fatal experience to the public. My story, combined with the knowledge I've gained from treating more than 20,000 patients, aims to reach the hundreds of thousands of people I couldn't possibly treat due to the limitations of my practice. My experience with Lyme+ was one of extremes on the wide range of possibilities for patients, but it's one that equipped me with the knowledge to ultimately help more people and have a highly attuned sense of empathy for those who do face worst-case scenarios with Lyme+.

We hope to change the status quo and rewrite the current narrative that does such a disservice to patients and their families.

IN THIS BOOK

We've organized this book into two parts. In Part 1: The Root, we cover the history, biology, and mythology of infections in the twenty-first century. Drawing from the latest science, we'll debunk commonly held myths, show how the medical world got the facts about Lyme+ so wrong, and turn medical dogma upside down. Among the questions answered, backed by science:

- Why are Lyme+ infections so misunderstood today? Why has the Lyme+ pandemic become so politicized?
- Why are tests for these infections so unreliable and why is diagnosing them so difficult?
- Why don't most health care providers know how to diagnose and subsequently treat Lyme+, especially difficult cases that do not meet the standards set by obsolete government guidelines? (And why are those guidelines obsolete?)
- What commonly happens upon infection with any of these vector-borne germs? What are the symptoms and how does such an illness progress?
- How did the medical world get this area of medicine so wrong?
- How can an infection cause an autoimmune disorder or psychiatric illness — or both? *Do we owe a good percentage of our chronic autoimmune illnesses and even forms of dementia to infections caused by bug bites?*

Then, in Part 2: The Remedy, we'll offer proven strategies for finding relief, which includes practical instructions on how to arrive at a proper diagnosis, how to interact with your medical team in a way that doesn't leave you feeling powerless, how to know which drug regimen is best, and how to deal with feeling worse before feeling better. We'll also explore supplemental techniques for healing while on the road to recovery, including advice for managing potential relapses and dealing with the trauma of chronic illness. The reasons this disease has generated such a fiery debate in the political-medical industry will unfold chapter by chapter.

Lyme and its associated diseases are typified by a waxing and waning of multi-system illness, which can be static over time, get worse, or even improve spontaneously, making these illnesses very difficult to diagnose. Vector-borne infections are exceedingly deceptive — regularly missed by even top doctors. And it's not because they aren't smart; it's because these avenues of research are usually not taught at the major teaching hospitals. Which is why, as this book will explain, you have to do a deep dive that goes far beyond traditional lab work. In many cases, you need to venture beyond the doctors who can't keep up with the newest research, who remain siloed by obsolete data and guidelines. Too many victims are suffering alone, in hazy despair.

We offer encouragement, hope, and help. You deserve to be healthy. The current medical dogma about chronic autoimmune disease is a crime against humanity. By the end of this book, we aim to leave you feeling empowered with the knowledge and strategies you need to move forward to reclaim your life. While at times you may feel like you're reading a mystery, there's no mystery here. May the truth prevail.

Do I Have a
Vector-borne Infection?

Below is a simple checklist of the most common symptoms of vector-borne infections. We'll be exploring potential symptoms in Chapter 2. Here's a helpful snapshot of what these infections can cause:

- ☐ Headaches
- ☐ Stiff neck
- ☐ Concentration/mood problems
- ☐ Sleep problems
- ☐ Heart palpitations
- ☐ Muscle pain
- ☐ Joint pain
- ☐ Fevers/chills/sweats
- ☐ Lymph node swelling/pain
- ☐ Numbness/tingling
- ☐ Belly pain/diarrhea/constipation
- ☐ Bladder frequency/pain

Note: There's no minimum number of symptoms required to suspect vector-borne illness. It often depends on how it impacts/disrupts daily living.

Diagnoses commonly caused by underlying vector-borne infections:

- ☐ Fibromyalgia
- ☐ Chronic fatigue syndrome
- ☐ Multiple sclerosis

- ☐ Rheumatoid arthritis
- ☐ Psoriasis
- ☐ IBS
- ☐ Migraines
- ☐ Heart failure
- ☐ Psychiatric and neurologic conditions
- ☐ Sarcoidosis[9]
- ☐ Sjogren's syndrome[10]
- ☐ Small fiber neuropathy[11]
- ☐ Adult-onset Still's disease[12]
- ☐ Complex regional pain syndrome
- ☐ Other autoimmune conditions

PART I

The Root

CHAPTER 1

A Wild Family of Infections

Wisdom begins in wonder.

—*Socrates*

F YOU COULD go back in time to the Middle Ages when the technologies we now take for granted were not yet in anyone's imagination, it would be next to impossible to explain computers, cars, X-rays, brain surgery, and space travel. But you could find common ground on the topic of death. Although there was no knowledge of germs or how infectious diseases were transmitted then, infections were among the top Grim Reapers — dysentery, cholera, typhoid fever, smallpox, diphtheria, and bubonic plague. We don't hear much about these ailments today; smallpox has been eradicated, and the others are preventable, treatable, and far less common than before. The World Health Organization (WHO) declared smallpox eliminated in 1980, just about the time HIV/AIDS began to garner attention and become one of the largest global pandemics.

Flash forward to the twenty-first century. Try having a conversation about Lyme and watch what happens. We have seen people dismissed, belittled, and told that they are misled by bad information — especially when chronic Lyme is mentioned. Challenge someone's autoimmune diagnosis by suggesting it could be rooted in an underlying infection and you may soon enter a tense, unending verbal spar. Unlike in the Middle Ages, we now have a huge arsenal of data and drugs. So why do so many continue to suffer? We can't think of any other modern-day plague that is shrouded by so much mythology in the lay public, and bitter, polarizing controversy in the medical community.

Most see it simply as a "tick-borne infection" akin to getting a sinus infection, that can be quickly and easily treated with a brief round of antibiotics. Done.

The vast majority of people also view Lyme as a problem confined to certain areas of the world, notably the northeastern U.S.

Wrong.

Wrong.

And triple wrong if you also thought that ticks carry just one germ. Or that these germs could only be transmitted by ticks. When people do speak of vector-borne illness, most people don't realize that Lyme is just the tip of the iceberg.

For starters, Lyme is not just an East Coast problem. While it was first named "Lyme" in honor of Lyme, Connecticut, it has been reported in all states except for Hawaii (where some people do have Lyme from infections they got elsewhere), with hot spots in the northern Midwest and northern California.[1] Infections now occur all around the world, with many areas in Europe and Asia having similar endemicity to the northeast U.S.

To say Lyme is a "tick-borne illness" overly simplifies the matter. As we began to explain in the introduction, the word "Lyme" has come to refer to a family of infections, referred to here as "Lyme+" — and the transmission of these germs is not just by ticks. In the case of *Bartonella*, they can be transmitted by other bugs like fleas, lice, sand flies, spiders, and ants, along with its stereotypical transmission via a cat scratch or bite.[2] And many of these infections have been proven to be transmissible from mother to child in utero.[3] We reiterate these basic facts because they are critically important. Remember them and then we can begin to dispel the many misconceptions that surround the topic.

Dr. Al Miller will not stop talking about Lyme and has no qualms about going up against the dogma of his own specialty: rheumatology. Although retired, he not only keeps abreast of the medical literature and the conversation, he starts the conversation. Born and raised in San Antonio, Texas, Miller received his medical degree from the University of Texas and went on to complete his residency in internal medicine and his fellowship in rheumatology at the Mayo Clinic. He practiced medicine in San Antonio from 1968 to 2008, and served on the clinical faculty at UT's medical school. In 2008, the same year he retired, Miller's daughter-in-law in Boston came down with a mysterious illness and was eventually diagnosed with amyotrophic lateral sclerosis (ALS), otherwise known as Lou Gehrig's disease—a devastating fatal illness with no cure, characterized by a progressive degeneration of the motor neurons of the central nervous system. It leads to the wasting of muscles, paralysis, and eventual death. She was only forty-three years old upon diagnosis and deteriorated quickly. Miller sprang into action, working his connections in the hopes of saving her life.

Although the MRI of her brain ordered by a neurologist at Harvard's Massachusetts General Hospital showed lesions consistent with multiple sclerosis (MS), her physical exam led doctors to diagnose ALS. A second opinion at Beth Israel Hospital confirmed the diagnosis. Miller sought further opinions from his former colleagues at the Mayo Clinic, who also believed that she had ALS. But Miller, convinced that something else was going on, needed to find the cause. He asked a single, significant question: What could look like MS in the brain but present as ALS on physical exam?

Looking to the medical literature, he found his answer: a neurological manifestation of Lyme disease caused by a systemic infection of spirochetes, the bacteria from the genus *Borrelia* responsible for Lyme disease.[4] He asked all three institutions, among the finest medical centers on the planet, about testing for Lyme. When the most basic test used came back negative, he sent another blood sample to a specialty lab that used more sophisticated technology. And that's when her test finally came back positive for Lyme. By then, his daughter-in-law's prognosis was poor. She was given four months to live. But instead of acknowledging Lyme as a possible cause of the ALS and prescribing antibiotic therapy as logic would dictate, her doctors refused antibiotic therapy, and advised her to go home and write essays to her four children that they could read later in life. Miller did not accept this, and rightly so. He began treating her with antibiotics for Lyme, which completely halted the progression of her ALS and extended her life by a stunning and odds-defying seven years. She died in 2015 of septic shock, unrelated to her Lyme treatment, at the age of fifty.

The Miller case reflects the mistreatment that so many patients go through when diagnosed with a disease of unknown origin. Are these misdiagnoses? It's really a matter of semantics. What happened to Miller's daughter-in-law highlights a particular area of human weakness: our herding instinct, in this case demonstrated by how tenaciously doctors were sticking to dogma over innovation, at the cost of human life. If a patient meets the diagnostic criteria for one of these ailments, and it's confirmed by several academic medical centers, but the individual has an infection causing it all along, does that patient have that mysterious disease? According to a survey of over 4,000 chronic Lyme+ patients, roughly 20 percent were initially misdiagnosed with one of the following serious neurologic diseases: MS, Parkinson's, ALS, or Multiple Systems Atrophy.[5]

Al Miller is now on a mission to shift the thinking in his field of medicine, rheumatology, that he calls "totally wrong." Fibromyalgia, chronic fatigue syndrome, rheumatoid arthritis, psoriatic arthritis, and others are frequently diagnosed conditions that can ultimately be attributed to an underlying hidden infection. Could his daughter-in-law's life have been saved if she'd been diagnosed sooner for Lyme and treated? We can never know, but he adamantly believes that every patient diagnosed with a chronic disorder of unknown cause should be properly evaluated for Lyme+. He goes so far as to suggest that Lou Gehrig himself, for whom the disease is nicknamed, might have been killed by Lyme. After all, he had a second home in Lyme, Connecticut, where he liked to garden.

Lyme, Connecticut. Is that where it all began? Is that ground zero? Not really. Let's look at a little history. Ticks and Lyme have been around for not just thousands, but millions, of years. Not only was Lyme found in a 5,300-year-old mummy,[6] ancestral *Borreliae*, the genus of bacteria that causes Lyme disease, were even discovered in a tick that was clutching a dinosaur feather, embedded in amber, 99 million years ago.[7] Ticks predate us by a long shot; they sucked the blood of our ancient ancestors and have adapted cleverly to our environment.

THE LYMELIGHT

The name "Lyme disease" was a stroke of marketing genius. Its stereotypical sentinel rash, technically called erythema migrans (EM), was originally discovered more than a hundred years ago in Sweden by dermatologist Arvid Afzelius.[8] Soon thereafter, it became known that a chronic neurologic illness could follow the rash, which in 1941 was termed Bannwarth Syndrome. But the disease did not gain public recognition until 1977 when Allen Steere, a young rheumatologist at Yale at the time, renamed the boring Bannwarth Syndrome as the media-friendly and memorable Lyme disease.[9] The rest is history. And history forgets. It forgets that the clinical characteristics of this multi-system illness were well documented in Europe for many decades before it became known as Lyme disease.[10] It forgets that it was Dr. Rudolph Scrimenti, a dermatologist in Wisconsin, who first discovered EM in the United States, described how it occurred after a tick bite, and recommended treatment with antibiotics.[11] He published these findings in the medical literature seven years before Steere, in 1970. Yet it was Allen Steere who came up with the sleek new name, and it's amazing what a good name can do. So despite almost a century of medical history already printed about this illness, he is now wrongly credited with discovering it.

The condition was first brought to Steere's attention by Polly Murray, who sounded the alarm about a sudden outbreak of fifty-one kids with arthritis — initially diagnosed as juvenile rheumatoid arthritis (JRA) — in and around Lyme, Connecticut.[12] In the early 1980s, Willy Burgdorfer, a medical entomologist at the National Institutes of

Health's Rocky Mountain Laboratories, determined that the infection was caused by a previously unknown bacterium, a *Borrelia* spirochete (pronounced *spy*-ro-keet) carried by ticks.[13] He wasn't studying Lyme at the time, but as with many scientific discoveries, he stumbled upon the groundbreaking finding unexpectedly. He'd been analyzing deer ticks from Long Island that were suspected to be causing spotted fever. Because he had studied spirochetes in graduate school, he knew what he was looking at when he peered into his microscope and saw the bacteria shaped like spiral corkscrews. In a 2001 oral history for the National Institutes of Health (NIH), he stated: "Once my eyes focused on these long, snakelike organisms, I recognized what I had seen a million times before: spirochetes."[14] Deer ticks had not been known to carry spirochetes, and more testing proved him right. In 1982, he and several colleagues published their findings in the journal *Science*.[15] As is standard in scientific practice, the newly discovered bacterium was named after him: *Borrelia burgdorferi*. This event reflects what the celebrated French biologist Louis Pasteur once said, "Chance favors the prepared mind." Dr. Burgdorfer admitted that his discovery was serendipitous, an accident that could have happened only to someone with more than thirty years of experience studying ticks.*

Actually, a spirochetal origin for this illness was first theorized even before Burgdorfer, by the physicians Garin and Bujadoux in France in the 1920s, when cases of Bannwarth Syndrome (also known as Garin-Bujadoux-Bannwarth Syndrome) were treated with penicillin, which was found to be effective.[16] Scrimenti also documented the

---

* Dr. Willy Burgdorfer had a history as a biowarfare researcher in addition to his work in medical entomology. Kris Newby's 2019 book *Bitten: The Secret History of Lyme Disease and Biological Weapons* takes readers on a riveting investigative tour of Willy's role in trying to weaponize ticks, fleas, and mosquitoes for the U.S. military's bioweapons program during the Cold War. The book provides evidence supporting the theory that the Lyme epidemic likely began around Long Island Sound in 1968 as fallout from a secret or accidental bioweapons release. This has not been definitively proven but the book raises important, albeit uncomfortable, questions we should be asking, and calls for more attention to Lyme+ victims; we need better science, advanced research, and proper funding.

clearing of EM with penicillin in the United States in his 1970 paper.[17] Yet despite decades of powerful evidence before Burgdorfer discovered *Borreliae* in ticks, Steere still posited that a virus, rather than a bacterium, caused Lyme disease, and wrote, "Symptomatic treatment only is advised, except in . . . rare instances."[18]

Fast forward almost forty years, and the fact that spirochetes cause Lyme disease is undisputed. But nearly everything else about Lyme — its clinical presentation, its diagnostic criteria, its effects in the body, its prevalence, its best treatment, and why antibiotic treatments often fail, leading to chronic illness — is bitterly debated. Ask ten different doctors how Lyme disease affects the body and why some patients fail treatment, and you'll likely get ten different answers. The most hotly debated aspect of this illness is chronic Lyme, a definition for which was published in late 2019 by me (Dr. Phillips).[19] The mainstream medical dogma evangelized by IDSA is straightforward: In most cases, the tick bite causes a skin rash (EM), which is easily identified by its bull's-eye appearance. If the illness persists for more than six weeks, the Lyme antibody tests will be positive by CDC criteria, a testing protocol that is so stringent that, by the CDC's own admission, it fails to capture 90 percent of Lyme cases. In fact, the CDC states: "This surveillance case definition was developed for national reporting of Lyme disease; it is not intended to be used in clinical diagnosis."[20] And yet IDSA continues to vigorously promote its use for diagnosing Lyme.

To make matters more complicated, there are many different strains of Lyme and many different tests on the market. Some will be more or less sensitive in detecting one strain versus another, which contributes to a high rate of inter-lab variability in test results. And studies going back decades show that we can be simultaneously infected with multiple strains,[21] as well as become repeatedly reinfected without ever developing immunity.[22] Although it would be beyond the scope of this book to go into the sheer volume of superb published medical data documenting the chronic and difficult-to-treat nature of a litany of zoonotic infections (that is, diseases that can be transmitted from animals to humans), suffice it to say that Lyme is but one of many that can be difficult to diagnose and cure, and which can cause chronic disabling mystery illnesses. Lyme and *Bartonella* are two of the most common, and are responsible for a large swath of the chronic illness that we come across, but they're by no means the only ones.

If left untreated, Lyme bacteria can spread to muscles, joints, the heart, and even the brain. Public-health officials assert that a few weeks of antibiotic treatment will almost always wipe out the infection, and that relapses are rare. In this view, put forth in guidelines issued by IDSA and parroted by the CDC, Lyme is considered easy to diagnose, easy to treat, and easy to cure. Nothing could be further from the truth. It's hard to believe that our most trusted medical and government agencies could be wrong, but they are not only wrong, they remain strident and unremorseful in their positions. The truth is that most people who have been infected with *Borrelia* don't develop or notice a rash. And most people never recall being bitten. A nymphal tick bite is generally painless and the bug delivering it is the size of a poppy seed. So despite the common belief that ticks are the size of a fly and easy to spot, nymphs are anything but. Of the four stages of their development (egg, larva, nymph, and adult), nymphs are the most likely to transmit disease. Because of their tiny size, they go unnoticed. The reported percentage of people who get the rash varies wildly; original data from Steere's published work in the 1970s showed only 25 percent of infected people get the rash.[23] Newer data is less reliable because the presence of EM is part of the CDC's reporting criteria; thus many studies use EM as an entry criterion into the studies, causing a skewing of statistics about prevalence of the rash. It's like concluding from a study that most people in prison have committed a crime, when committing the crime was the entrance criterion into the prison in the first place.

More troubling, many patients who are treated continue to suffer from persistent illness long after their conventional three- to four-week course of antibiotic therapy has ended. Or they feel fine for a while and then something crops up — some recurrent or new symptoms which their doctor describes as mystifying. This is what happened to each of us. Infectious disease experts refer to this chronic illness, which conservatively affects at least 20 percent of patients but has been reported to impact up to 61 percent of patients (according to a powerful study by Danbury Hospital, an institution at ground zero for Lyme in Connecticut), as "Post-Treatment Lyme Disease Syndrome (PTLDS)."[24] We strongly disagree with this term because we feel it implies that symptoms after short-term therapy are not attributable to an ongoing infection. In fact, we feel that it's extremely harmful to the public. Semantics guide care, so assigning the status of "post-infectious syndrome" to this chronic illness excludes the possibility that further treatment with antibiotics could help. We prefer the more accurate term "chronic Lyme," because the science is unequivocal: Lyme can certainly persist despite antibiotic treatment. Although it has been notoriously difficult to isolate live spirochetes from body fluids of even untreated, infected animals, it has been far easier to find them in body tissues. Thus, it's been relatively straightforward to demonstrate the persistence of infection despite antibiotics in diverse animal tissues, with many published studies proving this across many species.[25]

One extensive monkey study from Tulane University, for instance, published in 2017, demonstrated a zero percent cure rate after a one-month course of the commonly prescribed antibiotic doxycycline, which IDSA claims will cure humans.[26] Monkeys have a virtually identical disease course to humans and provide an ideal animal model. If this persuasive animal data weren't enough, in at least thirty different medical journal articles, live Lyme bacteria have been cultured from humans, despite both short- and long-term antibiotics, representing about seventy human cases of firmly documented chronic Lyme. It was even isolated from the knee tissue of a patient who had failed about one year of oral antibiotics and almost a year of IV and intramuscular antibiotics.[27] And in a revealing study, the NIH demonstrated that a tick, which was cultivated in a lab so as not to contain Lyme, became infected with the bacteria after it was allowed to attach to and feed on a patient with so-called PTLDS.[28] Obviously, the patient was still infected with Lyme, otherwise the tick couldn't possibly have become infected! In a final blow, major universities — including Johns Hopkins, Tulane, Tufts, and Northeastern — have all published data showing that the few antibiotics deemed "curative" by IDSA for Lyme in humans are all, every one of them, ineffective at killing *B. burgdor-feri* in the test tube.[29] If we can't kill it in the test tube, what chance do we have at a cure in the body? It's no wonder that researchers at Johns Hopkins reported that 39 percent of Lyme patients go on to develop chronic symptoms and/or functional impact after the standard few weeks of antibiotics for early Lyme.[30] In 2018, a headline from *Johns Hopkins Medicine* stated: "Study Shows Evidence of Severe and Lingering Symptoms in Some after Treatment for Lyme Disease."[31] And in 2019, a paper by a group of scientists including researchers from Columbia University found *Borrelia burgdorferi* antigens and their DNA in a fifty-three-year-old female who had received extensive antibiotic treatments over the course of her sixteen-year-long illness.[32] This was after the NIH had found live Lyme bacteria in her spinal fluid despite antibiotic treatment that was supposed to cure her. She died when her insurance company refused to cover more therapy. We shudder at the enormity of this problem: the massive number of patients diagnosed with "PTLDS" but still carrying an active infection. Instead of getting their infection treated, they're living a life sentence on pain meds, sleep meds, antidepressants, and tranquilizers. And as bad as this is, we shudder more at the thought of the majority who never even get diagnosed with Lyme or the other Lyme+ infections in the first place.

So anyone who has been told that there's no such thing as ongoing Lyme infection after treatment should feel much better after learning the results of these high-profile studies. And yet with the ineffectiveness of antibiotic treatments advised by the current IDSA guidelines, they might also feel a great deal of panic. Living in Connecticut, I (Dr. Phillips) see this everywhere. Recently, when I was waiting in line at the supermarket, a conversation broke out among the shoppers regarding the sad state of chronic Lyme and how patients can't get help. I said nothing, but I did continue to listen. A guy in his fifties was venting that he knew more about Lyme than his doctor, which brings us to our next point: One challenge going forward is accurate education. Sharing the truth with physicians and patients is easier said than done. The truth is so heavily varnished in the medical industry that it's almost unrecognizable. Don't be fooled into thinking that medicine is a squeaky-clean field; it's just as deceiving and corrupt as any other for-profit industry.

Two standards of care govern Lyme cases. One is best represented by the guidelines of the International Lyme and Associated Diseases Association (ILADS), a multidisciplinary medical society that favors a clinical diagnosis, supported by laboratory testing, but realizes the shortcomings of currently available tests. ILADS recommends treating patients with an individualized approach that is tailored to the severity and tenacity of each case, frequently resulting in long-term antibiotic therapy until they get better. The other is best represented by IDSA's recommendation, which is to diagnose based on meeting the CDC's reporting criteria, a threshold that fails to capture 90 percent of cases per the CDC's own admission, as we've said. These guidelines call for treating with two to four weeks of one of their recommended antibiotics, usually doxycycline. They call lingering symptoms "PTLDS" or diagnose these patients with another condition, frequently an auto-immune disease. Remember, most of the clinical features of Lyme disease are subjective — that is, symptoms that the physician can't see or measure. Such symptoms tend to be vague and varied, and could apply to many conditions. And although *Bartonella* and others in the Lyme+ group are more likely to produce clinical signs that doctors can see, like a swollen joint, inflammation of the eyes, or increased inflammatory markers in the blood, these patients are most often diagnosed with an autoimmune condition.

Despite all of the evidence, the term "chronic Lyme" is not considered mainstream, partly because clinicians are erroneously told by medical societies such as IDSA, or agencies such as the CDC, that it's extremely rare or nonexistent. And due to a lack of understanding of what the test results actually mean, many cases go undiagnosed, which increases the odds of developing chronic Lyme.

We should begin our explanation of Lyme testing by defining what an antibody test is. Antibodies are proteins manufactured by the immune system, which bind to bacteria, viruses, and other foreign invaders. The most common test for Lyme involves checking for these specific antibodies, which means that it's an indirect test. In other words, it doesn't represent the presence of the actual organism, but rather the body's *reaction* to it. Unfortunately, these tests are notoriously insensitive. Six studies showed an average of 56 percent overall sensitivity, but many researchers think that the true sensitivity is even lower.[33] A consequence of this finding is that there may be an antibody response that's not strong enough to meet the CDC's full reporting criteria for Lyme disease, which is more the rule than the exception. As previously stated, the CDC's overly strict criteria only capture 10 percent of Lyme cases. So, we ask, how can it be medically sound to make a diagnosis based on a testing criterion with only 10 percent sensitivity? HIV antibody testing is 99.7 percent sensitive.[34] If HIV tests were as inaccurate as Lyme tests, there would be rioting in the streets.

Patients are also becoming infected with other Lyme-like *Borrelia* species that cause the same symptoms as Lyme. These infections are common, but testing for them is either nonexistent or not readily available. Or the patients are infected with one of the relapsing fever *Borreliae*, which, although they have been known for decades and tests are available for them, usually don't come to the minds of doctors, even though it was probably on their medical board exam. Or they are infected by other vector-borne infections that are almost completely unknown to, and therefore almost never investigated by, their doctors. But these infections can cause severe and sometimes difficult-to-control illness — despite even very aggressive antibiotic therapy — because some are caused by inherently antibiotic-resistant microbes, such as *Bartonella*, *Brucella*, and *F. tularensis*. It's also important to note that, just as there are many species of non-Lyme *Borreliae* that cause disease and for which we do not have reliable testing, there are also many species of *Bartonella* that infect humans and for which we do not have *any* testing. Most doctors have heard of only two species, *Bartonella henselae* and *Bartonella quintana*, but there are many more that are human pathogens. This is a recurring theme among these kinds of infections. It would be a grave error of scientific arrogance not to acknowledge the probability that there are many additional species and strains of these organisms yet to be discovered. Nature isn't fickle — it tends to repeat things that work, and these pathogens work all too well. It comes as no surprise that new species of the family of Lyme+ are routinely being discovered in an almost limitless fashion, highlighting how little we know about these infections.

Bartonella is a different class of bacteria from Lyme, but causes many of the same symptoms. It is composed of a group of microbes that can cause anything from asymptomatic infection to virulent, nightmarish illness. The sickest "chronic Lyme patients" are usually infected with Bartonella. It's spread by the same tick, but other bugs can spread it as well, typically fleas and lice.[35] Published reports have even indicated infection via bites that are typically thought to be innocuous and therefore ignored, such as ant and spider bites.[36] It's a close cousin to the generally more serious Brucella, which causes a severe and often excruciating bacterial infection known as brucellosis. Brucella infections are less common in the U.S. than Bartonella infections, but they are underdiagnosed.

A frequent scenario is a Lyme+ patient being tested, being diagnosed with Lyme, and being treated with three weeks of antibiotics, yet the illness is not fully resolved. Their diagnoses are then defaulted to "PTLDS" as the cause of their persistent symptoms. Infectious disease experts claim that the lingering illness might be an "autoimmune response" to the original disease or residual damage to tissues caused by the infection. But if Lyme+ are real infections that manifest in real illness, then why does the medical community dismiss this subject area so vehemently? Why are these diagnoses frequently missed, and patients diagnosed with other ailments instead? Why do our most trusted public and professional health institutions, such as the CDC, the NIH, and IDSA, fail to acknowledge chronic Lyme? How can they not concede that treating the disease with long-term antibiotics — much longer than what current guidelines dictate — is a "best practice" in many cases when the available evidence (and common sense!) so clearly points to persistent infection?

In a world where doctors have been trained to require culture confirmation of a bacterial infection in order to prescribe antibiotics, it's no wonder that patients with Lyme+ go untreated — and mistreated — when their tests turn up negative or their symptoms don't fully resolve after a few weeks of antibiotics. In other areas of medicine, doctors are increasingly accused of overprescribing antibiotics, and yet with Lyme+, they under-prescribe, refuse to prescribe, or worse, make a diagnosis of a psychiatric disorder. We've heard from people so desperate to be properly treated that they have considered taking their dog's expired medications that were found in the back of desk drawers. You know you've hit rock bottom when you find yourself scrounging around for Fido's expired doxycycline. And did you know that expired tetracycline-class antibiotics, including doxycycline, can become toxic?

To get a sense of how dramatic and distressing the scenario can become, consider the case of Margaret, an alias we'll use for purposes of telling her tale as detailed by her father, whom we'll call Paul. The irony here is that Paul, like Dr. Al Miller, is no stranger to medicine. Paul is a pediatric anesthesiologist at an Ivy League medical center, where he specializes in critical care and pain medicine. Fighting back tears when he spoke with us, he said, "I wish it were my story; it'd be much easier to stomach if it weren't my daughter."

Margaret had recently been a healthy, thriving, thirteen-year-old girl preparing for seventh grade and figure-skating season. About four months before our interview with Paul, in the last week of July, she had attended an outdoor day camp on Cape Cod. A couple of weeks later, she came down with relapsing fevers, ear pain, and a sore throat. Paul chalked it up to an upper respiratory infection, but soon after, what was initially thought to be severe dehydration landed Margaret in the hospital. An initial workup demonstrated a low white blood cell count. The next day Margaret experienced dizziness, a slow heart rate, and trouble walking. She then developed debilitating headaches and soon needed a walker — when just a week previously she'd been figure skating. Nothing made sense.

A brain MRI and traditional Lyme testing were both negative. The doctors diagnosed her with a functional neurologic disorder triggered by a virus. In other words, they believed that Margaret had suffered a brain injury brought on by a virus (which didn't explain her persistently low white blood cell count). But an injury after a virus that had been cleared should not continue to worsen, and Margaret's condition got worse by the day. Doctors then labeled her as psychosomatic, which means they thought that mental or emotional factors were causing her symptoms. One doctor suggested to Paul that Margaret was "having some underlying stress issues causing these reactions." Margaret was now in a wheelchair and unable to go back to school. The concerned father looked further afield for help.

Additional testing revealed the culprits: multiple infections, including *Bartonella*, *Babesia* (a malaria-like protozoal infection), and *Borrelia miyamotoi*, one of at least fifty-two known species of *Borrelia*. (*Miyamotoi* is one of the few of the many newly discovered non-Lyme *Borreliae* that cause a Lyme-like disease, for which a test exists — for the others, there simply aren't tests available!). As we'll see later in the book, a chronically low white blood cell count is a common sign of a *Bartonella* infection. Paul had to catch up on his reading, as he'd never heard of some of these infections.

The treatment protocol was difficult to execute, not only because of potential side effects from antibiotics such as gastrointestinal distress, but because of Herxheimer reactions — a flare of underlying symptoms, and sometimes the development of new symptoms, in response to starting antibiotics. This only occurs in the context of an active infection with Lyme or another microbe that causes a Herxheimer (we'll explore this further in another chapter). Virtually all of Margaret's academic doctors dismissed her symptoms and accused Paul of "buying into the disease," "overtreating" with antibiotics, and "causing more stress." The family felt so intensely persecuted by the very people who were supposed to come to Margaret's rescue that Paul and his wife had serious concerns that they'd lose custody of their own daughter due to accusations of Munchausen by proxy, an exceedingly rare psychiatric condition in the caregiver of a minor where the caregiver is making the child ill. If that injustice were to occur, their daughter could end up in a psychiatric facility, as has happened with other children, most famously Justina Pelletier.

Justina was a Connecticut teenager who couldn't walk. Diagnosed with a mitochondrial disorder by doctors at Tufts University, she was then evaluated and admitted to Boston Children's Hospital, but the doctors there disagreed with her diagnosis. When her parents wanted to have her transferred to another medical facility, in a move that chills us to the bone, the hospital advised the Department of Children and Families in Massachusetts to take custody of Justina. She was then placed in a psychiatric ward at Boston Children's and kept in the hospital against her family's will for nine months. We wish we were making this up. In 2019, Justina celebrated the fifth anniversary of her release back to her family, who now have a well-justified mistrust of doctors.

Margaret's condition continued to deteriorate while her parents fought to get her proper care. She was eventually admitted to a children's hospital, where she lapsed into a coma-like state and remained so for almost ten months. The only time she woke up for any significant period was during a three-week course of antibiotics that the hospital agreed to give with outside medical input. Once it was discontinued, she lapsed back into a coma. For reasons we don't understand, the doctors taking care of her would not accept that her passing improvement was related to the antibiotics and they refused to treat her with them further. When Paul shared his experience with us, he spoke candidly: "As a pediatric anesthesiologist, I see a lot of hard stuff. But nothing like this . . . I'm a community guy. I teach lots of youth sports. I'm a doctor. When we bring up Lyme, people look at us like we're child abusers because they don't get it. They look at me like, 'What the hell are you talking about?' I feel like I'm losing my daughter and that no matter what I do here, I'm damned." Last we heard, Margaret was still doing poorly.

The experiences of these two families — the Millers and Margaret's — are not rare, outlier cases. We wish they were. They're all too common and represent how awful life becomes when a complicated, persistent infectious disease is ignored or denied. We must reiterate: The Lyme wars of the twenty-first century are the scourge of our time. We would venture to guess that fewer than 1 percent of doctors can treat complex cases of Lyme+, yet they affect millions worldwide. Too many patients' cries for help are ignored because modern medicine trivializes and, in many cases, ridicules chronic Lyme+ patients. Sadly, Lyme receives less than 2 percent of the public funding that West Nile gets and 0.2 percent of the funding that HIV/AIDS gets, despite the fact that the annual case count for Lyme dwarfs both diseases.[37] While CDC studies do show that the majority of doctors will treat for longer than IDSA mandates, they are clueless when a patient has chronic Lyme+. We keep finding ourselves saying to people who are struggling: *No, you're not crazy. You know your body. You know something is not right and you're not getting the right attention. Follow your gut.*

CHAPTER 2

The Myths That Get in the Way

Those who do not remember the past
are condemned to repeat it.

—*George Santayana*

L YME+ CAN CAUSE anything from long-term infection without symptoms to chronic illness ranging from mild to severe and
life-threatening. As mentioned, ticks and a host of other biting
bugs, known as arthropod vectors, can transmit many pathogens at
the same time; Lyme+ is our collective term for them. We don't like
calling non-Lyme infections "co-infections" because they can occur independently of Lyme and we don't want to minimize their own potentially devastating effects, but you are likely to hear that term used in the
media and literature.

Some common organisms that are considered part of the expan-
sive Lyme+ family include *Bartonella, Brucella, Babesia, Anaplasma,
Ehrlichia, Mycoplasma fermentans, Coxiella* (which causes Q fever),
Rickettsia (some species of which cause typhus and Rocky Mountain
spotted fever) and *F. tularensis* (which causes tularemia). Even though
Brucella, the bacterium that causes brucellosis, has historically been

said to be transmitted by eating infected dairy products, there is now persuasive evidence of vector-borne transmission, since it's been isolated from ticks, fleas, and lice, like its close cousin *Bartonella*. And most acute cases occur over the warm summer months.[1] In addition to these, borrelial infections can occur with bacteria that are cousins to Lyme but are technically not *Borrelia burgdorferi*. As previously mentioned, they can produce the same range of symptoms as Lyme disease, but testing for them is not routinely available.

Parasites, which are distinctly larger than bacteria, are another class of infectious organisms. They live in a host, such as a human, in order to survive and multiply. Members of this group range from microscopic single-cell creatures to multicellular animals that can be viewed with the naked eye. *Babesia*, a close cousin to the microbe that causes malaria, is an example of a parasite. Many chronic bacterial infections specifically suppress the immune response to ensure their survival. *Bartonella*, for example, will suppress the immune system against *Bartonella*; TB suppresses against TB. But parasites can cause more widespread immune suppression from an array of infections — from strep to the common cold. This is why people who have parasitic infections have more trouble getting over other infections. For example, *Babesia* dampens the immune response, which increases the burden of other infections, such as Lyme. We'll explore this phenomenon in much greater detail in a later chapter.

Willy Burgdorfer reported the presence of filaria, threadlike worms, in ticks from Shelter Island, New York, in the 1980s.[2] His visualization of filaria in *Ixodes* ticks led to his discovery of spirochetes in their midgut. We should note that the idea of parasitic worms as a potential member of Lyme+ is not on most people's radar, and certainly not in mainstream medicine. Some scientists have even suggested that *Borrelia* could be *inside* certain worms in a symbiotic relationship. The possibility of a systemic parasite needs to be fully investigated. Although we're trying to present the most common infections that can lead to chronic disease, parasites, some of which can be vector-borne and some of which are not, need to be considered. Remember, even if

a parasitic infection isn't causing symptoms, it may make it more difficult for the body to clear a bacterial infection due to the immune suppression from the parasite. This is well documented in the medical literature.[3] We've all wondered why some people get over Lyme+ with no
difficulty while others languish, disabled for years. Concurrent parasitic infections may be playing a larger role than anyone previously
thought. When I (Dr. Phillips) do a parasite workup, I order blood
tests looking for antibodies to a range of parasitic infections, as well as
a stool test looking for parasites.*

In 2017, another nightmarish tick-borne pathogen called the
Powassan virus† was reported to be spreading.[4] Though it's far less
common than other members of Lyme+, half of Powassan survivors
suffer permanent neurological symptoms such as headaches, memory
problems, and muscle wasting. About 10 percent of its victims die; in
October 2019, U.S. senator Kay Hagan from North Carolina died after
becoming infected in 2016. She experienced acute brain inflammation
(encephalitis) and other complications including pneumonia and neurologic decline. The scariest part of all is that Powassan can be transmitted within fifteen minutes of a tick bite and there's no treatment!
More recently, the Heartland and Bourbon viruses, which also have
high fatality rates, have been infecting humans via tick bites.[5] Most
cases reported to date have been in the Midwest and South. We suspect
the list of infectious agents in this realm will continue to expand. Per-

---

* Among the parasites tested for: toxocara, toxoplasma, filaria, trichinella, schistosoma, stronyloides, echinococcus, cysticercus, ascaris, entamoeba, giardia, cryptosporidium, and cyclospora/isospora.

† Viruses are not really organisms in that they're not alive. They're more like molecules than living creatures; they enter a host's cells and use the cell's machinery for survival. They do not eat food and cannot replicate outside of their host, though many
are known to live outside a host for a while (for example, a flu virus hanging out on a
countertop for hours awaiting its next host). Viruses are among the smallest agents of
infectious disease, while prions, infectious proteins without genetic material, are the
smallest currently known.

haps most troubling is the fact that all of these infectious agents — bacteria, viruses, and parasites — can be present simultaneously.

THE BIG LIST OF LYME+

Classic Lyme disease, as you know, is caused by *Borrelia burgdorferi*, a type of bacteria known as a spirochete. But other germs carried by ticks and other arthropod vectors can infect humans. Although the medical community calls these diseases co-infections, we again avoid the term because these other illnesses can develop with or without the presence of *Borrelia* and can often be worse than Lyme. Here's a partial list of these maladies:

Mycoplasma

This is a vast and ubiquitous group of intracellular bacteria, meaning they are capable of growing and reproducing within a host cell. They comprise more than 125 known species. They're the smallest of all bacteria known and lack a cell wall, making them naturally resistant to cell-wall-acting antibiotics like those in the penicillin and cephalosporin families. These organisms have been associated with a wide range of human diseases and are transmitted in many ways, including bugs. Some interesting facts supported by studies:

M. pneumoniae, which is airborne, is a common infection in the population. It's a frequent cause of pneumonia, even in healthy young people, and such patients are more likely than healthy controls to develop rheumatoid arthritis (RA).[6] It's also been shown to be in the lungs of 56 percent of asthmatics, but only 9 percent of people without asthma. It can cause neurologic symptoms including transverse myelitis, which is demyelination of the spinal cord that can lead to paralysis (though this outcome is rare).[7] It can also cause psychiatric symptoms such as psychosis.[8]

M. fermentans can be tick-borne, and has been isolated from the blood of RA patients who have higher rates of positive antibody tests than healthy controls.[9]

Multiple mycoplasma species were isolated from 69 percent of chronic fatigue syndrome patients versus 6 percent of controls.[10]

Multiple mycoplasma species have been found in patients with fibromyalgia and chronic fatigue syndrome at an overall rate that is five times higher than what's seen in the healthy population.[11]

M. hominis infection, which can be sexually transmitted, can lead to male infertility, with improvements in fertility after antibiotics.[12]

Chlamydiales, Including Chlamydia

Chlamydialis is composed of multiple bacterial families, including chlamydia and at least five others that are known as chlamydia-like organisms (CLOs). These bacteria can cause a range of chronic infections. Some interesting facts supported by studies:

Both chlamydiae[13] and chlamydiales[14] have been found in arthropod vectors, including ticks and fleas. Specific chlamydiales DNA has been detected in human skin which matches specific DNA from chlamydiales in ticks, implying tick transmission to skin.[15] Children have developed newly positive antibodies to chlamydia after tick bites.[16] It's not yet known if other members of chlamydiales will cause human disease in the way that we know chlamydia does.

C. pneumoniae, which is airborne like M. pneumoniae, is another common infection that causes pneumonia, even in healthy young people. It's also strongly correlated with atherosclerosis in large-scale analyses of data sets.[17] In addition, it's been found in the cerebrospinal fluid of MS patients and correlated with disease activity in those patients.[18]

Acute infection with C. pneumoniae has been shown to cause both new acute-onset asthma[19] and chronic asthma.[20] In placebo-controlled trials, asthmatics who tested positive for C. pneumoniae had their lung function improve with antibiotics but not placebo.[21] Steroids, a mainstay of asthma treatment by some doctors, make chlamydia infections worse.[22]

Chlamydial infections are suspected to contribute to autoimmune disease through molecular mimicry, whereby the foreign antigens on the bacteria are similar to the body's own antigens, confusing the immune system.[23] Even in its metabolically slowed but viable form, which persists inside cells, chlamydia releases a protein that's very similar to the human version of the same protein, which is what causes the reaction against our tissues.[24]

Tularemia (Rabbit Fever, Deer Fly Fever)

Francisella tularensis is the bacterium that causes tularemia, a potentially life-threatening disease spread to humans via contact with an infected animal or through tick, mosquito, deer fly, or horse fly bites.[25] Fleas also carry the organism, but have not yet been proven to transmit it. It only takes a small number of bacteria to cause an infection — as few as ten. In addition to causing flu-like symptoms, it can also attack the eyes, skin, lymph nodes, and lungs, depending on how and where the bacteria entered the body. There are also several types of tularemia, with each type having its own set of symptoms. Some people don't experience symptoms, while others suffer insidious, chronic illness. The average death rate for this disease without antibiotics may be 5 to 15 percent, and with antibiotic treatment, less than 2 percent. But like many infections listed in Lyme+, tularemia is usually only recognized by its more common signs and symptoms. Although the acute illness can carry a significant risk of death, the more chronic versions are less well defined but are published in the literature. Asymptomatic or minimally symptomatic infection rates are higher than many would expect. To put this in perspective, 12 of 132 (9.1 percent) healthy landscapers in Martha's Vineyard, Massachusetts, tested positive for tularemia.[26] Eight of them had no history of illness, two had a history of temporary fever, and two were previously diagnosed with tularemia and treated many years earlier. Most antibiotics are ineffective against *F. tularensis*, so it's important that this infection is diagnosed correctly and not missed.

Bartonella (Cat Scratch Disease, Trench Fever, and Carrión's Disease)

At least forty different species of *Bartonella* bacteria have been documented, more than twenty of which have been found to infect humans, causing bartonellosis. *Bartonella* species have been infecting humans for a very long time. *Bartonella quintana* DNA was demonstrated in a 4,000-year-old human tooth. *Bartonella* are mainly transmitted by ticks, fleas, lice, and biting flies, but transmission after ant and spider bites has been published in case reports as well.[27] *Bartonella* can cause a huge array of chronic illnesses, including neurologic conditions such as migraines and seizures, as well as rheumatic illnesses. Sudden onset of serious psychiatric conditions, including schizophrenia, can be caused by *Bartonella* infection, and its resolution with appropriate antimicrobial therapy has been published.[28] *Bartonella* is inherently antibiotic-resistant, can be difficult to treat, and Herxheimer reactions occur. Symptoms and signs of a *Bartonella* infection in my (Dr. Phillips') experience include depersonalization (loss of sense of identity), muscle or tendon pain with motion, fevers, back/sacroiliac/sternum/coccyx pain, large muscle jerking, breakaway weakness (where a muscle will just give out and then it's fine again), and a worsening of symptoms in the late afternoons into the evening. Signs that can be seen with *Bartonella* but also can be seen with other illnesses include chronically low white blood cell count, high C-reactive protein (CRP), hemolytic anemia (rapid destruction of red blood cells, causing anemia), and an enlarged spleen. Examples of other illnesses that must be ruled out in such cases include babesiosis (caused by *Babesia* parasites) and cancers of the blood, among other things.

Babesia microti and *Babesia duncani*

Babesia is a protozoan parasite of the blood that causes babesiosis. Over a hundred species of *Babesia* have been identified, and at least four infect humans;[29] in Europe, for example, *Babesia divergens* is one common species. In the United States, *Babesia microti* and *duncani* are the most common strains associated with humans; other species infect cattle, livestock, and occasionally domestic animals. People who contract babesiosis can develop anything from no symptoms to malaria-like symptoms with fever and anemia. As a result, malaria is a common misdiagnosis for the disease. Babesiosis can be dangerous in any age group, but is most likely to become life-threatening in the very young and very old, and in patients without a spleen. Herxheimer reactions upon treating babesiosis are not documented in the medical literature. If such a flare of symptoms develops, it's possible that the patient has another infection that causes Herxheimers, such as *Borrelia* or *Bartonella*, and that that organism is also sensitive to the medication for babesiosis.

Rickettsia, Including Rocky Mountain Spotted Fever (RMSF) and Typhus Fevers

These infections are caused by a diverse collection of bacterial species from the same larger family. (The term "Rickettsia" has nothing to do with rickets, which is a deficiency disease resulting from lack of vitamin D.) *Ehrlichia* and *Anaplasma* bacteria are often lumped into the same category; they are closely related but are not technically *Rickettsia*. The organisms tend to be very sensitive to doxycycline and clinical improvement is usually rapid once treatment is begun, but the mortality for untreated RMSF is 20 to 25 percent, so an accurate diagnosis and prompt treatment are imperative. As is the case for all Lyme+ infections, there are high rates of asymptomatic infection.

Brucella

Brucella bacteria, comprising many species and strains, have broad global distribution, and are close cousins to *Bartonella*. Like *Bartonella*, it's unusually resistant to most antibiotics and can be difficult to treat; relapses and chronic illness are common. Treating brucellosis can cause a potentially severe Herxheimer reaction, which can be fatal in rare cases. Brucellosis can be acquired by exposure to an infected animal via a cut in the skin, by inhalation of aerosolized bacteria, or by ingestion of contaminated food such as unpasteurized dairy or undercooked meat. In utero and sexual transmission have been documented. And like *Bartonella*, it's also been isolated from ticks, fleas, and lice. Arthropods can transmit *Brucella*, as researchers have now documented. In human brucellosis, acute illness has a marked seasonality, consistent with arthropod transmission, with higher numbers of acute cases occurring in spring and summer as opposed to fall and winter.[30] Arthropod transmission is now thought to occur.[31] One of the many names for brucellosis is undulant fever, because the symptoms worsen in the morning and then again in the late afternoon. Brucellosis is a highly debilitating condition, with extreme incapacitation being common. Patients frequently can't walk due to arthritis of the spine, and can experience severe rheumatic symptoms, anemia, fever, weight loss, inflammation of the eyes with vision loss, and depression. Mortality averages about 2 percent.

Relapsing Fever Spirochetes

Relapsing fever is caused by several species of *Borrelia* spirochetes that are transmitted by lice or ticks. The severity of illness and risk for fatality vary depending on which species of *Borreliae* cause the illness. Louse-borne relapsing fever is generally more serious than tick-borne relapsing fever, with untreated and treated mortality rates of 10 to 40 percent and 2 to 5 percent versus less than 10 percent and less than 2 percent, respectively. Symptoms include sudden chills, high fever, severe headache, nausea, vomiting, muscle and joint pain, delirium, and a rash on the trunk and extremities. Untreated patients can have two to ten recurrences of symptoms at one- to two-week intervals; these relapses manifest with a sudden return of fever and other symptoms. Herxheimers in relapsing fever, especially the louse-borne variety, can be very severe and even fatal. A strategy to make treatment safer is to use slowly increasing doses of antibiotics. Relapsing fever *Borreliae* can be visible in blood smears, in stark contrast to Lyme *Borreliae*.

Lyme and Lyme-Like Spirochetes

As already noted, there are numerous species of *Borrelia* (e.g., *burgdor-feri*, *afzelii*, *bissettii*, *mayonii*, *lonestar*, *miyamotoi*, etc.) with global distribution, and more species are discovered on a regular basis. There are commercially available tests for Lyme, Miyamotoi, and Mayonni, but at the time of this writing, it's next to impossible to find testing for the others. Although we have substantial data on the clinical manifestations of Lyme, much less is known about the closely related non-Lyme *Borreliae*. They're said to cause a Lyme-like illness, but there is insufficient research evidence to outline the extent of overlap and what key differences may exist. Lyme ranges from asymptomatic infection to a rapidly fatal illness, and typically includes flu-like symptoms, musculoskeletal pain, and cardiac and neurologic symptoms. Even in asymptomatic patients, there can be a late recurrence of symptoms similar to what occurs in syphilis. There are frequently Herxheimer reactions upon starting therapy, which, although potentially severe, are usually less severe than some other Lyme+ infections. Lyme *Borreliae* cannot routinely be visualized in body fluids, and antibody tests are notoriously unreliable. Lyme *Borreliae* are not inherently antibiotic resistant, but they become persistent in response to antibiotics, which is a different mechanism. Resistance is the ability to actively grow in the face of antibiotics, whereas persistence is the ability to morph into metabolically slowed-down organisms, which survive or, as the name implies, persist, despite antibiotic therapy, and then return to normal growth characteristics when the environment is more favorable. Therefore, Lyme's course is typically plagued by frequent relapses.

Coxiella *(Coxiella burnetii)*

This bacterium causes Q fever, which is shortened from its original name, "query fever,"[32] so named because of its inexplicable nature.[33] It's one of the least understood infections in Lyme+. It naturally infects farm animals, such as goats, sheep, and cattle, but is not limited to them, and is found in the placenta, amniotic fluid, urine, feces, and milk of such animals. Humans can become infected by inhaling dust that has been contaminated by infected animal body fluids and tissues, by eating contaminated, unpasteurized dairy, or through blood transfusion. In utero and sexual transmission have also been documented. Tick bites are another potential source of Q fever transmission, which has been documented in animal studies. Like all infections in Lyme+, the spectrum of illness runs the gamut — from asymptomatic to life-threatening. The symptoms of early Q fever are non-specific flu-like symptoms, which makes it difficult to diagnose and easy to miss. Untreated, it's estimated by the CDC that about 5 percent of infected individuals go on to develop chronic Q fever with high levels of bacteria in the bloodstream, which is hard to treat.[34] Treatment recommendations vary widely depending on the stage of illness, but the illness stage is not easy to identify, which makes trying to understand Q fever a puzzle.

Other important parasites, many in the U.S. and some more common elsewhere in the world, that can both cause multi-system illness and potentially worsen the outcome of other Lyme+ infections are listed below.

- **Filaria,** a threadlike worm, is transmitted by biting flies and mosquitoes.
- **Toxocara,** a parasitic roundworm transmitted from a dog or cat by handling their feces, is not able to complete its life cycle in humans, so baby worms never grow to adulthood and lay eggs, but they can cause disease in their juvenile state.
- **Toxoplasma,** a single-cell parasite, spread by eating undercooked meats, exposure to cat feces, or in utero, can cause severe illness in pregnant and immunosuppressed patients.
- **Strongyloides,** a roundworm whose larva can infect humans by penetrating skin when a person is walking barefoot, can complete its life cycle within humans, unlike many of the

parasites that can infect us. This can result in a loop of reinfection from our gastrointestinal (GI) tracts, called hyper-infection.

- **Trichinella,** a parasitic roundworm spread by eating undercooked contaminated meats, particularly pork, can cause a multi-system illness, whose severity is linked to how many parasites are consumed.

- **Echinococcus,** a tapeworm whose larval forms cause human disease, is spread by ingesting food contaminated by dog feces. Even petting an infected dog carries a risk, because eggs from feces can be caught in the fur. In humans, cystic disease develops and sometimes requires surgery in addition to medication.

- **Cysticercus,** the larval form of *Taenia solium*, the pork tapeworm, can be ingested on fecally contaminated foods and cause cysticercosis, a potentially severe disease where cysts form throughout the body, including the brain. Whereas cysticercosis is *only* acquired from ingestion of eggs, *not* by the ingestion of cysticerci (which are, again, larval forms of *Taenia solium*) in undercooked pork, ingestion of cysticerci from undercooked pork can infect humans with adult tapeworms that live in our intestines.

- **Schistosoma** are parasitic worms that can penetrate the skin of persons swimming in bodies of fresh water. The resulting disease is called schistosomiasis. Species of these worms that cause severe disease are present in seventy countries. Although we don't have the worms that cause schistosomiasis in the United States, we have cousins to those worms, other schistosomes, which penetrate skin, causing swimmer's itch when they typically die in the skin, but they sometimes penetrate other organs as well.[35]

- **Leishmania** is a mostly tropical parasite spread by the bite of sand flies. It's present in over ninety countries. It is uncommon in the U.S., although it's been acquired in Texas and Oklahoma. In early stages leishmaniasis can cause skin and mucous membrane lesions. It can be difficult to diagnose and treat, and in untreated advanced cases it is usually fatal.

- **The GI parasites** include giardia, entamoeba, cryptosporidium, and cyclospora/isopora.

Note that even for the infections that are more endemic in certain parts of the world, the nature of travel today make them all potential next-door neighbors.

The complexity of Lyme+ is partly why so many misconceptions and myths can perpetuate. We're going to cover the main ones below. This information will help you gain the most from our book.

MYTH: It takes 24 to 48 hours of attachment for ticks to transmit Lyme or other infections.

FACT: Some authorities state that it takes the tick at least thirty-six hours to transmit *Borrelia*, but this is not the case. There is no safe time for a tick to be attached since the minimum attachment times for transmission of almost all of these pathogens is unknown; however, there are studies that indicate rapid transmission of some. Colorado State University's Gregory Ebel and Laura Kramer of the New York State Department of Health were the first to demonstrate that Powassan virus infection can happen within fifteen minutes of tick attachment, publishing their findings in 2004.[36] Although Brazilian researcher Danilo Saraiva and his colleagues found that transmission of *Rickettsia rickettsii* by unfed *Amblyomma aureolatum* ticks required more than ten hours' attachment time, they also found that transmission could occur in as little as ten minutes with engorged ticks.[37] In a 2014 medical journal review article looking into tick duration times to transmit Lyme, British scientist Michael J. Cook reports a paper from 1987 in which data from rodent studies showed that the longer a tick was attached, the higher the risk of infection.[38] But the timing was mixed. One of the rodents became infected in less than twenty-four hours while others took longer. When the scientists calculated the probability of transmission within twenty-four hours, they came up with a percentage as high as 20.37. In his own paper, Cook writes: "The claims that removal of ticks within 24 hours or 48 hours of attachment will effectively prevent Lyme are not supported by the published data, and the minimum tick attachment time for transmission of Lyme in humans has never been established." *Borreliae* are present in the salivary glands of even unfed ticks about 20 percent of the time, which could make transmission of Lyme more rapid from those ticks.[39] And some studies in the past didn't take into account the length of time that ticks crawl around before biting, which can be substantial, amounting to an overestimate of the tick attachment time required for transmission.

MYTH: Tick bites only happen to people who are outdoorsy, have pets, and do a lot of hiking and camping.

FACT: You can pick up a tick by taking even one step through short grass. It happened to Dana twice! After strolling from the curb into a restaurant and brushing against a few blades of cut grass along the walkway in Sag Harbor, New York, I picked up a sneaky tick that tried to emb itself between my toes. And twenty-four hours after a concert at Jones Beach in which I took one step on a short patch of grass, I found an engorged tick embedded in my thigh, in spite of wearing long pants and copious amounts of DEET (diethyltoluamide) all over. This bite required two weeks of prophylactic antibiotics. You can even get bitten on a beach or in your sleep! And remember, ticks aren't the only culprits — they're just one of many disease-carrying bugs.

MYTH: People with early stages of Lyme disease typically get a rash, and that rash looks like a classic "bull's-eye" (a red circular rash that's clear in the center).

FACT: The most common appearance of erythema migrans (EM) is a solid pink circular-to-oval rash. Remember, the initial published findings by Dr. Steere documented that only 25 percent of patients had a history of rash compatible with EM. Other published research has pegged the rate of prior EM in late Lyme patients at 22 percent.[40] Part of the problem with arriving at an accurate percentage is that the CDC's statistics on the rates of EM in early Lyme may be inherently skewed higher. It may be likened to publishing a study about how many moviegoers purchase tickets, when the ticket purchase is required for entrance in the theater in the first place.

MYTH: You would know if you were bitten.

FACT: Ticks and tick bites are tiny, frequently occur in hidden places such as within hair on the scalp or in body crevices, and often go unnoticed. Most Lyme patients don't recall having a tick bite. The distinctive bull's-eye rash is an *atypical* presentation, and other symptoms like fatigue, joint pain, and fever mimic many other illnesses.

MYTH: Diagnosing Lyme is easy.

TRUTH: Diagnostic failures cause much of the confusion around Lyme and associated diseases. The widely used diagnostic for Lyme is the two-tier blood test, which measures the presence of antibodies against the pathogen and, as mentioned, misses most cases of Lyme. It also does not reveal the presence of the bacterium itself. Because it can take two to four weeks for the body to generate antibodies, too-early testing has been shown to miss up to 60 percent of acute (early-stage) Lyme cases. Sadly, detection of late-stage cases doesn't fare much better. Lyme antibody testing also does not detect related *Borrelia* species (e.g., the Lyme-like *Borrelia miyamotoi, bissettii, mayonii,* or *lonestari*), or any of the other infections such as *Bartonella, Babesia, Anaplasma, Ehrlichia, Rickettsia, F. tularensis, Brucella,* or filaria, among others. They also have high variability between labs and cannot be used to assess treatment response following antibiotics. Also notable is the fact that this kind of testing cannot differentiate between active infection and a previous one. (Much more on testing later.)

MYTH: If you test negative for Lyme using bodily fluids such as blood, spinal fluid, urine, and/or tissues to detect *B. burgdorferi* and/or its components, and if you fail to have the objective signs outlined in the CDC case criteria, such as EM, Bell's palsy, arthritis, or atrioventricular heart block, then you can't have Lyme disease.

FACT: As mentioned, Lyme antibody testing is abysmal. There are over fifty medical journal articles documenting active Lyme disease despite negative antibody tests.[41] Even a normal spinal tap doesn't rule out Lyme; intact live bacteria and their DNA have been found in normal-appearing spinal fluid.[42] This research spans all stages of illness. In terms of objective signs (what doctors can see and prove) versus subjective symptoms (what patients feel but can't prove), volumes of published data show that subjective symptoms of Lyme such as fatigue, headache, muscle pain, and joint pain outnumber the objective signs by significant numbers.[43] So to restrict clinical diagnosis to those patients who have the few objective features (e.g., positive Lyme test along with usual clues like the rash) that comprise the CDC criteria reinforces a medical paradigm of dismissing patients and leaving them undiagnosed. Remember that the CDC admits that their criteria fail to capture 90 percent of Lyme cases!

MYTH: Direct testing, which uses special technology to detect DNA from an invading germ, rules out the presence of Lyme disease when negative.

FACT: Unfortunately, direct detection of the infection has proven challenging due to a number of complicating factors and cannot be relied upon when results are negative. Newer, more accurate detection approaches are being developed, but despite good research supporting their validity, they have not yet become publicly available.

MYTH: Neurological problems from Lyme disease are not common.

FACT: Neurological problems resulting from Lyme disease are extremely common, much more so than arthritic issues, which typically affect the knees and are associated with positive Lyme antibody tests. But neurologic features, especially later into the illness, are associated with fewer positive Lyme tests, making late-stage neurologic Lyme symptoms more difficult to diagnose than Lyme arthritis. (*Bartonella* is far more likely to be associated with a widespread inflammatory arthritis than Lyme.)

Studies have shown that within two weeks of entering the body, Lyme *Borreliae* can invade the brain and spinal cord.[44] At this stage, some patients develop meningitis (inflammation of the lining around the brain), but it's often asymptomatic. Lyme meningitis isn't the acutely life-threatening kind like the ones caused by fast-growing bacteria. A rarer but potentially more serious manifestation of brain infection with Lyme *Borreliae* is encephalitis (inflammation of the brain itself). Once inside the central nervous system, the organism can wreak all kinds of havoc, ranging from mild to severe, including headaches, sleep disturbance, sensitivity to light and sound, cognitive dysfunction, numbness, weakness, abnormal muscle movements, and even mental illness. Common psychiatric manifestations include depression, anxiety, and OCD (obsessive-compulsive disorder). Less common psychiatric outcomes include bipolar disease and psychosis.

MYTH: It's not Lyme, it's MS, and we can always tell the difference.

FACT: The tail of *Borrelia* spirochetes contains flagellin, which appears nearly identical to myelin to the immune system. Myelin is the protective sheath surrounding nerves. During the immune system's response against Lyme, and probably non-Lyme *Borrelia* spirochetes as well, there can be collateral damage to myelin, the medical term for which is *demyelination*, the hallmark of multiple sclerosis (MS). Back in the early MS literature, researchers found spirochetes in the brains of MS patients on autopsy.[45] So convinced were they that it caused MS, they called it by a Latin name that meant "myelin destroyer." The causal relationship of spirochetal infection, likely *Borreliae*, to a significant percentage of relapsing MS is well documented in the medical literature and explored in later chapters. We can't tell you how many times patients have been diagnosed with MS when, in reality, they had an underlying Lyme infection causing their demyelinating disease. It is never normal for your body to start attacking itself for no reason. There is always a reason, and if we don't find it, lives can be lost. Multiple sclerosis was definitively thought to be an infectious disease before the concept of autoimmune illness sprang up with the discovery that steroids could temporarily suppress symptoms.

Despite their toxicity, immune-suppressing drugs (like the ones in numerous TV commercials) have become commonplace treatments. They can sometimes temporarily suppress symptoms but they do not get to the root of the problem in people who have an underlying infection. When the immune system is suppressed, the bacteria are able to go deeper and become more entrenched in the body, while patients are also made vulnerable to other serious infections. This is why giving steroids before, and even with, antibiotics increases the risk of antibiotic treatment failure in Lyme. If that's not enough to make you think twice about immunosuppressants, tune in to the disclaimers for these exorbitantly priced drugs and see for yourself: Their toxic side effects involve almost every organ while Big Pharma gets filthy rich. Ocrevus, for example, is a drug for MS and costs $65,000 per year. But that's just the price of the drug. It doesn't include all the associated fees involved with administering it.

One of my (Dr. Phillips') patients was paralyzed on the left side of his body with a diagnosis of multiple sclerosis (MS) at the age of thirty-eight after he had Lyme. With antibiotics, his paralysis resolved, as did most of his eleven brain and spinal cord lesions. Because he responded more quickly than average, it only took a month for the paralysis to get 90 percent better, and within seven months, he was 95 percent back to normal. Over twenty years have passed and he's not relapsed, though he still gets the occasional minor symptom. His protocol includes pulsing — going on and off antibiotics intermittently. (More on treatments in Chapter 7.) Generally, it involves three weeks of oral antibiotics about six times per year because relapses are very common when severe central nervous system illness has become established. Most of my MS patients come to me already on standard MS drugs and not doing well. If I find evidence of Lyme, I add in combinations of oral, pulsed antimicrobials centered on a backbone of tetracycline-class antibiotics and the large majority see their symptoms improve, along with about a 50 percent rate of lesions disappearing on MRI. However, it usually takes twice as long to treat these patients as the average Lyme+ patient. I've had other doctors tell me they think it's a coincidence when my patients get better after a decade of illness. I'll never cease to be amazed by the power of bias.

MYTH: PANS isn't a real illness.

FACT: Children and teens can develop a neurological form of Lyme+, which seems to be mostly due to *Bartonella* infection, that manifests as acute behavioral or emotional disturbances, termed PANS (Pediatric Acute-onset Neuropsychiatric Syndrome). These kids experience a range of symptoms that can include immediate, dramatic personality changes, most notably OCD, tics, and sleep disturbance. PANS can range from mild to severe, frequently resulting in withdrawal from social activities and worsening school grades, and even the inability to attend school at all. The stress and trauma, for both the patient and the family, that a severe case of PANS can produce is beyond words. Parents become prisoners to an illness that doctors are clueless about. Imagine your darling fourteen-year-old daughter, on the honor roll, well behaved, funny, the apple of everyone's eye, who in the span of two months turns into a terrorizing, cursing, raging stranger with narcolepsy. A stranger who spits at you, screams that she hates you, throws dishes at your head, sleeps all day, and sneaks out of the house in the middle of the night to find trouble. Welcome to PANS.

One case in particular that hit home for us is the story of a bright young man starting college. Eric was a freshman at a college in Southern California in the fall of 2017 when, two months into the semester, he developed flu-like symptoms, followed by two asymptomatic weeks, and then three weeks of severe vertigo. He then suddenly developed severe anxiety and derealization, which is a feeling that one's surroundings are not real. Depersonalization and derealization are common neuropsychiatric symptoms of bartonellosis in my (Dr. Phillips') experience.

Eric had never had a psychiatric disturbance in his life. Panicked, he asked his parents to find local doctors. He saw five who came up empty and eventually referred him to a psychiatrist, whose treatments were unsuccessful. So many doctors, no answers, yet the medical literature is rife with studies documenting that psychiatric illnesses can be linked to common infections like Lyme+. The fact that it came on so abruptly made it all the more suspicious for infection. How did the doctors miss this? They probably just didn't know; many general doctors and even psychiatrists don't know the breadth of what these infections can do, and dismiss them out of sheer ignorance. After spending $5,000 on psychiatrists, Eric experienced no relief, and his anxiety and derealization worsened to the extent that he could no longer leave his dorm room. Desperate, he dropped out of school and flew home to be evaluated by a Lyme doctor. His *Bartonella* and Lyme tests came back positive and he started antibiotics. He had a rocky beginning and experienced only limited benefits after several months of uninterrupted antibiotic therapy focused on *Bartonella*. He finally came to me (Dr. Phillips) and I made some simple adjustments to his regimen, both in the individual drugs and by changing them to a pulsed schedule.

He improved and only required a couple of additional months of treatment before he felt fully recovered. He was able to return to school and now, at the time of this writing, he reports feeling great.

MYTH: Long-term antibiotic therapy for Lyme is an unproven treatment that's highly dangerous.

FACT: Of course, we want to minimize risks to patients from treatments and maximize benefits. Therapies for most serious diseases can have serious side effects, but the risk of fatality from long-term antibiotic therapy is quite low. Far more deaths have been caused by Lyme+ than by its treatment. The risk of fatal outcomes in the treatment of inflammatory diseases with immunosuppressive agents, and cancer with chemotherapy, is far higher than for antibiotic therapy, but the difference in those diseases is that they are accepted by the CDC as legitimate, therefore the risk is deemed justifiable. But high rates of treatment failures using short-term antibiotic therapy are well documented in the medical literature.[46] It has been clearly demonstrated in study after study that short-term antibiotics are simply not effective in many cases.[47] This, coupled with published research proving bacterial persistence despite short-term antibiotics, makes the case for longer treatments until better treatments come along.

One of the earlier case reports revealing how Lyme disease can survive antibiotic treatment was published by the University of Chicago's *Journal of Infectious Diseases* in 1988. A group of Swiss scientists successfully grew *B. burgdorferi* from joint fluid three months after a fifteen-year-old girl was treated for Bell's palsy (facial paralysis) due to Lyme disease.[48] She'd been bitten by a tick in Austria but experienced none of the typical symptoms — no rash, malaise, fever, or musculoskeletal pain. It wasn't until one side of her face drooped that doctors suspected Lyme, after which she underwent the conventional, two-week antibiotic treatment. After initially improving, she relapsed a couple of months later, developing sudden, unexplainable arthritis in her right knee. Her doctors finally found *B. burgdorferi* in her joint fluid and ordered another round of antibiotics, concluding that a two-week course of antibiotics for Lyme was inadequate.

In 1993, a more dramatic report was published out of the Department of Medicine at Fitzsimons Army Medical Center in Aurora, Colorado.[49] There, a twenty-four-year-old patient with Lyme arthritis continued to relapse when the antibiotics were stopped. Despite *years* of oral and IV antibiotics, the researchers found *B. burgdorferi* in the patient's joint tissue and joint fluid—proof again that the bacteria can escape the assault of antibiotics. But the IDSA guidelines fail to take studies like these into account.

To understand the importance of considering novel treatments to address complicated health challenges—in this case, long-term antimicrobial therapy for Lyme+—it helps to consider other areas in medicine where out-of-the-box thinking eventually revolutionized the field, but only after hard-won battles. It was long thought, for example, that stomach ulcers were caused by diet and stress, for which bland foods, antacids, and meditation were prescribed, without benefits. Such patients went on to suffer, some requiring surgery, and some dying from bleeding ulcers or stomach cancer. In 1982, the Australian physicians Robin Warren and Barry Marshall found a link between *Helicobacter pylori* infection and ulcers, concluding that the bacteria—not spicy foods and a mean boss—were to blame. In 1983, they presented a paper to the Australian Gastroenterological Society, but never finished their presentation because they were laughed off the stage.[50] Barry Marshall took drastic steps. He had a baseline endoscopy of his stomach performed, which was normal, and then drank a batch of *H. pylori*. Soon after, he developed severe gastritis that was documented by another endoscopy. He then took antibiotics, which resolved his condition, documented again by endoscopy. It was because of this desperate tactic that Marshall and Warren were able to turn around medical dogma within fifteen years, which is light speed for a complete about-face in medical doctrine.[51] In the past, other physicians had tried to change medical dogma but couldn't break through the medical community's wall of arrogance.[52]

For example, in 1940, Dr. A. Stone Freedberg, of Harvard, found the spiral-shaped bacteria in the stomachs of ulcer patients, but wasn't believed. In 1946, Dr. Constance Guion presented a paper on treating stomach ulcers with the antibiotic chlortetracycline, but her colleagues at Cornell Medical School denounced her so mercilessly that she ditched her thoughts of treating ulcers with antibiotics. And then there was John Lykoudis, a physician from a small town in Greece, who developed a bleeding ulcer and cured himself with antibiotics. Since they worked for him, he treated his ulcer patients with antibiotics too, and found they were effective. He soon had patients flying in from all over the world to have him treat their stomach ulcers with antibiotics. In the 1950s, he presented his work to professors at several Greek medical schools but was met with laughter. He then contacted the Greek minister of health, the prime minister of Greece, and eventually the chairmen of the department of medicine at Athens Medical School, to no avail. He was treated like a pariah. Unable to get his work published, he died without vindication, never getting to see Drs. Marshall and Warren win the 2005 Nobel Prize for their discovery.*

The state of medical dogma today regarding Lyme+ is worse than it was for stomach ulcers before Marshall and Warren took the stage. The Lyme+ doctrine is similarly based on obsolete, erroneous data, but far more riddled with financial conflicts of interest, as follows:

1. Big Pharma sells few cures, but it sells lots of bandages — very expensive bandages that require lifelong refills. No pharmaceutical company is interested in finding the cause of autoimmune disease and eradicating it. That wouldn't be profitable.[53]

---

* In 1997, the CDC, with other government agencies, academic institutions, and the medical industry, launched a national education campaign to inform health care providers and consumers about the causal link between *H. pylori* and ulcers. Until word got out, millions suffered needlessly, including family members of our own, having no idea that their cure was an inexpensive prescription away. At the time the national education campaign spread the news, nearly 90 percent of patients were still subscribing to the old dogma and relentlessly popping antacids and avoiding their favorite foods to no avail.

2. Obsolete, inaccurate Lyme blood tests still bring in big money for their patent holders, so why would they want to improve them? Why not just control the conversation, keep saying that they work fine?

3. The now defunct Lyme vaccine lined the pockets of certain physician researchers who continue to espouse the same medical doctrine that was required to get its FDA (Food and Drug Administration) approval (perhaps in the hopes that it would clear the way for a second Lyme vaccine). The belief that Lyme is easy to diagnose and easy to cure was a necessary prerequisite for vaccine approval because administering the Lyme vaccine to someone who still harbors *B. burgdorferi* in their body could be dangerous.

MYTH: The medical establishment has no idea what causes Post-Treatment Lyme Disease Syndrome or what the best treatment for it is.

FACT: If you've been dealing with chronic Lyme+, then chances are you've heard this statement. As previously noted, PTLDS is a misleading term given the wealth of published information that these organisms can persist — and indeed continue to thrive — despite drugs that were initially thought to kill them but don't. It's an illogical construct. Think about it: What are the chances that a second disease of mysterious origins (i.e., PTLDS or an autoimmune disease), but with the same symptoms as the first disease, would come and replace the first disease? What are the odds, in light of published evidence that the pathogens that cause the first disease survive after both short- and long-term antibiotics? Consider also that there are numerous other chronic bacterial infections that require long-term combination antibiotic therapies: tuberculosis, leprosy, chronic coxiella, brucellosis, and Whipple's disease, to name a few, some of which are included in what we term Lyme+. Many of the other members of Lyme+ are no different and should be included in the same category.

The consequence of referring to patients with persistent symptoms of Lyme disease after a short course of antibiotics as having Post-Treatment Lyme Disease Syndrome is a *fait accompli*, in that such patients, now desperately searching for answers on the CDC website, may feel that antibiotics can't possibly help them. You may already believe this if you've ever gone to the CDC's website. But if someone with Lyme+ is led down the path of PTLDS, this will only delay care further and increase the likelihood of subsequent antibiotic treatment failure. Late-stage Lyme+ is difficult to treat. Because semantics guide patient care, we believe the term Post-Treatment Lyme Disease Syndrome is harmful, and in some cases fatal, and it should not be used.

MYTH: Reports of cases of Lyme being mistaken for other diseases are rare.

FACT: There are many published cases where Lyme has been mistaken for other diseases, which prompted the nickname "The Great Imitator." Of course, in these cases the diagnosis of Lyme was eventually made, hence the ability to have the published reports. The natural question that follows is how many patients never get appropriately diagnosed with Lyme, never get treated, and remain in the category of "other disease"? This is why we refer to Lyme (but really Lyme+) as "the great cause." In my (Dr. Phillips') clinical experience of treating more than 20,000 patients, I see people come in with diagnoses of fibromyalgia, rheumatoid arthritis (RA), chronic fatigue syndrome, GI disorders, cardiac symptoms, and MS on a regular basis. When I find evidence for Lyme+, the large majority of these patients markedly improve with antimicrobial therapy.

Take the case of Suzie, a fifty-year-old woman with no significant medical history. Unlike most patients, Suzie knew she got a tick bite and immediately called her primary care doctor to get prophylactic antibiotic treatment. But he refused, advising her instead to watch for symptoms. Within a week, she developed rapidly progressive and severe arthritis, a condition she'd never previously experienced. At that point her doctor prescribed doxycycline for a few weeks, but it only had a minimal impact, and he refused to refill the prescription. She became markedly worse, with her joints swelling to literally ten times their normal size. She had elevated levels of inflammatory markers in her blood, indicative that her body was fighting something. If you consider the elevated inflammatory markers from a Lyme+-centric view, most likely *Bartonella*-centric to be precise, you'd think of infection. But if you're a rheumatologist, you might be inclined to see these test results and symptoms as consistent with rheumatoid arthritis.

Turns out Suzie was referred to a rheumatologist, who diagnosed her with rheumatoid arthritis. She pleaded that her symptoms arose following a tick bite, but the rheumatologist insisted that it wasn't related and strongly advised her to begin a course of immunosuppressants. Suzie refused. By the time she came to see me many months later, her ankles were the size of soccer balls and she had similar inflammation in most joints. She couldn't move without intense pain. After a year and a half of aggressive treatment using multiple rounds of antibiotics, she was strikingly better and never needed to go on immunosuppressants. Although she still has some mild arthritic symptoms, she is now fully functional. This all would likely have been avoided had her primary care doctor treated her bite with a few weeks of doxycycline before she developed symptoms.

MYTH: *Bartonella* only appears as cat scratch fever and will go away on its own without treatment.

FACT: Cat scratch fever constitutes only a small fraction of the many manifestations of *Bartonella* infection. The disease got its name because someone contracted it from a bite or scratch from a cat infected with *Bartonella henselae*, but in reality, arthropod bites are responsible for the large majority of *Bartonella* infections. Hence the term "cat scratch fever" is misleading. As we have seen, *Bartonella* is a class of bacteria that cause an enormous range of human chronic disease. Illnesses known to be caused by *Bartonella* species include trench fever and Carrión's disease. Trench fever, also known as five-day fever, is caused by *B. quintana*, and named for its original discovery when the infection was spread through body lice among soldiers in the trenches in World War I. At that time, up to one-third of ill British troops had the disease, which can consist of periodic fevers at five-day intervals along with a multi-system illness similar to most *Bartonella* infections. Carrión's disease is an often acutely fatal illness, caused by *B. bacilliformis*, named after the medical student who discovered it. In 1885, Daniel Carrión inoculated himself with *B. bacilliformis* to prove the cause of the infection, which is spread through the bites of certain sand flies. Twenty-one days after becoming infected, at the age of twenty-eight, he died of the illness that now bears his name. Carrión's disease has been reported to have a fatality rate as high as 88 percent in the acute phase in patients who aren't hospitalized. Many patients who survive *B. bacilliformis* infection go on to develop a chronic form of the disease, *verruga peruana*, meaning "Peruvian warts," whose hallmark is large disfiguring skin lesions. So we see that *Bartonella* infections can cause everything from acute life-threatening illness to debilitating, chronic disease.

A case to illustrate the reality versus the myth of *Bartonella*:

Two months before twenty-year-old Justin Soriano came to see me (Dr. Phillips) he developed acute-onset eye irritation and left-sided Bell's palsy (the left side of his face drooped). A blood test for Lyme was positive, but not strong enough to meet the CDC diagnostic criteria. He was seen by a major university-based neurologist who is well published in the field of Lyme. Despite the Bell's palsy and the positive Lyme test results, two indications that he had Lyme, she did not offer him antibiotics because he failed to meet the stringent CDC criteria. Instead, Justin was treated with steroids, which made him much worse. He developed a new right-sided Bell's palsy to match his left-sided one, headache, inflammation of his optic disc (the exit door for nerve fibers to go from the eye to the brain), and pan-uveitis (inflammation of the entire uvea or middle layer of the eye, which is vision-threatening). He was admitted to the hospital, where a spinal tap tested positive for Lyme. The doctors didn't tell him he had Lyme, though Justin's dad overheard one doctor outside the room say, "I bet this kid has Lyme disease." In the hospital, he was kept on steroids and also treated with IV ceftriaxone (an antibiotic frequently used in hospitals for Lyme) for four weeks, with significant but incomplete resolution of the uveitis and no change in his optic disc swelling.

Upon stopping ceftriaxone, but staying on the steroid prednisone, Justin's illness became far worse. He developed hearing loss, tinnitus (ringing in the ear), lower back pain, ankle and knee pain, and rashes on the tops of his feet, sides of fingers, and wrists. He was seen by a rheumatologist, who didn't appear to recognize the important fact that his symptoms improved on ceftriaxone and worsened upon stopping it. Instead of pursuing an infectious cause for his illness, he diagnosed him with a "non-specific autoimmune" condition and started him on the chemotherapy drug methotrexate to suppress his immune system. His levels of inflammation, measured with a blood test, skyrocketed. This prompted the doctors to give him higher doses of this already toxic chemotherapy drug. Even though that didn't work, he was kept on methotrexate, and was then started on the popular immunosuppressant drug Humira, which didn't help either. Other, increasingly toxic chemotherapy drugs were suggested.

Three months later and rapidly deteriorating, his parents brought him to me. I immediately suspected bartonellosis from his clinical features. His *Bartonella* test was blaringly positive, but his uveitis specialist dismissed the diagnosis after Justin wasn't fully cured with a few weeks of Zithromax, which helped, but not completely. This doctor had the false impression that bartonellosis is always easy to treat. In total, it took eight months of intermittent antibiotic treatment to get him fully recovered. Justin's eye problems resolved and signs of inflammation completely abated. He has now been completely off of antibiotics for two years, takes no immunosuppressants, and still enjoys excellent health. It's scary to think about what would have become of Justin had his parents not questioned the advice of their first team of doctors and brought him to me. It's even scarier to think of all the Justins guided down the path of long-term chemotherapy and other immunosuppressants by their academic physicians, curing nothing, killing them slowly.

MYTH: Lyme disease cannot be transmitted in utero.

FACT: Studies dating back to the 1980s describe maternal-fetal transmission of Lyme disease.[54] Intact *B. burgdorferi* have been documented in stillborn babies, but somehow this transmission route remains contested. At first the WHO recognized congenital Lyme, but then removed it from their listings six months later, amid suspicions of political pressure.[55] The American Academy of Pediatrics (AAP) refuses to acknowledge the mounting evidence, some of which was recently published.[56] According to the AAP, "Lyme disease is not thought to produce a congenital infection syndrome." We know many patients who have had children infected transplacentally, documented by Lyme DNA in the cord blood, placenta, or foreskins. Transplacental transmission can cause miscarriage, stillbirth, and multiple, potentially serious developmental problems, which actually happened to one of my (Dr. Phillips') patients. She had been sick for a short time but had a serious case. This stage of illness, called *acute disseminated*, is associated with the highest risk of transplacental transmission if not treated with antibiotics, so I advised her to treat through the pregnancy. She was treated for a few months without incident and then moved away, to an area of the country not considered endemic for Lyme. Her new doctors told her that there was no such thing as transplacental Lyme and to stop antibiotics, which she did. Her son was born with birth defects, seizures, and fevers from day one, only to be diagnosed with Lyme by his pediatrician when he was a year old. The question of whether Lyme can be transmitted congenitally can also be addressed within the context of the other Lyme+ infections that are known and accepted to cross the placenta, many with less overwhelming evidence than

Lyme. So, why is Lyme being held to a higher, unrealistic standard of proof? Even the relapsing-fever *Borreliae*, which are Lyme's close relatives, are accepted to cause transplacental transmission. It's also accepted that *Babesia, Coxiella, Bartonella, Brucella*, and tularemia bacteria can cross the placenta.

Another infection to which Lyme can be compared is syphilis. Most people don't realize that syphilis and Lyme are cousins. Their culprits (*Treponema pallidum* and *Borrelia burgdorferi*) belong to the same group of spiral-shaped bacteria (spirochetes) that move like corkscrews, and they're both highly invasive. Syphilis is the poster child for congenital transmission, yet scientists claim that its cousin — *Borrelia burgdorferi* — has been transmitted in only "isolated case reports," which means that they're acknowledging that it happens. The truth of the matter, we reiterate, is that both animal and human congenital transmission of *Borrelia burgdorferi* have been repeatedly documented in the peer-reviewed medical literature, similarly to the many other Lyme+ infections currently accepted as being transplacentally transmitted.[57] And yet the reality of congenital Lyme is being denied.

Sue Faber, RN, is among Canada's most vocal advocates for Lyme+ patients based in Ontario; she co-founded LymeHope (LymeHope.ca) in 2017 following a harrowing experience with Lyme herself and with her three infected children. LymeHope is a not-for-profit dedicated to education and outreach on the subject of Lyme and related diseases in her country — a place where Lyme was unheard of two decades ago. Sue is on a mission to spread the word about congenital Lyme. According to her, the transmission of Lyme disease from mother to child in pregnancy drastically challenges and deconstructs the status quo — from a purely zoonotic disease to a disease that can be transferred from human to human, mother to baby. It only makes rational sense that these infectious bacterial microorganisms would be transferred in utero and follow patterns similar to other well-established TORCH infections. (TORCH refers to a group of infectious diseases that are known to cause problems in a developing fetus because they can be transmitted from mother to child. TORCH stands for: Toxoplasmosis;

Other agents including HIV, syphilis, varicella zoster, and fifth disease; Rubella; Cytomegalovirus; and Herpes simplex.)

In Sue's words: "Acknowledging and confronting this reality head-on opens up a Pandora's box that will undoubtedly result in upheaval, re-thinking, reordering, reinvestigating, and re-prioritizing. However, we have no choice but to act with the highest integrity, impartiality, and honesty. Maternal-fetal transmission of Lyme disease turns the current case definition of Lyme disease on its head, because congenitally infected babies obviously won't have a requisite tick-bite from an endemic area with an expanding EM rash. Standard blood testing may not be an appropriate diagnostic tool to determine if the baby has been exposed/infected with *B. burgdorferi* due to an immature immune system and reliance on blood tests may result in misdiagnosis of congenitally infected infants." She's right. What's more: "The limited published scientific and medical literature that exists on in-utero transmission identifies issues with striking significance that should be raising red flags and ringing the alarm bells."

Among the most pressing facts to address are that infected mothers can be asymptomatic (without recollection of a tick bite or typical Lyme symptoms) and yet still transmit Lyme bacteria to their baby, that mothers can test negative and yet still transmit Lyme bacteria to their baby, and that babies can be infected and asymptomatic at birth, only to develop progressive illness later. There have been reported cases where mothers were treated for Lyme disease with antibiotics and yet transmission of the organism to their baby still occurred. Sue also makes parallels to Lyme's relative, syphilis, when she calls for more research into transplacental transmission. The reason that women are universally screened for syphilis in pregnancy is because it is well known that women can be asymptomatic and still transmit *Treponema pallidum* to their baby, with devastating consequences. It is also widely known and accepted that up to 60 percent of syphilitic babies are asymptomatic at birth and only later develop signs and symptoms.

Sue's favorite quote, which she believes applies to what is happening with congenital Lyme borreliosis, comes from thought leader Margaret Heffernan: "The fact is that most of the biggest catastrophes that we've witnessed rarely come from information that is secret or hidden. It comes from information that is freely available and out there, but that we are willfully blind to, because we can't handle, don't want to handle, the conflict that it provokes. But when we dare to break that silence, or when we dare to see, and we create conflict, we enable ourselves and the people around us to do our very best thinking."* Out in western Canada, Dr. Ralph Hawkins at the University of Calgary in Alberta can no longer accept new patients because his wait list is at least three years long — too long for anyone to wait for treatment, given the gravity of this disease. He, too, is one of Canada's leading voices in the fight against Lyme+ disease and hopes more doctors have the courage to do what is, in their conscience, the right thing rather than to stick with the herd and be bullied into behaviors that don't help people who are suffering. He says, "When the system is in the way, you have to go through the obstacles."

Another area of denial is sexual transmission of Lyme. Again, it's similar to its cousin syphilis. Along with recovery of live *Borrelia* spirochetes from human semen and vaginal secretions, identical strains were recovered from sexually active couples, providing supportive evidence of sexual transmission. Given the wide array of borrelial strains, which number in the hundreds, the chances of isolating the exact same strain from sexual partners would be remote. Both congenital Lyme and sexual transmission of Lyme are hot-button topics, with far too little research being done to clarify these important issues and too much effort going into blanket denialism.

---

* If you have not watched Margaret Heffernan's 2012 TED talk, "Dare to Disagree," we highly recommend you check it out. In it, she chronicles the story of Alice Stewart, a pioneering British doctor in the 1950s who studied disease patterns and discovered that the children of women who were X-rayed during pregnancy were at a much higher risk of developing childhood cancers than those of expectant mothers who were not irradiated. At the time, this flew in the face of conventional wisdom, which held that X-rays were safe. Stewart rushed to publish her preliminary findings in *The Lancet* in 1956, but it took fully twenty-five years for the British and American medical establishments to abandon the practice of X-raying pregnant women.

SCIENCE IS PROVISIONAL

As the old saying attributed to philosopher George Santayana goes, "Those who do not remember the past are condemned to repeat it." As an analogy to Lyme+, consider the following historical context. In the vast territories of the British Empire in the nineteenth century, the most dangerous place to be was not some primitive land in British-controlled Africa or the wilds of a jungle. In the filthy, squalid confines of a Victorian teaching hospital, patients entered with trauma wounds and were carried out as corpses after developing what was called "hospital gangrene." Wound infections were common, and there was no such thing as hygiene as we know it today. At the time, the prevailing theory said that infections came from "miasma"—poisons in the air that originated from rot and decay. For Joseph Lister, however, a serious surgeon with a curious nature, this didn't make sense. If miasma was the culprit, then why did wounds not become reinfected after the rotten tissue was scoured out and the remaining tissue was doused with mercury pernitrate? (This was a form of mercury used at the time to treat an array of diseases.)

Lister's ideas coincided with Louis Pasteur's experiments that suggested that germs—not bad air—were the cause of infections. Cue the proverbial light bulb over Lister's head. He proposed that the culprit was not miasma but a lack of cleanliness, and that treating infected wounds with chemical agents that killed germs could prevent them altogether. Lister experimented with carbolic acid, a derivative of coal that sewage engineers used to deodorize the human waste that was recycled for fertilizer. His experiments led to dramatic reductions in infection rates. But teaching his newfound wisdom about antisepsis was difficult. Harvard's renowned Henry Jacob Bigelow, a dominant figure in Boston medicine, called it "medical hocus-pocus." Slowly but surely, however, doctors and scientists around the world began to adopt his antiseptic methods and Lister won over his detractors (and would forever be immortalized by the popular mouthwash that bears his name: Listerine). His persuasive weapon? Relentless focus on data and results. His warm and friendly personality earned him points, too. Lister was smart to target audiences of medical students—the next generation of physicians whose young minds were not yet ossified.

This approach predated what German physicist Max Planck would later observe in his own attempts to convince his colleagues of his radical ideas about quantum mechanics: "A new scientific truth does not triumph by convincing its opponents and making them see the light, but rather because its opponents eventually die, and a new generation grows up that is familiar with it." In other words, change does not occur because scientists with incorrect opinions change their minds in response to sound evidence, but rather because younger generations of scientists are more open to new ideas. This appears to be a recurring and sad truth across all the sciences—including medical science. We'd like to think that the truth is the truth and that's all there is to it. But that's not how it works. We're all shaped by what we have already learned, and our biases are far more powerful than we realize. Max Planck said it so eloquently in the past, but now it's been reduced to the very famous and to-the-point quote, "Science advances one funeral at a time."

Planck's remarks are perhaps more relevant today than ever before. A 2019 study coauthored by MIT economist Pierre Azoulay, an expert on the dynamics of scientific research, confirmed that Planck was right.[58] It often takes the death of star scientists for new scientists—and their perspectives—to gain attention and respect. Azoulay's research actually calculated the difference: the deaths of prominent researchers are often followed by an 8.6 percent increase of articles by those who did not previously collaborate with earlier, big-name scientists. These newcomers to the field are also more likely to publish papers that become heavily cited and influential.

The idea that we need a new generation of thinkers in the realm of Lyme+ is one that we not only strongly believe ourselves, but so do all the people we've encountered in researching and writing this book. In the words of psychiatrist Dr. Preston Wiles, Professor of Student Psychiatry at UT Southwestern Medical Center and Director of the Student Wellness and Counseling program there, "Doctors are fast learners, but they have a very difficult time when what they've learned has changed . . . Science is always provisional."

In order for real change to occur in the Lyme+ world in the next ten years, we need a concerted multi-pronged effort. We're writing this book in an effort to spread awareness, so please share it with your friends and loved ones! We're also working with our good friend Neil Spector, a Duke University oncologist and professor, on developing a more effective antimicrobial therapy for Lyme+, one which is designed to have broad activity and gets around the resistance mechanisms of these pathogens.

CHAPTER 3

Bitten and Broken

It is foolish to be convinced without evidence, but it is
equally foolish to refuse to be convinced by real evidence.

—*Upton Sinclair*

A JULY 2014 WEDDING on Long Beach Island, New Jersey, was the start of my (Parish's) nightmare. It was a beautiful weekend filled with love. There was lobster and champagne and a crazy Gordon Gekko–style house on the beach. I sang a few songs, made a toast, and cried happy tears for my dear friends tying the knot.

Two days later, I woke up back home in New York City with a crushing head and neck ache. It was weird but I figured that I'd sleep it off. After a few days, I felt better.

That weekend, when I got out of the shower, I saw a faint red circular rash on my shoulder with a bug bite in the middle. My knees buckled. I called for my husband, Andy. "HUNNEEEE! I have LYME!" He really didn't think so, because the rash didn't look like a stereotypical "bull's-eye." But I knew, and walked to the ER, where the fresh-faced doctor took a quick glance at my shoulder and said it looked like Lyme. The tiny bite surrounded by the rash that's diagnostic for Lyme was enough for her to arrive at the diagnosis. The doctor also said to be glad I caught it quickly. I took the twenty-one days of doxycycline as prescribed, following up with an infectious disease specialist a few days later, to be safe. He reassured me that I would have no complications since I caught the bite within a week. Though I still felt uneasy, I decided I was being overly cautious, and convinced myself to move on.

A month later, I woke up with my breast swollen and painful. Fearing that this could be a symptom of a deadly cancer, I rushed to my long-time internist, Dr. K, who looked scared, and said my breast tissue felt "like tons of little beads." Dr. K stepped out of the exam room and called an oncologist, who was kind enough to make room for me that day. He did not know why I had these strange symptoms ("too much soy, hormonal, maybe") but was certain it was not cancer. I saw him two more times to be sure. He was puzzled by my fixation and panic since he had ruled out the worst. But I know my body, and none of this felt right.

By October, my arms were profoundly, alarmingly weak. A fork felt like a bowling ball after my normal workout at the gym. I noticed my heart was palpitating and racing at night, and I could barely fall or stay asleep. When I did, drenching sweats startled me awake. Every time I closed my eyes, I saw horrifying faces melting into each other. I told Andy I was seeing monsters. My brain felt hazy and unfamiliar, and I was suddenly scared to be alone.

For the weakness, Dr. K sent me to a sports medicine doctor, who barked, "You're weak! You need to lift weights!" I told him my sternum ached. And my ribs. My bones. I feared I had lymphoma. I was so weak from the five-pound weights I lifted in his office that the next morning I couldn't wash my hair. I whispered to my sister-in-law, "Something is very wrong."

From there, I had burning rashes coming and going all over my sternum and traveling down my arms. I went to a second infectious disease doctor at NYU. I asked if all of my symptoms could still be from Lyme and he said no. When I pressed, he told me he was sure because he "went to medical school" and "Lyme is killed 100 percent of the time in the test tube with doxy." His flip answer unnerved me, so

I asked if he could send me to a Lyme specialist. He laughed and said, "Oh God. A bunch of shysters!" Instead, he sent me to an allergist who detected no allergies, yet prescribed me a strong antihistamine anyway. It didn't work.

I returned to the infectious disease doctor and asked him to check my inflammatory markers, which he thought was a "great idea." I wondered why he didn't think of it himself, especially when the results turned up a high rheumatoid factor, which means I had signs of autoimmunity, as can be seen in rheumatoid arthritis. He had no explanation or remedy.

In the midst of this, another NYU infectious disease doctor I knew joked about my spiraling health, asking, "How does your husband take it?" That outrageous comment sent a wave of shock through my system that solidified my determination to get to the bottom of my illness and share my story with everyone who'd listen.

By Thanksgiving, on the cusp of signing my new deal with Sony, I was relentlessly short of breath. It was my most terrifying symptom, and there was no way I could sing or write songs with it. I went to a cardiologist, who performed an echocardiogram and said my heart function was at 40 percent, like "a seventy-year-old man's." She used the words "heart failure" and said she was not sure why. Tears streamed down my face as I lay there gasping for air. The cardiologist paged Dr. K, who worked at the same hospital, to come and console me.

During Christmas week of 2014, I was in California with Andy, resting at our friend's beautiful farm. I was too weak and short of breath to walk from the bed to the car. I couldn't sleep and stayed up all night crying. I asked Andy to do an online search of all my bizarre, disparate symptoms and tell me what was wrong. I believed I was dying. He pulled up a comprehensive online checklist written by a well-known Lyme specialist, Dr. Joe Burrascano. I had thirty-seven of the sixty symptoms. Full-blown Lyme. I was enraged, overwhelmed, and afraid.

Luckily, my friends knew a specialist—a Lyme-literate doctor in San Diego, four hours away—who mercifully agreed to see me over the holiday if I could get to him. He examined me, took some blood, and listened to my story. He calmly said, "You have Lyme. Lyme does all kinds of weird things, but you'll get better. Amazing that I am only the twelfth doctor you've been to. Most find me somewhere between twenty and a hundred."

I flew home feeling terrified but took some solace in the fact that I finally had an answer and a plan. But I was not at all comfortable starting such a potentially grueling treatment with a doctor on another coast. After furious research, a last-minute email to friends led me to Dr. Phillips. I got in on a cancellation in January 2015 and began treatment with him. He clinically suspected that I also had *Bartonella*, which, he explained, complicates Lyme. He ordered a blood test that was positive for *Bartonella henselae*. To my detriment, all the others had missed it, delaying my life-saving treatment by five months.

I started on the pulsed, rotating course of long-term antibiotics he prescribed, along with a Chinese herbal protocol by Dr. Qing Cai Zhang of New York City's Zhang Clinic, and a strict paleo (anti-inflammatory) diet. In days, my muscles and joints calmed down. Within eight weeks, my brain fog lifted and the nighttime visions of melting faces stopped. My heart recovered normal function (70 percent) by April.

At this writing, it's been five years since I started proper treatment for Lyme and *Bartonella*. Although I still take short courses of antibiotics when I begin feeling symptomatic, I'm generally about 97 percent better and have been for about four years.

Now I look back on a childhood marred by chronic, excruciating bladder pain and inflammation (my urologist said my bladder looked like "a bloodshot eye") that was later diagnosed as the idiopathic "interstitial cystitis." I also suffered strange facial tics, and recurrent strep throat and congestion resulting in the removal of my tonsils and adenoids at age twelve. I also experienced sudden allergic reactions, intermittent anxiety, and panic attacks that my pediatrician called "generalized anxiety disorder." I now recognize that I likely had some strain of Lyme or a similar infection for most, or all, of my life. And now, with treatment under Dr. Phillips' care, all of those earlier symptoms, including interstitial cystitis and anxiety, are gone, too. I didn't know who I was until I treated Lyme.

I (Dr. Phillips) came down with my first case of *known* Lyme while backpacking across Europe between my first and second years of medical school. It should have been a straightforward diagnosis: a history of rashes compatible with EM followed by flu-like symptoms, then cardiac, neurologic, gastrointestinal, and musculoskeletal symptoms. But it was missed by a team of academic doctors in New York City. It wasn't until six months later, after learning about Lyme in med school, that I demanded a Lyme test, which luckily enough was positive at a local lab.

By then, however, Lyme was entrenched. Although antibiotics helped greatly, I experienced multiple relapses with each attempt to stop them, which prompted even more doctor visits. I ended up seeing about fifteen specialists, about half of whom re-treated me with antibiotics, frequently intravenously as was the preference among infectious disease doctors and rheumatologists in the early 1990s. The other half told me Lyme was gone, and that I was having "after-effects" of the infection (which just happened to get worse not only when antibiotics were discontinued, but also temporarily upon restarting them, consistent with Herxheimers).

Growing up, I had no health problems. I did great in school, was athletic, slept well, and was happy. But then a one-time episode of lightheadedness at age seventeen prompted a cardiologist visit and I was diagnosed with mitral valve prolapse. This is a common, largely innocuous heart condition, but in my case it was associated with advanced degeneration of my heart valve. My cardiologist estimated that I'd need heart valve surgery by the age of fifty. Nothing changed for seven years until I was diagnosed with Lyme and started long-term antibiotics. After that, my mitral valve started gradually healing on its own, which was demonstrated by yearly sonograms of my heart. By the fourth year of treatment, I had no heart valve disease, and at the time of this writing, at age fifty-four, my heart is still normal. What was the connection?

While I'm certain that I got a new Lyme infection during medical school, it's also possible that, despite being otherwise healthy, I got a weak strain of Lyme, or Lyme+, early on in life, as several of these infections have been shown to cause heart valve disease. It's been extensively documented in the medical literature that mild versions of these infections are common. By the end of my medical training, my health was good, despite chronic Lyme. At that point, my goal wasn't to be a Lyme doctor. That all changed when I realized my father had been suffering with undiagnosed Lyme for twenty years. His Lyme diagnosis was missed by the heads of cardiology in multiple teaching hospitals in New York City, which eventually culminated in life-threatening heart problems. By the mid-1990s, he was given six months to live unless he had a heart transplant, which was the next planned step. Since Lyme is a known cause of dilated cardiomyopathy, my father's condition, I asked his cardiologist about the possibility that he might have Lyme-induced heart failure, but he wouldn't even entertain the notion. To make a long story short, I diagnosed and treated my father with Lyme when his cardiologists scoffed, and his heart function began to normalize. About a year later, my father's heart failure had resolved, and antibiotics were continued for two more years. At the time of this writing, my father is eighty-seven, and not only has he never needed a heart transplant, he still doesn't have heart failure.

In August 2010 my own story took a darker turn. Over several weeks, I developed excruciating neck, back, and shoulder pain. I have no other way to describe it apart from saying that it was shockingly severe. I'd never experienced anything like this with my prior Lyme and several rounds of oral antibiotics brought only minimal and temporary improvement, leaving me baffled and scared.

In the weeks that followed, my sternum became visibly swollen, the pain intractable. My Lyme doctor, assuming this was due to Lyme, prescribed the intravenous antibiotic ceftriaxone (Rocephin), which had never cured my Lyme in the past but at least used to help. On a grey day in November 2010, three months after I first woke up with neck pain, I had to leave work because of wrenching sternum pain, canceling a full day of patients. I remember texting my brothers as I got into my car to drive home, barely able to lift my arms to the steering wheel, "I don't know what's happening to me. Getting worse every day. Leaving work to go home. I'm so scared."

Desperate, I restarted ceftriaxone that day. Within hours, all my joints were screaming in pain, which never happened in the past on that drug with my prior Lyme. But within a few days, my sternum swelling and pain improved. I stayed on it longer, thinking the joint pain a Herxheimer that I had to see through, which I did for several months, but despite the improvements to my sternum, everything else continued to worsen. And within two days of stopping it, my sternum pain crept back.

My symptoms expanded to include a piercing pain in the bones of my sacroiliac (SI) joints, which are the main joints connecting the lower spine to the hips. The pain was so extreme that I couldn't stand, let alone walk, for more than a few minutes. My doctors couldn't help me. The antibiotics that had worked best in the past to buoy me from the depths of Lyme were failing miserably. A functional medicine doctor couldn't help me either, despite strict adherence to her restrictive diet and faithfully taking all her supplements. Connective tissue throughout my body became so tight and injury-prone that simply straightening my legs was torture, resulting more than once in internal bleeding, with blood pooling in my calves. And like clockwork, all symptoms worsened markedly in the late afternoons, associated with severe flu-like symptoms forcing me horizontal and under blankets. I mentioned this afternoon worsening to every doctor I saw but it rang no bells.

I saw a rheumatologist soon after. The furrowing of her brow while performing a very thorough physical exam spoke volumes. By that time, the areas behind both knees were so contracted that they stayed bent after getting up, forcing me to walk like a crab for a few minutes. During the exam, while lying on my back, I couldn't raise my legs off the table due to the pain in my knees and SI joints. Unsolicited, she told me that I was fully disabled, incredulous that I was still working. That was January 2011, five months following the first surge of pain.

She was the first doctor to accurately describe what was going on with my back: spondylitis, which means arthritis of the spine, which is not a diagnosis that explains the origin of the problem. It's descriptive only, a label. She held my hand, looked me in the eyes, and said, "We can cure this," later recommending Enbrel, a powerful immunosuppressant, which was the "cure" to which she referred. I immediately wondered: To cure something, isn't it important to know its cause and get to it, rather than mask its symptoms?

I didn't want palliation. I wanted to get to the root. I refused Enbrel and requested a trial of rifampin, an antibiotic with activity against *Bartonella*, despite my numerous negative *Bartonella* tests. One day into rifampin, malaria-like symptoms emerged: chills and malaise so profound that I could do little else other than lie down under covers and suffer. My sternum pain spiked so intensely that I could barely breathe and couldn't speak in more than a whisper. Without a pain doctor, I had to stop rifampin after only two days. It was then that I woke the beast. Within weeks I became extremely anemic and developed recurrent fevers to 102°F every night. My spleen enlarged, and my C-reactive protein levels (CRP), which measure inflammation, were off-the-charts high. My late-afternoon flares forced me to be horizontal from about 3:00 pm to 9:00 pm, unable to sit up without passing out. Within six months I lost forty-five pounds, down from 180 to 135. A parchment tracing of my former self, I couldn't believe how broken I'd become.

Over a more than two-year period, I saw about twenty-five doctors and it became painfully clear how little they knew. Autoimmune and chronic illness is a gaping black hole in medical science, and I was sucked in.

I filed for disability with a target closing date of June 15, 2011, but by June 4, I couldn't take a single step on my own, and was forced to leave the office. I was taken home to bed, and there I stayed, confined to my memory-foam mattress prison for a full year, ultimately requiring twenty-four-hour care, unable to turn over in bed or sit up on my own, unable to raise my arms against gravity, losing vision from an inflammation of my eyes called uveitis, and indeed coming very close to death. I had failed one and half years of antibiotic treatment prescribed by several leading Lyme doctors, including many months of various intravenous antibiotics — all of which stirred up symptoms but never eased them. These long-term flares were described as Herxheimers by some doctors I saw, but that's not correct — they weren't followed by improvements. (This phenomenon is called blebbing, and we'll elaborate on that in another chapter.) It was only when I took my care into my own hands that I turned around, ultimately saving my own life and bringing myself back to good health and vitality. Many lessons learned, the very hardest of ways.

Getting back to a normal life took a combination of luck, skill, hard work, and logic. First, the luck part: I got a chance email from an old patient, asking if I knew anything about brucellosis, as her friend's daughter was critically ill in the hospital and she had tested positive for it. Although I'd heard the name in med school, I wasn't familiar with it either, so as sick as I was, I looked it up, hoping to help if I could. As I read down the list of clinical features, my heart dropped: arthritis of the spine and elsewhere, fevers that are worse in the late afternoons to evenings, anemia, enlarged spleen, high C-reactive protein, weight loss, uveitis, and profound disability — all of my own symptoms. I started to cry as I dared to hope again.

Then came the skill and hard work. Thankfully, I already had the expertise to understand the published medical data on brucellosis. After scouring the literature and writing to *Brucella* researchers around the globe, I formulated a plan. Despite my repeatedly negative brucellosis testing at U.S. labs, I shared with my Lyme doctor my ideas for an aggressive combination antibiotic treatment against this infection. Nothing else was working, so my doctor agreed to the plan, and by the second month of treatment I started to improve.

Lastly, the logic part. If there are two lessons I've learned from my experience, the first is to give each treatment both "the fair shake" and "the expiration date." The fair shake is the minimum time period an antibiotic treatment regimen should be used to begin to see benefits, and it varies by treatment. The expiration date is the maximum time period a treatment should be used without success, after which it can be considered a failure and it's time to move on, which also varies per regimen. A big part of the reason I was sick for so long is that I stayed on ineffective medications far longer than I should have, on the advice of my doctors.

And the second lesson is that if it walks and quacks like a duck, it's probably either a species of duck or at least another water bird. My *Brucella* tests ultimately came back negative even from an esteemed university-based research center in Europe. I received the email congratulating me on my lack of brucellosis after I was already starting to improve on its specific treatment. Either my tests were falsely negative, or I had a new species of *Brucella*, or I had a species of *Bartonella*, *Brucella*'s very close cousin, or I had some other closely related bacterial infection. These are the choices that most logically explained my symptoms, my resistance to many aggressive antibiotics, and my ultimate improvements with directed therapies against these classes of organisms. An eye-opening article in the *Proceedings of the National Academy of Sciences* in 2016 estimated that 99.999 percent of microbes on our planet are yet to be discovered. It's a humbling reminder of how little is known about the microbial world.

After months of effective treatment and considerable improvements, I revisited two of the three rheumatologists I'd seen before, to update them, thinking they'd change how they view their other patients with rheumatologic diagnoses. To my surprise, the first one said she was very familiar with brucellosis, that she actually trained under an expert in the field. And then she congratulated me for figuring it out, saying, "You did it!" But it would have saved me two years of pain and suffering if she'd pointed me down the right path when I'd first seen her. I told her that maybe her rheumatology patients had something similar and that maybe they could get better too, but was met with a blank expression. When I updated the second rheumatologist, she just looked at me in disbelief, finally admitting that both my exam (apart from the persistence of rheumatoid nodules) and my blood tests were immeasurably better, but then tried to attribute these benefits to the anti-inflammatory effect of antibiotics. Good grief, not that tired old line again. (Some antibiotics have anti-inflammatory effects and some don't, but even in the ones that have them, it's weak compared even to ibuprofen.) She then said that, in addition to spondylitis, she could also diagnose me with rheumatoid arthritis. No, thank you. I had been labeled enough, and it nearly cost me my life.

Preston Wiles' experience with Lyme was totally different, but tormenting nonetheless. We introduced Dr. Wiles a few pages back: a first-rank psychiatrist with training from Baylor, Harvard, and Yale. He went on to further training in child and adolescent psychiatry at the internationally renowned Yale Child Study Center. Now back in his native Texas, he is a recognized expert in the treatment of young people with neuropsychiatric disorders, including autism spectrum disorders, ADHD, and learning disabilities. In addition to his duties as the Drs. Anne and George Race Professor of Student Psychiatry at UT Southwestern Medical Center and Director of the Student Wellness and Counseling program there, he served as Medical Director of the UT Southwestern/Children's Medical Autism Center.

You'd think that someone already within the medical community could receive immediate treatment and never be second-guessed. But as happened to me (Dr. Phillips), even when you think you've got the keys to the proverbial kingdom, you can meet a wall of animosity, cynicism, doubt, and ignorance. Training for triathlons in his forties while living in Connecticut and working at Yale, Dr. Wiles was in the best shape of his life when his symptoms first appeared. "Oh, you're training too hard . . . oh, you're fine," people said. He developed Raynaud's syndrome, a condition in which extremities of the body feel numb, cold, or painful with exposure to cold. For Wiles, this seemed logical given his outdoor runs in the near-freezing temperatures of the Connecticut winter. But his instincts told him he should be tested for autoimmune disorders. Everything turned up negative, including a test for Lyme, not that he really thought he had it. Over the next two years, his symptoms continued, and included joint pain, brain fog, dry eyes, dry mouth, and sinus infections. He went on and off the popular antibiotic Zithromax over the next several months to deal with the recurrent sinus infections; eventually he said to his doctor, "Every time I come off the Zithromax, my joint pain and brain fog come back." That was a huge clue.

But his doctor didn't want him to be taking long-term antibiotics, concerned that their chronic use would lead to *C. diff* colitis, which is a potentially serious infection caused by an overgrowth of a resistant bacterium in the colon. By now Wiles couldn't exercise and was gaining weight. His commute to his office was only three blocks from home but the walk was daunting. His condition continued to worsen, with migraines added to the joint pain and brain fog. He saw ENTs (ear, nose, and throat doctors) and ophthalmologists, who treated him symptomatically. A visit to a rheumatologist led to a diagnosis of osteoarthritis and a call to his internist saying that Wiles was depressed. All the doctors avoided the conversation about Lyme, as if it were taboo. A psychotherapist left him with the following absurdity: "I think you have middle-aged life crisis depression thing."

Meanwhile, his wife was Googling his symptoms and Lyme disease kept coming up. Wiles finally decided to "go off the medical grid" and see a doctor who specialized in complex cases of Lyme. This doctor ordered a commonly used test for Lyme (the Western blot—more on this shortly) and it came back positive. He went back on antibiotics and began to feel better. Although more strange episodic symptoms followed, such as the sensation of full-body internal vibrations in the middle of the night accompanied by profuse sweating, it marked the beginning of a path to healing. Wiles's recovery—including getting on his bike again—would take place back in Texas after he'd been sick for four years. He continued the aggressive treatment started by a physician in New York and found relief within six months. Although he remains much better, he continues to treat as needed today. Finally he could turn his full attention to what he does best: treating kids with neuropsychiatric disorders. As we'll see in a later chapter, Wiles now has an informed view of the cause of many children's seemingly unexplainable psychiatric challenges. "When kids experience weird psychiatric things, you need to consider Lyme. Sudden onset of tics, OCD, bipolar disorder, and so on, you need to think of Lyme."

While Preston was still in Connecticut, kids with complex presentations involving physical and neurologic symptoms were often sent to him for psychiatric evaluation by doctors who didn't take Lyme seriously. Knowing there was often an infectious cause for their symptoms, Preston would refer these patients to Dr. Charles Ray Jones, a New Haven pediatrician who is renowned for treating the most difficult cases of pediatric Lyme disease. His long-term antibiotic approach, however, is reviled by some of the doctors who sent the children to Preston in the first place, as they "don't believe in" chronic Lyme or the subsequent long courses of antibiotics it generally takes to get patients well. When the Yale doctors learned that Preston's patients were getting better, they sent him even more patients, having no idea that it was actually antibiotics prescribed by Dr. Jones and others that were giving them back their lives. Due to the contentious landscape, parents were often afraid of telling their pediatricians that they'd consulted Lyme doctors. As a result, the pediatricians had no idea of the treatment the children had undergone and what the cause of their improvement was.

Our experiences with Lyme+ are in some way unique to each of us, but they share a commonality: infection. Dr. Wiles never saw a rash on his body; he never considered Lyme until his internist mentioned it. Currently, the clinical "signs" most doctors look for when diagnosing Lyme disease are a history of a tick bite with the appearance of that telltale bull's-eye rash around it, and a positive blood test for Lyme antibodies. But as we've said repeatedly, most people with Lyme either don't recall a tick bite, didn't see a rash, or the rash wasn't a bull's-eye. Even worse is the overreliance on blood tests, which are false-negative more than half the time. The same is true of blood tests for *Bartonella* unless they're sent to a lab with specific expertise in *Bartonella*, such as Galaxy Diagnostics in North Carolina.

The reality of the infections in Lyme+ is far from the "textbook" stereotypes; unlike most other medical conditions, which have limited numbers of potential symptoms, the symptoms of Lyme+ are typically multi-systemic and varied. They show up differently in different people and most of the clues are subject to interpretation (in other words, if you have fatigue, joint pain, and dry eyes, those symptoms do not define a single illness).

Here are some of the more common symptoms that Lyme+ can cause. Then we'll explain why this list is so breathtakingly long and inclusive.

Symptoms, Signs, and Descriptive Diagnoses:

GENERAL
Fatigue
Fevers
Flu-like symptoms
Night sweats
Chills
Sore throat
Swollen glands
Shortness of breath
Cough
Weight loss or gain
Menstrual irregularity
Need to sit or lie down
Hair loss

NEUROLOGICAL/NEUROPSYCHIATRIC
Headaches, migraines
Memory and concentration problems, confusion, "brain fog"
Difficulty with speech, writing, reading
Mood swings, irritability
Depression, anxiety, OCD, bipolar disorder, psychosis
Eating disorders
Seeing flashing faces/melting faces when eyes are closed
Vertigo, defined as a sense of external motion (not just spinning),
     increased motion sickness
Problems with coordination

Ringing in the ears (a.k.a. tinnitus)

Meniere's disease (some combination of ringing in ears, hearing loss, ear pressure, vertigo)

Meningitis

Encephalitis

Hearing loss

Difficulty walking

Sudden severe anxiety in the middle of the night (waking up with a bolt of fear)

PANS (Pediatric Acute-onset Neuropsychiatric Syndrome), characterized by sudden onset of behavioral/emotional changes, including OCD, tics, and narcolepsy in children (although similar symptoms can sometimes be seen in adults)

Small-muscle twitching, like an eye twitch, but elsewhere

Large-muscle jerking; can be worse upon being surprised by sound or touch, and sometimes worse when falling asleep

Tremors

Seizures

Abnormal sensations, i.e., tingling, burning/cold feelings, vibrating like a cell phone in one part of the body, numbness

Chronic muscle weakness

Intermittent muscle weakness, a.k.a. breakaway or giveaway weakness, which is rapid-onset, rapid-resolution weakness that produces a shakiness or buckling of legs and dropping things from hands

Facial paralysis/drooping (Bell's palsy)

Internal vibrating sensation of the whole body

Sound sensitivity

Hypersensitive skin (including sensation of bugs crawling on skin)

Difficulty falling asleep and/or staying asleep

Sleeping too much

MUSCULOSKELETAL

Pain in a specific tendon or muscle with motion

General muscle pain at rest

Stiff neck
Pain in the back, SI joints, tailbone, breastbone, or ribs
Joint pain
Arthritis
Joint laxity (loose joints)

GASTROINTESTINAL
Heartburn
Irritable bowel syndrome, constipation, or diarrhea
Nausea, vomiting
Abdominal bloating/pain

CARDIOVASCULAR
Chest pain
Heart palpitations
Heart failure
Low blood pressure
New or labile (fluctuating) high blood pressure
Feeling lightheaded, close to fainting, as in getting up too quickly
    from a squat
POTS (postural orthostatic tachycardia syndrome), which means
    poor control over blood pressure and heart rate upon standing;
    can be severe, leading to inability to stand

GENITOURINARY
Bladder frequency, incontinence, difficulty urinating, bladder pain
    (a.k.a. interstitial cystitis)
Genital irritation/inflammation
Sexual dysfunction, poor libido
Pelvic or testicular pain
Infertility, miscarriage

OPHTHALMIC/OCULAR
Conjunctivitis (pinkeye)
Sensitivity to light

Dry eye

Blurry or double vision

Increase in floaters (floaters are common in healthy people)

Visual snow (described as "static" in the visual fields)

Inflammation of the optic nerve (optic neuritis) or optic disk
   swelling (disk edema)

Inflammation of the retina (retinitis)

Inflammation of the uvea, the middle part of the eye (uveitis)

Inflammation of the cornea, part of the outer coat of the eye
   (keratitis)

Inflammation of the iris, the colored circle around the pupil
   (iridocyclitis)

Inflammation of the choroid, a layer of blood vessels in the eye

Inability to move eye normally due to oculomotor nerve palsy
   (damage to third cranial nerve, which supplies the majority of
   the muscles controlling eye movements)

Loss of vision

Ophthalmic migraine, partial loss of vision, blind spot

MISCELLANEOUS

Fissures in the corners of the mouth (also called angular cheilitis;
   other less common but still not uncommon locations for
   fissures: fingertips, behind ears, anus, vagina, and edge of
   nostrils)

New allergies (to foods and/or medicines; "multiple chemical
   sensitivities")

Breast pain

Alpha-gal syndrome (see below)

Morgellons (see below)

UNUSUAL CONDITIONS

Two of the more unusual conditions associated with Lyme+ are
alpha-gal syndrome and morgellons. Alpha-gal syndrome is a red meat

allergy, which can range from mild to severe, and can cause mouth or facial swelling, itching, wheezing, shortness of breath, GI distress, anaphylaxis, and other symptoms. In the U.S., alpha-gal often results from the bite of a Lone Star tick when it injects the sugar galactose-alpha-1,3-galactose, abbreviated alpha-gal, thus causing an allergic sensitization to it. This allergy has been caused by other types of ticks in Australia, Asia, and Europe. Because alpha-gal is present in many of the animals humans consume, some people with unexplained, frequent anaphylaxis and who test negative for food allergies are thought to have alpha-gal syndrome and are told to avoid red meat. There is currently no official treatment or guaranteed cure, but effective desensitization to beef has been published.[1] Note that symptoms often don't appear for three to six hours after eating meat, so it can be hard to connect the dots. Doctors feel that the delayed onset of allergic reaction is one reason why the discovery of alpha-gal syndrome wasn't made sooner. Large chain labs, for example Quest and Labcorp, both offer a blood test for alpha-gal allergy.

Morgellons is a condition linked to Lyme whose manifestations include skin lesions containing fibrous material. There is considerable debate and controversy about the condition but it continues to be reported around the world.[2] Some researchers believe that these patients suffer from delusional parasitosis[3] and recommend antipsychotic medications, whereas others have documented infection with B. burgdorferi and H. pylori in their skin samples.[4] I (Dr. Phillips) have seen a great number of patients with a range of skin lesions, but less than a dozen who have reported fibers coming from their skin. Those who did report fibers responded to antimicrobials in the same fashion as patients without the skin condition. In regard to the claims of delusional parasitosis, I haven't seen any evidence of delusional thinking in the patients that I saw, but my experience in this area has been limited.

Non-Lyme+ Infections That Share Similar Symptoms

Among the other chronic infections that can have overlapping symptoms with Lyme+ are the following:

- **Tuberculosis:** *Mycobacterium tuberculosis* is the bacterium that causes TB, which usually affects the lungs, but can spread throughout the body and become life-threatening. In fact, TB is the tenth leading cause of death worldwide. It's spread by airborne droplets that come from an infected patient who has a mass of live bacteria (which is like an abscess) in the lungs so that it's aerosolized with coughs or sneezes. Most people exposed to the bacteria do not develop symptoms or active disease. But some patients require aggressive, long-term, combination antibiotic treatment. Cases of treatment-resistant strains of the bacterium are on the rise.

- **Syphilis:** This bacterial infection, caused by the spirochete *Treponema pallidum*, has been recognized for centuries and, as previously stated, is a cousin to *Borrelia*, coming from the same family of spiral-shaped bacteria. It's typically spread sexually and is often characterized by four stages: primary, secondary, latent, and tertiary. The primary stage frequently involves a painless sore on the genitals, rectum, or mouth, but 40 to 85 percent of women and 20 to 65 percent of men report not having had one, reminiscent of the EM rash seen in Lyme patients that's sometimes reported, sometimes not. After the initial sore heals, the secondary stage can be characterized by a multi-system illness, including sore throat, fever, swollen lymph glands, headaches, fatigue, joint pain, muscle aches, loss of appetite, and a patchy flat rash on the trunk and extremities, including palms and soles, which can become extensive and sometimes form wart-like patches around skin folds or genitals. Then there are often no symptoms for many years—on average fifteen but which can be in excess of forty—characterized as the latent stage, until the final stage, which may occur years later. This tertiary stage can result in damage to the brain, nerves, eyes, or heart and be both life-threatening and difficult to treat. Syphilis is also spread congenitally from mother to fetus, 60 to 80 percent of the time in primary or secondary syphilis and about 20 percent of the time in latent or tertiary syphilis.[5] Although syphilis causes fetal death in a significant portion of cases, most syphilitic babies are born without symptoms, only to appear over months to years. Lessons learned in congenital syphilis should be applied to other spirochetal infections, like Lyme.

- **Leptospirosis:** Caused by bacteria of the genus *Leptospira*, another spirochete related to *Borelliae*, this disease is uncommon in the U.S. but cases have been reported. I (Dr. Phillips) test for it frequently in people who've lived in Africa or Southeast Asia. Humans can get leptospirosis through direct contact with urine from infected animals or through water, soil, or food contaminated with their urine. Some people do not experience symptoms, but left untreated, it can lead to kidney and liver damage, inflammation of the brain, bleeding from the lungs, even death. Among those with severe illness, the fatality rate is 5 to 15 percent. Congenital transmission is known to occur.[6]

NO TWO PATIENTS ARE ALIKE

Some people experience the sudden onset of severe symptoms (the "Runaway Train"), while in others they build more slowly (the "Slow-Boiled Frog" that doesn't jump out of the pot as the water temperature increases). And many people — us included — can have episodic bouts of illness that are at times fast and furious like the runaway train, and at other moments resemble the slow-boiled frog. Once you surrender to medicine, and doctors, and specialists, and prescriptions, and recommendations, and naysayers along the way, it can be terrifying, confusing, and lonely. And not every remedy comes in a pill.

Children and Adolescents versus Adults

Sometimes there's a difference in how Lyme+ presents in children versus adults (children under the age of fifteen account for 25 percent of reported cases of Lyme disease, with boys from five to nine years old the most commonly affected group, presumably because they spend a great deal of time in outdoor activities).[7] Many children develop sleep problems with nightmares and/or bedwetting, tics, and gastrointestinal (GI) symptoms that get diagnosed as reflux, gastroparesis, irritable bowel syndrome (IBS), ulcerative colitis, or Crohn's disease. More troubling is that they're also more likely to experience neuropsychiatric symptoms that can arise suddenly and be misdiagnosed as a purely psychiatric illness without infectious cause. Earlier we defined PANS (Pediatric Acute-onset Neuropsychiatric Syndrome). An older term for essentially the same thing is PANDAS (Pediatric Autoimmune Neuropsychiatric Disorder Associated with Streptococcal Infection), because doctors initially thought the condition arose specifically after strep infection. Now they realize that a broader variety of infections may play a role, hence the more inclusive PANS designation.

Child psychiatrist Dr. Rosalie Greenberg, who is a Distinguished Fellow with the American Academy of Child and Adolescent Psychiatry and was trained at Columbia University's College of Physicians and Surgeons where she served as Chief Resident in Child Psychiatry, has been treating kids for nearly forty years. Over her decades in private practice in New Jersey, she began to recognize that infections were playing a role in her patients who weren't improving. She started to add testing for Lyme+ and found that many came back positive, most of whom hadn't seen a tick bite, let alone a rash. The more she learned about vector-borne diseases, the more fascinated she became with their various manifestations. Once her patients with psychiatric symptoms were properly treated, many of them improved—some quite dramatically. For others, many of whom had gone undiagnosed for years, their ailments lingered.

As she described it to us, "Parents need to understand that

the immune system is capable of causing neuropsychiatric symptoms. A hot temper and a hot knee are the same. In all my years of practicing, I have never seen so many kids with so much encephalopathy and multi-systemic illness. We have a rise of PANS and PANDAS—all these kids whose immune systems are off, with suicide as the leading cause of death since 2014 in kids ages 10 to 14."

Children with PANS/PANDAS are likely to complain of headaches and may also have problems with speech, motor skills, and sensory processing that ultimately impact their ability to learn and stay in school. They're also prone to developing OCD and narcolepsy (a tendency to fall asleep easily in a relaxed setting). In 2019, reports of kids with ticks on them who suddenly experience paralysis were reported in the media. This is what's called tick paralysis, which is rare and more likely to occur in children. But it does not trigger chronic infection if the tick is removed and has not transmitted bacteria (if it has any). The paralysis is not caused by an infectious organism; it happens as a result of the tick transmitting a neurotoxin that's in its saliva. Luckily, once the tick is removed, the person can recover within a few days.

Charlotte Mao is the leading pediatric infectious diseases physician at Harvard's Dean Center for Tick Borne Illness/ Spaulding Rehabilitation Hospital in Boston. She received her medical degree from Harvard Medical School and spent twenty-five years treating kids with HIV/AIDS and other complex infections at Boston Children's Hospital. She has seen a lot of infection-induced neuropsychiatric symptoms in kids, rampant anxiety being among the most pervasive. According to her, "Outside of PANS and PANDAS specifically, I do think that there's an epidemic of anxiety among children and young adults, and I have a lot of suspicion that Lyme and *Bartonella* could be playing a role." When asked if she sees a rise in tick-borne disease, her response was unequivocal: "Absolutely." She also worries about other means of transmission besides ticks. "There are other insects—I worry about other vectors and non-vectors of transmission, such as congenital transmission. We need to learn more about other possible modes of transmission. There potentially is a number of ways that Lyme and *Bartonella* can show up in children and adults. And there are many, many unanswered questions." Dr. Mao has much to contribute to this field, and we'll come back to her wisdom later in the book. For now, let's turn to some basic biology.

THE BODY'S COUNTERATTACK

To understand how symptoms develop, it first helps to gain an understanding of how the body handles infections. The human body is constantly under siege. It must defend itself from a whole host of bacterial, parasitic, and viral invaders, not to mention rogue cancerous cells. The immune system is the primary line of defense in this game of chess, recognizing and ignoring our own chemical structure, known as "self antigens," while vigorously attacking foreign ones.

Most everyone has experienced a bacterial infection for which a seven- to ten-day course of antibiotics is prescribed. What is it about Lyme+ that can be so different from your run-of-the-mill infection like staph? Why are Lyme+ infections so stealthy, so persistent despite antibiotics and the immune system?

For starters, unlike other infections, most of the infections included in Lyme+ can affect just about any organ, cell, or system in the body —from your brain and nervous system to your muscles, joints, bones, intestines, eyes, skin, and heart. The result is that your immune system finds itself up against an entrenched army. When the tick punctures your skin, bacteria are released within a coat of saliva. Tick saliva contains immune-suppressing proteins which prevent the tick bite from being painful or itchy, allowing the tick to stay attached longer and therefore increasing its survival, but this also serves to prevent the invader from being detected by the body's immune system. Even weeks after the tick transmits the infection, the body may still be unaware that there's been an invasion. If the immune system hasn't become fully alerted to the infection at the outset, the infections themselves induce an immune suppression called anergy. Anergy is defined as the lack of immune response to specific targets. So in the case of Lyme, *Borreliae* lull the immune system into not attacking *Borreliae*, and in brucellosis, *Brucellae* stop the immune system from attacking *Brucellae*, and so on with most other chronic bacterial infections. Since anergy is a fairly specific process to one particular bacterium, other infections can still be identified by the immune system. But parasitic infections are different: They cause a more global immune suppression, which can worsen the outcome with a range of other infections. Some of this immune suppression is at least partly responsible for false-negative testing, but some of it, for example with Lyme, is also due to poorly designed tests.

Even though the immune system can detect certain microbial proteins, it cannot effectively attack the incoming infections. Keep in mind that these Lyme+ infections have been around for millions of years. They've had plenty of time to figure out how to outsmart and adapt to our complex immune systems. An abnormal inflammatory response follows, which can cause damage to the body's tissues. What's sneaky about *Borreliae*, in particular, is that they can change their outer surface proteins to confuse and further evade the immune system. These proteins — antigens — are what the immune system needs to identify the invader and effectively attack it. Another way that many Lyme+ bacteria, including *Borrelia*, *Bartonella*, *Brucella*, and *F. tularensis*, can protect themselves is through the formation of a biofilm — a slimy substance consisting of bacteria in an extracellular matrix that allows them to evade the immune system and resist harsh environmental conditions such as antibiotic treatments. Biofilms are what help bacteria remain in a slowed-down, but still disease-causing, metabolic state for periods of time until the environment is favorable again, after which they can come out of hiding, back to their normal faster metabolism, and relaunch a full-onset attack.

The way Lyme+ can attack the brain is particularly interesting. We'll be exploring Lyme+ and psychiatric manifestations in more depth later in the book, but it's worth noting here that these infections can attack the brain due to the brain's special immune system, which, when activated, can damage nerve cells. To make matters worse, the brain's immune cells aren't very effective at recognizing and eliminating infections. For all of these reasons, a multi-system, integrated treatment approach is required, using medications that cross into the brain.

Here's where the story gets even more complex. As we've previously mentioned, parasitic worms may be able to hitch a ride through a tick, or other arthropod, bite and complicate the infection. On top of this, a wide range of parasitic infections are transmitted in many in other ways besides arthropod bites. It's surprising just how common these parasitic infections are in the healthy population. Let's do a deep dive on one of them to give you an idea of what a parasitic infection can look like.

Toxocara is an example of a common parasitic infection that's spread to humans from dogs and cats, which have a 30 and 25 percent rate of being infectious, respectively.[8] The infection is transmitted via microscopic eggs in the dog's or cat's stools. Most of us grew up with dogs, cats, or both. As kids, did we really wash our hands properly after cleaning up dog poop or emptying the litter box? Do adults even wash properly? These infections are much easier to acquire than commonly thought. For example, in the U.S., rates of positive *Toxocara* antibody tests in healthy people are as high as 14 percent, and in regions of some developing countries it's even been reported as high as 65 percent.[9] For *Toxocara* and many other parasites, humans are paratenic hosts, which means that the baby worms, or larvae, can't mature to adults inside us. This means that humans are not routinely infectious to others because no eggs are laid in our stool. It also means that after a course of treatment for *Toxocara*, the portion of infection which is destroyed can't come back because the larvae don't multiply. They can, however, migrate through our tissues if left untreated. For many patients, this infection doesn't cause symptoms that are ever linked back to it, but it can cause serious symptoms in some, including infection of the brain, with dementia and neurologic damage. There may also be psychiatric illness related to *Toxocara* infection, as a higher rate of positive tests for it is well known to occur in a range of psychiatric conditions,[10] especially schizophrenia.[11] Cases have been documented where psychosis has fully resolved after treatment for *Toxocara* infection.[12] It would be beyond the scope of this book to unpack each of the many parasitic infections in detail, but it's important to note that although most can't replicate within humans, some can, like *Strongyloides*, which requires immediate treatment.

But even if the parasitic infections, including both single-celled organisms and worms, aren't causing symptoms themselves, they can still make it harder to recover from other infections in Lyme+. This phenomenon has been well documented in many parasitic infections that are concurrent with bacterial and viral infections.[13] A full discussion of the immunologic relationship of parasitic infection to other infections would be very complex, but to simplify, the immune system's response to parasites is distinct and, in some ways, opposite to its response to viruses and bacteria. Parasitic infections can result in a mild but pervasive immune suppression, making it challenging to get over a variety of other infections. Parasites don't trigger the same inflammatory pathways, and in fact trigger some anti-inflammatory pathways, which results in immune suppression. The global immune suppression they induce can have the effect of worsening other infections. In effect, the immune system's powers are subdued by the parasite's presence.

THE IMMUNE SYSTEM'S COMPLEXITY

The immune system is a very complex and nuanced organ, but in broad strokes, there are two arms: the antibody-mediated and the cell-mediated. The cell-mediated arm can further be subdivided into two general classes of immune response. Type 1 is associated with T helper 1 cells (TH1), and type 2 is associated with T helper 2 cells (TH2). TH1 responses are more pro-inflammatory, focusing on intracellular spaces (the spaces inside cells), whereas TH2 responses are anti-inflammatory, focusing more on the extracellular spaces (spaces outside or between cells). TH1 is geared toward the clearance of most pathogens, but can worsen the outcomes of infections with large helminths, or worms. TH2 reactions are associated with clearance of helminth and other parasitic infections. A specific type of immune cell called a mast cell is frequently activated as part of this immune response and is beneficial in the clearance of parasites.

However, parasitic infections are not the only thing that can push the immune system toward a TH2 response. Severe stress, immunosuppression, or any severe infectious burden can prompt the immune system to develop a TH2 response to an infection that is normally best controlled by TH1 immunity.[14] TH2 responses are associated with the new development of allergic phenomena. I (Dr. Phillips) have seen patients who have developed extreme allergies in the context of Lyme+. For example, I've seen two patients develop multiple episodes of spontaneous, life-threatening anaphylaxis. I remember that the first of these patients was so desperate to get to the root of her problem that she and her husband stocked their car up with Epi-pens and drove across the country to see me. I've also seen a broad range of other more common allergic phenomena in patients with TH2 responses and associated mast cell activation. Such patients can develop flushing, spontaneous hives, low blood pressure, and new or worsening food, medication, or environmental allergies. In extreme cases, some patients are diagnosed with multiple chemical sensitivities, where common odors such as cologne or shampoo become intolerable. Studies have demonstrated that these patients have a considerably reduced quality of life.[15] Once considered a dubious diagnosis, it's now more accepted, but women who have the condition are still being especially stigmatized by the medical community.[16] Despite the abundance of good published literature on the topic,[17] in my experience these patients are still routinely ignored.

MOLD

We're exposed to mold, a multicellular type of fungus, every day of our lives, with every breath, and with every morsel of food we eat. Some fungi are benign and we even incorporate them into our food purposely, like bleu cheese. Others, like the "black mold" *Stachybotrys chartarum*, express a powerful toxin which has been known, rarely, to kill people. Molds reproduce by setting free microscopic lightweight spores that float around and can survive harsh conditions. When they land in a suitable environment, such as one with high enough humidity and temperature, they begin to grow. Over time, evolution has gifted us with mechanisms to manage mold exposure, so much so that even coming in contact with a moderate amount of *Stachybotrys chartarum* spores is unlikely to be fatal. But if there is a severe mold exposure, a toxic immunologic reaction can occur which overwhelms our defenses. Common reactions to severe mold exposures in people with normal immune systems include respiratory ailments with asthmatic features.

For patients with Lyme+, toxic mold exposures should be especially avoided. There's a lot of discussion about mold in patient forums, with diverse opinions. Some claim that it causes an illness virtually identical to that of Lyme+. I (Dr. Phillips) don't think this is a coincidence, for the following reason: Although I think that exposure to toxic molds can be a serious issue and should be avoided, I don't think that mold exposure, on its own, is the primary cause of most cases of autoimmune and chronic illness. For example, I had a patient who was doing great after five years of antibiotic therapy. He got a job working in a moldy building, and within a few months, started to feel that his Lyme+ symptoms were returning. Did exposure to mold cause a new illness with the same symptoms as his prior Lyme+? Or was the mold exposure a stress to the body, analogous to sleep deprivation, taking steroids like prednisone, emotional stress, or poor diet? It is the unfortunate probability that even in Lyme+ patients who feel perfectly normal after antimicrobial therapy, some infection remains that doesn't cause symptoms. I've seen many situations where there have been relapses of Lyme+ illness in association with all of the above-mentioned stresses, including mold exposure.

A word of warning about mold remediation companies: This can be a poorly regulated industry in many states, often with no rigorous training required by state law on the part of those who claim to be mold experts. I've seen patients taken advantage of, having spent in excess of $20,000 in order to get their houses remediated for mold, at times when they're especially vulnerable, both emotionally and financially. It's imperative to get a well-vetted contractor to stop the source of water first, then to remove the contaminated materials. There are other steps the contractor may also take if it's indicated, such as fogging the environment with an enzyme-based product to destroy mold spores circulating in the air. An example of this type of product can be found at https://usenzyme.com/shop/mold-toxin-klear/moldtoxinklear/.

VIRUSES

A healthy human harbors untold numbers of microbes, including many chronic viruses, which have found a permanent home within us. Among them, herpes viruses, which constitute a large family of viruses, can pose a significant human health risk. Some herpes viruses are ubiquitous in the population, such as Epstein-Barr virus (EBV), which is best known for causing mononucleosis (mono), and the virus that causes chickenpox and shingles, varicella zoster virus (VZV). Others are common, infecting large swaths of the population, such as cytomegalovirus (CMV), which can also cause a mono-like illness; herpes simplex 1 (HSV1) and herpes simplex 2 (HSV2), which cause oral and genital herpes, respectively; and herpes 6 (HHV6), which is well known for causing roseola. And there are many others, all of which persist in the body, and many of which can lead to serious illness in the longer term. For example, EBV is very efficient at creating lymphomas, a cancer of the white blood cells, most of which, thankfully, are destroyed by the immune system before they have a chance to take hold. Other herpes viruses, including HSV1, have been repeatedly demonstrated in the brains of Alzheimer's patients, and treatment of HSV1 has been associated with a decreased incidence of dementia.[18]

Because herpes viruses are chronic infections, they can recur during periods of immunosuppression in the same way that symptoms of Lyme+ can recur. Unfortunately, infections with Lyme+ can be immunosuppressive themselves and can therefore be associated with reactivation of these opportunistic herpes viruses, which can then in turn cause problems — a vicious cycle.

I (Dr. Phillips) believe that HSV1, HSV2, and VZV outbreaks should be treated with prescription antivirals because these medications are relatively safe and effective against these viruses. However, I don't feel the same for EBV, CMV, and HHV6, except in extreme circumstances. This is because we don't have safe, effective antivirals for these infections. The only effective antivirals we have for these herpes viruses are very toxic, which means that their use must be justified by a significant risk from the virus — for example, post-transplant lymphoproliferative disease due to EBV in organ transplant recipients, which has a high mortality.

There are researchers who believe some of these herpes viruses, especially HHV6 and EBV, may cause chronic fatigue syndrome (CFS). There was even a study in 2013 demonstrating that treatment with one of the above-described toxic antivirals can reduce some symptoms.[19] Although I believe that reactivation of both HHV6 and EBV due to Lyme+-induced immunosuppression can cause problems, I don't believe that these viruses are the primary causes of CFS. In my opinion, there's better evidence that Lyme+ itself induces the syndrome.

The questions I have are: How effective is treatment with the toxic antivirals? Is it worth the risks? I've personally seen a number of patients take these treatments over the years but I've never seen a single one materially improve, despite long-term therapy and the risk that it entails. There has been little in the way of persuasive follow-up scientific evidence since the 2013 study that this line of treatment is prudent. Another potential treatment for herpes viruses is monolaurin, which acts against enveloped viruses, and is generally extremely safe. In sum, I've seen far greater improvements in CFS patients when they're evaluated and treated for underlying Lyme+, rather than only treating herpes viruses. Once Lyme+ is under control, I've seen many instances in which recurrent herpes infections, such as cold sores and shingles, are markedly reduced.

The Impact of Heavy Metals

Heavy metals like lead, mercury, arsenic, cadmium, chromium, aluminum, and others can add another layer of insult to that already caused by Lyme+, or cause damage themselves. Heavy metal toxicity can cause fatigue, headache, bone marrow disease, gastrointestinal and neurologic dysfunction, and other symptoms. A standard way to test for heavy metals is a twenty-four-hour urine sample. Some physicians, primarily those in alternative medicine, feel that a more sensitive method is to draw metals out of the body tissues with a chelating agent, such as oral DMSA in advance, and then collect the urine for testing. This is called a stimulated test. The issue I (Dr. Phillips) have with this method of testing is that for every test result I've seen to date, the reference ranges have been for non-stimulated urine samples. I don't have an opinion on whether the urine tests should be unstimulated or stimulated, but I think that the results of a stimulated urine sample should be judged based on a stimulated reference range, and the results of an unstimulated urine sample should be judged based on an unstimulated reference range. Please note that DMSA should not be used during pregnancy.

Prevention of heavy-metal exposure is the most effective way to avoid heavy metal poisoning. Simple steps like testing your well water and avoiding too much predator fish, for example tuna and swordfish, can go a long way. However, if such poisoning has already occurred, it can be treated by a variety of chelating agents that cause metals to bind with them, which will then be excreted in urine. These chelating agents can have side effects, so it's best to work with someone who is experienced and highly skilled in the field.

THE CASCADE

Further complicating this picture are the effects of the ongoing infection on multiple systems. The body's inflammatory processes against the invader can create mayhem and stir up symptoms. Those inflammatory chemicals that are released can cause fatigue, aches and pains in joints, muscles, and nerves, sleep and mood disorders, and cognitive difficulties. In a vicious cycle, the sleep disturbances that often result from these infections can cause secondary problems. Without restorative sleep, the body suffers multiple consequences, from hormonal imbalances that involve the adrenals, thyroids, and sex hormones to cardiovascular health, brain functioning, and overall metabolism. So, in addition to treating the infections, you must also address their fallout.

Justin's story from the previous chapter illustrates the complexity of Lyme+. As happens in far too many cases, doctors write a flurry of prescriptions that include strong steroids and then ever-stronger immunosuppressants in a misguided attempt to quell symptoms of an underlying problem whose cause they can't identify. When Justin's doctors prescribed intravenous ceftriaxone for twenty-eight days, they did not officially say it was for Lyme, calling it instead a "broad-spectrum antibiotic." When Justin partially improved, that should have been a clue. But after the treatment stopped, all of his symptoms came back with a vengeance. That should have been another clue. But after those clues were missed, even more drugs were prescribed, including the immunosuppressive and toxic chemotherapy drug methotrexate, which is a known carcinogen, as many chemo drugs are. (While we believe it's wrong and harmful to prescribe a chemotherapy drug for someone who does not have cancer, methotrexate is a standard therapy used by rheumatologists to control some symptoms of rheumatoid arthritis such as joint pain, because it suppresses the immune system.)

In multiple published clinical trials for rheumatoid arthritis, antibiotics work and placebos do not.[20] When antibiotics were added to immunosuppressants, RA patients did remarkably better than when they were just treated with methotrexate or even methotrexate plus steroids.[21] Why are antimicrobials not being promoted as a treatment option for RA patients? Shouldn't patients be given another choice that doesn't include immune suppression and toxic, cancer-causing chemotherapy drugs?

Meanwhile, Justin's dad kept doing his own research because he couldn't get a definitive diagnosis out of the doctors. They kept telling him that Justin had a non-specific autoimmune condition, which is why he had uveitis, but none of that made sense. He was the same kid he was a week before his illness began. How could his immune system just go haywire? Doctors who support the autoimmune theory posit that maybe a virus triggers the dysfunction, but that wouldn't explain the multitudes of research papers documenting that antibiotics resolve so-called autoimmune disease. Lyme kept cropping up when he Googled his son's symptoms but the doctors dismissed that diagnosis. Instead, a world-renowned uveitis specialist at Mt. Sinai suggested Vogt-Koyanagi-Harada (VKH) disease, a rare autoimmune inflammatory disorder involving multiple systems including the eyes, ears, skin, and central nervous system. The treatment plan was horrific, consisting of even more toxic immune suppressants and chemotherapy drugs.

About this time, Justin's father came across me (Dr. Phillips) in his desperate online search for help, but was shattered to hear that the waiting list was over a year long. He pleaded with my secretary to get his son in sooner and, as luck would have it, a last-minute cancellation got them an appointment. By then, however, Justin was in tough shape. When his Lyme and *Bartonella* tests both came back positive, he began eight months of treatment that entailed five and a half months of antibiotics, and finally regained his health to 100 percent. When his dad went back to the rheumatologist and told him what Justin had and that he'd gotten better on my protocol, the doctor retorted, "Sounds like voodoo medicine." And so it is in medicine, as in other areas of life, that arrogance frequently goes hand in hand with ignorance. It's a wonder medical science makes any progress at all.

CHAPTER 4

How the Medical World
Got It So Wrong

Truth is incontrovertible. Malice may attack it,
ignorance may deride it, but in the end, there it is.

—*Winston Churchill*

NOBODY SHOULD GO through the suffering that so many of us have endured. Unbearable, unending pain, along with a litany of bizarre and all-consuming symptoms, brings us to the breaking point, only to find no relief, let alone a cure. Then we lose again when the institutions we once held up as the Holy Grail of healing provide no true answers or real healing. We know what it's like to be given the runaround. Anyone who has gotten caught in the confusing, draining maze that constitutes our modern medical system understands that the "First, do no harm" oath is tenuous today, at best. At worst, which is the case far too often, real harm is being done in the name of the scientific process, hidden behind claims of "evidence-based medicine." We've been there, which is why we're going to take you on a tour of the science and story behind this tragedy and share empowering insights. Our hope is that this will guide you to appreciate where medicine fails, and show you how to fill in the gaps in order to help yourself.

Most of our doctors are doing their best with good intentions and using the evidence they have to make informed decisions. But they can only do so much, because a primary care doctor can see twenty-five patients or more in a day. Can they actually make sound clinical decisions in the few minutes they have with each patient? Or are they blindly following an algorithm designed for expediency? In order to efficiently care for this many people, doctors commonly follow guidelines on how to diagnose and treat various conditions and are looking for quick instructions from the NIH and the CDC. But there are often problems with the accuracy, or lack thereof, of their advice. Misinformation and conflicts of interest abound. Here, we give you the facts in layperson terminology with the scientific evidence to back it all up. And if you're reading this book having already received a diagnosis — perhaps you've been told that you have fibromyalgia, rheumatoid arthritis, multiple sclerosis, or some other autoimmune ailment, all of which describe symptoms but none of which speaks to a root cause — you've come to the right place.

HISTORY REPEATS ITSELF

"Even in its rapid advancement the science of medicine may repeat the past," was written in an article called "Medical History Repeats Itself" in 1941.[1] It only takes a quick trip through history (and history does repeat itself) to see that medicine and doctors can be horribly wrong. Some gems include narcotic-rich "soothing syrups" given to fussy babies and disobedient, cranky children in the nineteenth century; in the mid-twentieth century doctors claimed the "ice-pick-to-the-freaking-eye" method of lobotomy could cure depression and anxiety (and moody teens); bloodletting was one of the most enduring and popular medical practices in history, originated by the Greeks and used up until the nineteenth century for, well, basically everything. If you were feeling under the weather back in the day, perhaps it was because you had too much blood. (Although leech therapy is still used today, it's not on par with bloodletting. Leeches secrete peptides and proteins that work to prevent blood clots; they are used in parts of Europe to prevent complications during some surgeries.) And let's not forget that cigarettes were once "physician approved" and we were all told to use "healthy" trans-fat-heavy margarine instead of butter. And those are just some of the more innocent medical blunders.

Other, more sinister examples abound, such as the Tuskegee syphilis study. In 1932, hundreds of impoverished black men from Alabama with syphilis were enrolled in a study without ever receiving adequate information about the nature of the study or providing informed consent.[2] The patients were followed over time to document the natural course of untreated syphilis and not offered antibiotics. This study was sponsored by the U.S. Public Health Service, a division of the Department of Health and Human Services, and was supported by the CDC and the American Medical Association (AMA). Despite the fact that penicillin was accepted as the treatment of choice for syphilis eight years after the study began, and despite the fact that penicillin treatment was demonstrated to prevent the incurable later-stage manifestations of syphilis, which result in dementia and death, such treatment was never offered to these study participants. The study went on for forty years, and was still being championed by the CDC and the AMA thirty-seven years into it. On May 16, 1997, President Clinton apologized on behalf of the nation for this human atrocity.

Granted, certain medical blunders were perpetuated because doctors truly believed them to be beneficial, but eventually the science spoke and practices changed. Yet, sadly, to this day the denial of absolute truth abounds — that HIV/AIDS doesn't exist, that the Holocaust never happened, that smoking does not cause cancer, and that no one ever landed on the moon. Denialism is a sport that seems to come easy for narrow minds. In their fascinating 2009 paper titled "Denialism," published in the *European Journal of Public Health*, the former WHO economist and long-time anti-tobacco activist Pascal Diethelm and his colleague Martin McKee, of the London School of Hygiene and Tropical Medicine, define denialism as "the employment of rhetorical arguments to give the appearance of legitimate debate where there is none, an approach that has the ultimate goal of rejecting a proposition."[3]

They identify five characteristics common to most forms of denialism, crediting earlier groundwork on the subject done by Chris and Mark Hoofnagle, American brothers — one a Berkeley law professor and another a surgeon in Maryland. The five features:

1. *Conspiracy theories*: When scientific data demonstrates that something is true, the denialist won't admit scientists have independently studied the evidence to reach this conclusion. Instead, they claim scientists are engaged in a complex and secretive conspiracy. Those who deny the existence of chronic Lyme ignore irrefutable evidence. According to IDSA guidelines, for example, "Lyme disease lacks characteristics of other infections that justify longer treatment, such as . . . infections caused by an intracellular pathogen,"[4] yet multiple studies — not cited by IDSA — show that *B. burgdorferi* is an intracellular pathogen. (Intracellular pathogens are organisms that can multiply in cells.) IDSA also states that the cystic, round-body forms of the bacterium (now called persister forms) that can survive in the body are of no concern. IDSA ignores studies that prove otherwise. These studies (not cited by IDSA), dating back decades, have shown the importance and impact of the bacterium when its structure takes on a round (cystic) appearance, which can not only cause infection, but shape-shift back to its spiral form, which can move around easily.[5] In 2019, it was reported by researchers from Johns Hopkins and Tulane, among others, that these persister forms cause more severe disease in mouse models of Lyme arthritis.[6] Back when *Treponema pallidum* — the spirochete bacterium that causes syphilis — was a public health threat, round spirochetal forms were identified as important hallmarks of spirochetal infection.[7]

2. *Misinformed experts*: These are individuals purporting to be experts — and they may very well be in one particular field — but whose views on a certain topic are inconsistent with up-to-date knowledge and science. Their ignorance combined with arrogance leads them to discredit even the results of solid studies,

labeling the findings as "junk science." Some rheumatologists and neurologists, in whose offices many Lyme+ patients wind up, for example, who don't know the complex science of vector-borne infections, are frequently ready to dismiss an infectious basis and refuse to treat such infections to get to the root cause. Instead, they push powerful drugs to cover up the rheumatic and neurological symptoms while the infection continues unchecked. The damage this has caused patients around the world is enough reason to have written this book.

3. *Cherry-picking*: You can make any argument work in your favor if you cherry-pick the science, which involves selectively drawing on isolated papers that challenge a scientific truth and neglecting more persuasive research. In the Lyme world, legitimate, well-performed studies show the persistence of spirochetes in patients despite what IDSA deems "appropriate" antibiotics, but these have been ignored in their Guidelines, or, when referenced, have had their critical findings omitted. In 1994, Dr. Alan Steere and colleagues published cases of chronic Lyme despite treatment in the *Annals of Internal Medicine*.[8] Tests on patients given less than a month of antibiotics and even those who received multiple courses of antibiotics showed they still had Lyme. Such pertinent findings in studies like these are often ignored, sadly even by the studies' own authors — deleted from the science in favor of other cherry-picked data.

4. *Impossible expectations of what research can deliver*: If you change the expectations or the rules that govern how research is conducted, then you can change the outcomes of that research. Case in point: The tobacco company Philip Morris tried to promote new rules for conducting epidemiological studies. But these new guidelines would have invalidated in one sweep a large body of research on the health effects of cigarettes. (We know cigarettes are bad for us, but Philip Morris didn't want the research to show that.) An example in the Lyme world would be when Boston University's Mark Klempner and his colleagues

used an unreasonable expectation for the level of improvement antibiotics could offer patients. In their clinical study, published in 2001, chronic Lyme patients would have had to improve to an average level of health high above that of the American public in order to demonstrate an antibiotic treatment effect.[9] It's reasonable for antibiotic therapy to bring patients back to, or close to, normal, but not reasonable to expect them to make patients feel better than normal. It's like expecting patients to be able to play the piano after antibiotics when they never did before.

5. *Misrepresentation and logical fallacies*: Here an opposing argument is misrepresented and thus easier to refute. An example of this from the Lyme world would be the claim that the treatment of chronic Lyme patients with long-term antibiotics will give rise to antibiotic-resistant superbugs, but they don't blink an eye at the long-term antibiotic treatment of acne in teenagers or infections such as tuberculosis, Whipple's disease, Q fever endocarditis, and leprosy, just to name a few. And they never mention the animal farming industry, where about 80 percent of our antibiotics are used to keep the animals healthy in overcrowded, unsanitary conditions, when what would best create healthy animals is to let them roam free on pastures. It's from the scandalous livestock industry that the vast majority of the superbugs are born.[10] And lastly, they paint long-term antibiotics and long-term antimicrobials with the same brush. In my (Dr. Phillips') experience, many patients can get better with a minimum amount of antibiotics in conjunction with non-antibiotic antimicrobials; the latter don't cause antibiotic resistance, and will be discussed more in a later chapter.

Due to the colossal numbers of people affected and how deeply they're impacted, nowhere is contemporary scientific denialism more calamitous than in the area of vector-borne disease. The infection, or germ, theory of disease is gravely due for a rewrite. Germ theory was first proposed in the sixteenth century, though it would take more than three hundred years for us to understand that many diseases are caused by microorganisms. These microbes, which include bacteria, viruses, fungi, protozoa, and some baby helminths (i.e., worms, which can grow to be quite large), invade living hosts in whom their growth and reproduction can cause disease. Around the turn of the twentieth century, microbiology enjoyed a "golden era," during which the germ theory quickly led to the identification of bacteria and other microbes that cause many ailments. *Mycobacterium tuberculosis* causes tuberculosis (and still kills about two million people per year globally), certain species of *Plasmodium* parasites cause malaria (which kills over one million people per year worldwide), and *Streptococcus* and *Pseudomonas* cause pneumonia and many other infections (three million people per year die from pneumonia alone; it's the single largest infectious cause of death in children worldwide).

Many outbreaks throughout history owe their origins to some virulent germ, even if at the time nobody knew what, exactly, was the culprit. In the Late Middle Ages, the bubonic plague, for example, which by some estimates wiped out more than half of Europe's population, was caused by the bacterium *Yersinia pestis*, typically transmitted by fleas (it took two hundred years for the world population to recover to its previous level). Nobody yet knew that microorganisms existed. Today we know otherwise. We also have remedies to combat many known infections, plague and TB included. And when it seems we're on the cusp of a new outbreak, the media are quick to report the urgency of getting ahead of it and finding a cure if none yet exists.

When we began hearing terror-stirring facts about Zika, influenza, whooping cough, and measles — all of which have been making headline news in recent years due to outbreaks — government leaders called for emergency funding. In fact, in May 2016, at the height of the Zika outbreak, President Obama urged Congress to release $1.9 billion to fund a response, including preventing its spread and researching its cures. Obama called it a "pretty modest investment." He told reporters, "This is not something where we can build a wall to prevent it; mosquitoes don't go through customs. To the extent that we are not handling this thing on the front end, we are going to have bigger problems on the back end."[11] Well, ticks, fleas, lice, biting flies, and spiders don't go through customs either.

Why, then, is the truth about Lyme+, a pandemic caused by other vector-borne microbes that have shattered the lives of millions of previously healthy children and adults, pathologically ignored? Why is it that Lyme research is only given a paltry $30 million per year in funding by the NIH?[12] Why isn't it worth the same "pretty modest investment"? Why has it taken decades for this conversation to reach the proverbial fever pitch? Why the denial?

A question you might be asking right now is why the recommendations of ILADS are not embraced by mainstream medicine (and, by extension, why it cannot come to an agreeable consensus with IDSA on the science and guidelines). This has been a classic David versus Goliath story. IDSA is an old, private society, at least ten times larger than ILADS, with long, cozy ties to the CDC, the NIH, and insurance companies. ILADS, on the other hand, has no ties to the CDC, the NIH, or insurance companies and has been around for only about twenty years. Both societies hold Continuing Medical Education–approved medical conferences and both have published peer-reviewed medical guidelines on how to diagnose and treat Lyme. These guidelines had been accepted by the National Guideline Clearing House, which, until its recent closure due to lack of funding, had been under the auspices of the Department of Health and Human Services, and was the nation's key source for evidence-based scientific guidelines. (They're trying to find funds to get it back up and running as we write this.) The key difference is that both the NIH and the CDC actively promote IDSA guidelines while negating ILADS.

Shockingly, the CDC advises against using polymerase chain reaction (PCR) testing for Lyme. PCR is an extremely well-established, reliable method for amplifying, or duplicating, DNA in a sample, and can be very helpful in demonstrating the presence of an active infection. It's *the* standard for virtually every other infectious disease out there, as many, like Lyme, can be very difficult to culture, or grow, in the test tube. PCR is the next best thing to culture — finding a microbe's DNA equates with finding the live microbe, because in general, dead

DNA doesn't stick around for very long. So why the double standard for Lyme? Likewise, insurance companies frequently deny coverage to Lyme patients for antibiotics beyond thirty days. This is slowly changing, but these changes are hard-won not only in response to the science from respected, high-profile institutions, but also the result of laws passed to protect Lyme+ patients.

Until research documenting chronic Lyme is accepted without bias, IDSA will continue to call it a dubious diagnosis not based on scientific fact. Unsurprisingly, this stance was shared by the American Academy of Neurology (AAN), which sought to offer "independent corroboration." Disgracefully, IDSA and the AAN were not as independent as they appear. The AAN guidelines panel consisted of nine members, three of whom also served on the IDSA Lyme guidelines panel, including the chairman of each. In allowing its panelists to serve on both groups at the same time, IDSA violated its own conflicts-of-interest policy. Not surprisingly, the AAN guidelines concluded that "the diagnosis is suspect, and treatment with antibiotics long-term is unsupported and risky."[13] These statements flatly refute scientific evidence dating back to the 1980s in the peer-reviewed medical literature proving otherwise from well-regarded institutions and publications. According to then-Attorney General of Connecticut, Richard Blumenthal, "My office uncovered undisclosed financial interests held by several of the most powerful IDSA panelists. The IDSA's guideline panel improperly ignored or minimized consideration of alternative medical opinion and evidence regarding chronic Lyme disease, potentially raising serious questions about whether the recommendations reflected all relevant science."[14]

More alarming, IDSA is conducting another review of its guidelines, but with an important caveat, according to Dr. Paul Lantos, Associate Professor of Medicine and Pediatrics at Duke University, who is heading the review. In an email to the writer David Conner on September 19, 2016, he stated, "One thing I should point out is that the guideline being written now is not an 'IDSA' guideline and you won't hear any of us refer to it that way. This guideline is a joint and equal effort of the American Academy of Neurology (AAN), the American

College of Rheumatology (ACR), and IDSA. I am co-chair on behalf of IDSA, but there are co-chairs from the AAN and the ACR, and a methodology co-chair from the GRADE consortium.

"There are also official representatives on our panel from numerous major specialty societies, including the American Academy of Pediatrics (both the Section on ID [infectious diseases] and the Section on Emergency Medicine), the American Academy of Family Physicians, the American College of Physicians, the Entomologic Society of America, the Pediatric Infectious Diseases Society, the American Association of Child Neurologists, the Association of Medical Microbiology and Infectious Diseases (Canada), and the European Society of Clinical Microbiology and Infectious Diseases. Additionally, we have two clinical microbiology/lab diagnostics experts and a cardiologist on the panel. There are no representatives from any state or federal agency (no one from NIH, CDC, or any other public entity)." And, apparently, nobody from ILADS.

Why were so many medical societies recruited to buy in to these "re-branded" guidelines? It's much harder to attack a large group with extensive combined resources. It's typical pack mentality, but convincing more people to affirm specious arguments doesn't make it right — it just makes it that much more wrong. We remind you that in 1969, the CDC doubled down on its unethical, harmful stance on the decades-long, disgraceful Tuskegee Syphilis Experiment by gaining support from the American Medical Association and the National Medical Association. Similarly, we feel that the efforts by IDSA will result in further marginalization and harm to Lyme+ patients in need of long-term antibiotic therapy.

"THE WHEELS ARE OFF THE BUS"

Lorraine Johnson, JD, MBA, is the Chief Executive Officer of LymeDisease.org, a well-respected non-profit that advocates, informs, and conducts big data research through its patient registry, MyLymeData, which has enrolled over 12,000 Lyme disease patients. A major proponent of quality healthcare, she has spent the past decade focused on the medical, legal, and ethical aspects of evidence-based healthcare in the context of Lyme and has over forty publications in the peer-reviewed literature related to this topic. According to Johnson, "the wheels are off the bus" when it comes to difficult cases of Lyme+. She notes that although Lyme+ is a common disease, it is also a "research-disadvantaged disease." Johnson states, "The financial incentives for conducting research are not aligned with patient care." Big Pharma, which usually develops treatments to cure disease, is not incentivized to do so in Lyme disease because the antibiotic market is not seen as profitable.

She further states, "There are also structural barriers to care that exist because the guidelines developed by a highly influential medical society, the IDSA, leave patients undiagnosed and undertreated. Patients seek out more effective care under the ILADS guidelines but are essentially caught in a turf war between the two medical societies as the IDSA seeks to drive out its competitors from ILADS. Our patient surveys show that very few patients (<10%) elect to be treated under IDSA guidelines because the poor quality of care leaves them sick and without treatment options."

She also observes that "research has not been occurring that should be." One particularly important but underestimated issue is the lack of research into differences between men and women when it comes to Lyme disease. Put another way, the sexism. For example, women tend to elicit 4 positive bands on the Western blot, while men elicit 6. The CDC requires 5 bands for a positive test. This means that women are less likely to test positive for Lyme disease or get treated.[15] The testing for Lyme disease relies on the body's immune response. There is a growing awareness that women may have different immune responses from men because they are hard-wired biologically to bear children.

I (Dr. Phillips) knew a husband and wife who fell ill within two months of each other. The man received immediate antibiotic treatment from his infectious diseases physician while the wife was recommended Prozac by the same doctor. Over the next year, she lost some of her vision until she was finally diagnosed properly and treated. Medically negligent? I think so.

Breast cancers used to be treated mostly with radical mastectomy. Women were not given the right to choose a lumpectomy with radiation even though research was beginning to show these therapies conferred the same survival benefit for women without metastatic disease. Women's health advocacy groups and some clinicians/researchers motivated the passage of legislative mandates regarding breast cancer treatment in twenty states between 1979 and 1999, insisting on patient informed consent and forcing the old guard — the surgeons who'd perform the radical mastectomies — to shift their focus. So yes, the battle we're fighting now in the Lyme+ world has precedents in other fields of medicine.

UPENDING DOGMA

The myths and misinformation that swirl around the topic of Lyme+ do nothing but cloud the field, prolong suffering, and prevent new science from revising archaic ideology. This brings to mind one of Dr. William Osler's most famous contributions to medicine more than a century ago: "The greater the ignorance, the greater the dogmatism." Dr. Osler is revered as the father of modern medicine.

One physician we spoke with only agreed to offer her input off the record, due to the politics involved in speaking on behalf of an ivory-tower institution. This woman, whom we'll call Dr. X, is not only working and teaching at one of our nation's oldest and most respected Ivy League institutions, but she's on the front lines of the public-health battle against Lyme+ and challenges the conventional diagnosis and treatment of vector-borne diseases. Like us, Dr. X questions a lot of the conventional, outdated Lyme dogma — that it takes a tick forty-eight hours to inject Lyme bacteria, that tests are reliable, and that a short course of antibiotics will eradicate the bacteria. She understands how crafty a spirochete can be. She explains that it can corkscrew into tissue as well as travel in the bloodstream. "It can do whatever it wants. It's twice the speed of a white blood cell, which is our fastest cell. It's so strong it can swim against the flow of the bloodstream." As if playing hide and seek, a spirochete can escape the pursuit of the immune system and drill into tissue and conceal itself. There are videos showing this incredible feat.

Dr. X doesn't blame doctors for their shortcomings. She acknowledges a gap: "All physicians want to help people. There's so much misunderstanding because there's not enough education." But she also admits that ego can be a problem when it comes to learning new facts that replace established wisdom. "Doctors don't want to embrace a new way of looking at this disease. Most doctors will change their minds when presented with new data, but some just won't. You have to be a good politician and then a good scientist to make change. Still, the CDC needs to update its data and position and stop disseminating thirty-year-old information."

What's more, scientists like to hide behind this veil of high and mighty, while acting like roving gangs — leveraging fear and intimidation. Many patients she sees have been suffering the physical, mental, and emotional effects of the disease for so long, they have lost the will to live. The first thing she does is validate their experience, telling them, *I believe you.* "Sometimes they start crying because somebody finally listened. Some patients show symptoms of post-traumatic stress disorder because they've been ignored for so long. Marriages dissolve all the time because one spouse thinks the other is being lazy. Many chronically ill patients end up alone." Dr. X is particularly interested in the effects of tick-borne diseases on the brain. Some of her most remarkable cases have been people diagnosed with serious brain-related ailments that come on abruptly and mysteriously: the kid with major behavioral problems that appeared overnight; the twenty-something-year-old with acute-onset schizophrenia; those with sudden-onset dementia.

Although he was not her patient, Dr. X likes to mention how the actor, singer, and songwriter Kris Kristofferson reversed his dementia once he was properly diagnosed with Lyme disease. "That should be a lesson for medical professionals on how pervasive the disease is, and how often it is overlooked." Sudden-onset dementia should always be a red flag for Lyme+, among other infectious or toxic etiologies. I

(Parish) wrote about Kristofferson's experience with long-diagnosed Alzheimer's disease (along with fibromyalgia, heart arrhythmias, and anemia) for the Huffington Post after interviewing his wife, Lisa Meyers. In Lisa's words: "When I look back, his symptoms really should've caused his doctors to test him for Lyme and they missed it. Most doctors are just not looking for it . . . I don't understand the stigma or lack of awareness. It's like doctors don't wanna touch it. I think what I am teaching doctors now is that there is no downside in testing for and treating for Lyme when you can't find anything else that makes sense. Because not acknowledging Lyme can be so devastating."[16]

Kris Kristofferson's Story

This Country Music Hall of Famer has a long list of credits to his name, from Rhodes scholar to acclaimed actor and Grammy winner. But he was no match for Lyme disease, which almost took his brain away from him. His symptoms began more than a decade ago when he was diagnosed with fibromyalgia and was experiencing large, painful spasms all over his back and legs. He tried acupuncture, heat and massage, a cortisone shot in his spine, and a low-dose antidepressant. He'd also been diagnosed with sleep apnea and anemia, and had been given a pacemaker for heart arrhythmias. Three years before he was finally diagnosed with Lyme, two different neurologists had diagnosed him with Alzheimer's and were treating him with drugs. At the time, he had symptoms consistent with Alzheimer's, such as memory lapses and a loss of sense of smell. He'd also had fainting spells. In early 2016, his wife took him to a new doctor, who finally ordered a blood test that came back positive for Lyme. Soon after starting treatment, he began to improve and came off all the other drugs he'd been taking. Lyme disease explained his medical mystery. His symptoms of fibromyalgia, sleep apnea, cardiac issues, and twitching are now gone, and his dementia is far improved thanks to the Lyme treatment. And he's back on the road, touring again.

THE POWER OF BIAS

The last diagnostic guidelines for Lyme disease were issued by IDSA in 2006,* yet even before then, and especially since, there has been significant scientific data to further document the chronic nature of Lyme+ and refute their obsolete statements. What is very clear is that *B. burgdorferi* has been isolated alive from both animals and humans *despite administration of antibiotics that are deemed curative by IDSA and the CDC.* The number of studies demonstrating the persistence of the bacteria in the body, as already described, is copious, convincing, and compelling. Equally persuasive are the multitude of published reports demonstrating vast improvements among chronic Lyme patients who manage to receive long-term antibiotic treatment when symptoms recur.[17] This needs to ring loudly in the ears of people who feel that they have been misdiagnosed or mistreated by the medical system. To reiterate, this organism has also been isolated alive from humans after antibiotics were given for many months and even years, which is far in excess of what is declared curative by these same agencies. The antibiotics sanctioned by IDSA and the CDC as the cure for Lyme are now proven by several prestigious universities, including Johns Hopkins, to be incapable of killing the organism even in the test tube.[18] If they can't kill it in the test tube where there's no place to hide, what are the chances that these same antibiotics will work in the body, with all of its hiding spots, such as within cells or across the blood-brain barrier? All of this makes the IDSA and CDC position untenable at best.

It all speaks to the sad, ubiquitous, and inescapable nature of bias.

---

* The Infectious Diseases Society of America, American Academy of Neurology, and American College of Rheumatology issued new draft guidelines in mid-2019 but they have not been formally published yet and they do not change the recommendations much. By some accounts, they make matters worse by further discouraging the use of long-term antibiotic therapy in chronic cases and even suggesting against routine testing in children who show behavioral or psychiatric disorders. Many experts agree that these newly proposed guidelines only engender more controversy.

For example, the IDSA Guideline authors state that Lyme disease is easy to cure. Yet their own studies prove otherwise. They demonstrate that Lyme bacteria can be isolated from patients who received "appropriate" (meaning IDSA-recommended) antibiotic therapy. These medical journal articles were either not referenced in the IDSA Guidelines, or when they were, they did not specifically refer to the aspects that document persistent Lyme infection despite antibiotic therapy. In other words, they even *censored their own previously published data*, redacting any evidence that went against their guidelines. They cherry-picked and misrepresented. This is a flagrant act of obfuscation.[19]

We are all, unfortunately, victims of our own biases and even intelligence. Confirmation bias refers to the tendency to interpret new evidence as confirmation of one's existing beliefs or theories. Published evidence documents that confirmation bias is universal and can lead to faulty decision making. Call it part of the human condition, but it's all too easy for intelligent individuals in large groups to fall prey to these biases. This is true even with the best intentions. We shudder to think what occurs when intentions are less than honorable.

Dr. Kenneth Liegner, in Pawling, New York, is a board-certified internist with additional training in pathology and critical care medicine, who has treated thousands of patients with chronic and neurologic Lyme+. He has been actively involved in the diagnosis and treatment of Lyme disease and related disorders since 1988. He emphasizes the urgent need for widespread clinical availability of improved methods of diagnostic testing and for the development of better treatment protocols for Lyme+ in all its stages.

"I've given it deep thought," he said, when discussing the controversy and misinformation that swirls around vector-borne diseases. "[Our adversaries] have a belief system that they are committed to. You don't want to assume they are nefarious. You want to assume they are trying to do good. But they are committed to a certain paradigm — that core belief that enables them to conduct themselves without guilt . . . It's a very complicated situation. I still don't completely understand it. They have seized on this very simplistic notion. They've resisted the data and their position coheres with the consulting work that they've done, both with the insurers and as expert witnesses, and that has enriched them . . . The power of bias is really strong." Dr. Liegner went so far as to call one known physician in the other "camp" a "therapeutic nihilist." He told us, "The best thing you could hope is that these physicians really believe what they are saying, but are in error. At least, then, they would be 'honestly' wrong. But there is clear evidence of duplicity on the part of some of them as is demonstrated in their own publications and patents, so that raises the questions of whether or not they 'know better' but, for improper motives, have forsworn their own prior work. And that raises the question of corruption . . . That's the only way to explain the behavior. It's like Big Tobacco. You lie, you lie, you deny."

He also thinks the denial of the existence of chronic Lyme disease has set the research back by three decades, and we agree. "You can't solve a problem you don't acknowledge," he says. "Private funding is making a difference now. I'm optimistic but it's not over. It is a 'battle ongoing.'" In a lengthy letter to the Institute of Medicine dated September 2010, shortly before it convened a panel of physicians and scientists on Lyme disease and other tick-borne diseases, Liegner wrote: "In the fullness of time, the mainstream handling of chronic Lyme disease will be viewed as one of the most shameful episodes in the history of medicine because elements of academic medicine, elements of government and virtually the entire insurance industry have colluded to deny a disease. This has resulted in needless suffering of many individuals who deteriorate and sometimes die for lack of timely application of treatment or denial of treatment beyond some arbitrary duration."

In a 2017 paper for Oxford Academic's *Open Forum Infectious Diseases* journal, Dr. Jaan Peter Naktin, an infectious-disease expert in Allentown, Pennsylvania, wrote: "Throughout its history, Lyme disease has been a slow burning public health crisis. There can no longer be two systems of diagnosis and treatment; it is time that all levels of care are held equally accountable and transparent at a statewide and national level."[20] We couldn't agree more. Time is of the essence, because for many, the progression from infection to an explosion of illness can happen overnight, and in some cases, is life-changing and even life-ending. Interestingly, a study *funded by the CDC* and published in 2015 demonstrated that the majority of U.S. physicians polled treat Lyme disease with antibiotics for longer than four weeks, which is in excess of what the IDSA Guidelines recommend.[21] If someone with a CDC/IDSA-centric view were to have confirmation bias, they may interpret this data as a wake-up call to better educate physicians on the proper way to treat Lyme disease. However, a more neutral approach might be to ask oneself why most physicians aren't following the IDSA Guidelines. Perhaps it's because they don't work well in curing patients.

It's crucial to point out that twelve of the fourteen IDSA Guidelines authors have egregious conflicts of interest, many with financial ties to pharmaceutical companies pushing for Lyme vaccine development, whose sordid history and murky value we'll get into later in the book.[22] Some of the CDC's own employees have filed patents related to Lyme diagnostics. Emails obtained through the Freedom of Information Act by the producers of the Oscar-shortlisted documentary *Under Our Skin* show a scheming collaborative effort forged between IDSA and the CDC to go to "war" against Lyme activists.[23] The time has come to end this war and give this infection the respect and attention it demands. We cringe when we see aggressive advertising for drugs to treat autoimmune disorders that very likely have their roots in a covert infection — often bartonellosis — not a wayward immune system in need of dangerous suppression. We have to ask the question: Why are immunosuppressants the subject of so many TV commercials churned out by the pharmaceutical industry? What are the costs of these drugs and the profit motives? More important, what are their risks? The increase in the rate of autoimmune disease diagnoses is fueling an ever-skyrocketing immunosuppressant drug market.

One of the most popular immunosuppressants, Humira, has sold upwards of $130 billion since 2010.[24] Another lucrative example, Enbrel, garners Amgen and Pfizer, the pharmaceutical giants who co-market the drug, nearly $5 billion in revenue annually.[25] According to the American Autoimmune Related Disease Association (AARDA), in 2017, the most recent analysis, there were 50 million people suffering from autoimmune diseases in the United States.[26] That's 20 percent of the population, or one in five people. And because none of these conditions are cured with these treatments, symptom suppression over the remainder of a patient's life amounts to an annuity for Big Pharma. How many of our immune systems are being disrupted primarily by a common infection that the CDC and IDSA refuse to acknowledge and address?

The Duke University oncologist Dr. Neil Spector, who lost his heart to long-undiagnosed Lyme and is now the recipient of a heart transplant, states, "It's always been felt that infections are underlying triggers for autoimmune diseases. Sadly, the development of expensive drugs to mask symptoms has overshadowed efforts to identify root cause of autoimmune diseases." Neil wrote about his near-death experience in his 2015 memoir *Gone in a Heartbeat: A Physician's Search for True Healing.* Here again we find someone within the medical community needlessly suffering because the diagnosis takes far too long. His symptoms started in the early 1990s with heart arrhythmias and, later on, arthritis pain. Doctors told him he was just stressed with his busy career. Although he'd lived in an area endemic for Lyme, he never recalled getting a tick bite or seeing a rash.

His diagnosis was finally confirmed in 1997, after which he received antibiotic treatment, but his heart had already been severely damaged by the illness. He received a life-saving heart transplant nearly twelve years later for dilated cardiomyopathy. After that, he could finally reclaim a largely normal life and heal from the damage that Lyme had done to his body. Today, as a cancer doctor, he draws a lot of parallels between the two maladies, calling Lyme the infectious-disease equivalent of cancer. "We don't talk about cancer as just one disease any more, and we should stop talking about Lyme this way." We agree, as there are so many strains and other infectious agents that ride with Lyme.

Lyme+ infections of the heart can cause a range of heart muscle diseases, including dilated cardiomyopathy (a type of Lyme carditis), which is the type from which both Dr. Spector and Dr. Phillips' father suffered. And it may be far more common for infection to be the root cause of these conditions than most doctors realize. A study of 110 patients with dilated cardiomyopathy demonstrated *B. burgdorferi* DNA in 20 percent by heart muscle biopsies.[27] The patients were treated with antibiotics and their heart failure resolved. Alarmingly, 64 percent of the patients who tested positive by heart muscle biopsy tested negative by blood Lyme antibody tests and none had stereotypical clinical manifestations of Lyme, such as arthritis or Bell's palsy. In sum, the correct diagnoses for these patients would have been missed if the endorsed diagnostic criteria from virtually every medical society that makes recommendations about Lyme were followed, with the only exception being ILADS. Accurate and prompt diagnosis and treatment is crucial, as sudden death can occur.[28] This has become such an urgent matter that the CDC has advised that if Lyme carditis is suspected, it should be treated with antibiotics immediately—don't wait for test results to come back.[29]

In addition, some patients with Lyme+ develop the inability to control blood pressure and pulse, a condition called dysautonomia, which in severe instances can reach the threshold to be defined as postural orthostatic tachycardia syndrome (POTS), where the heart rate increases by more than 30 beats per minute,[30] or stays above 120, upon standing for 10 minutes. IBS, food intolerances,[31] allergies, and neuropathy[32] are frequently associated with POTS. This comes as no surprise to Lyme+ patients because these are all conditions that are frequently associated with Lyme+.

Published research has shown that Lyme can cause POTS.[33] There is no similar research for *Bartonella*, but in my (Dr. Phillips') experience, it's actually patients infected with *Bartonella* who generally have the more severe POTS presentations. Keep in mind that much of the medical literature on Lyme disease never investigates *Bartonella* infection, which is an important oversight, as the two frequently go hand in hand. Treatments for POTS include graded exercise programs,[34] fluid and salt loading,[35] and prescription medications, such as fludrocortisone, beta blockers, and midodrine, each of which can have side effects. Generally, clinical improvements in POTS are tied to clinical improvements in Lyme+. In my experience, when patients improve across other fronts, their POTS symptoms improve as well.

The idea of an infection causing serious heart problems is more recent to the medical literature, but the link between infections and autoimmune disease is nothing new. In 1917, the German researchers Philalethes Kuhn and Gabriel Steiner injected guinea pigs and rabbits with spinal fluid, spinal fluid mixed with blood, and blood from patients suffering from multiple sclerosis.[36] They then found spirochetes in some of the rabbits, supporting the theory that a spirochetal infection likely caused the multiple sclerosis in those human donor patients. These animals even showed signs of the disease similar to those seen in humans, such as difficulty with movement. Later researchers had similar findings. As we'll cover in the next chapter, the infection theory of Alzheimer's is also gaining momentum. Ailments like MS and Alzheimer's may very well strike when infectious, genetic, and environmental factors gang up to eventually impair the function of nerve cells in the central nervous system.

If we can acknowledge and put significant funding into researching the infectious causes of autoimmune disorders, and create better diagnostics and treatments, imagine how many lives we can save. As we grow older, our overall viral, bacterial, and parasitic loads increase due to cumulative exposures over time. You can never know how a particular infection you contract will affect you in the months or years to come. Multiple forces are at play, from the genetically programmed strength of your immune system to non-genetic environmental factors that can change how your DNA behaves and expresses itself—a phenomenon called epigenetics. We'll be getting into those details in the next chapter, where we continue to turn medical dogma upside down.

Immanuel Kant, an eighteenth-century German philosopher, is regarded as one of the most influential thinkers of modern Europe and of the late Enlightenment. One of his most memorable quotes we find particularly relevant: "The death of dogma is the birth of morality."

CHAPTER 5

Modern Plagues Caused by Underlying Infection

The only thing that interferes with
my learning is my education.

—*Albert Einstein*

A L MILLER FIRST learned about Lyme disease at a medical conference in 1977, when he heard Dr. Allen Steere describe his finding: an epidemic of arthritis in children near Lyme, Connecticut. Five years later, Dr. Wilhelm Burgdorfer identified a tick-borne species of *Borrelia* as the causative agent of what came to be known as "Lyme disease."

Dr. Miller says he's rarely encountered a case of MS, ALS, or Parkinson's in a patient who doesn't test positive for Lyme. He believes all patients who have been given a diagnosis of a neurodegenerative or autoimmune disease—including ALS, Alzheimer's, Parkinson's, MS, RA, lupus, and fibromyalgia (the latter of which is not technically autoimmune but is a common and painful condition often treated by rheumatologists)—should be evaluated for Lyme+. For reasons science is still trying to figure out, women are twice as likely to be diagnosed with fibromyalgia. Interestingly, women are also more prone to false-negative testing for Lyme, leading to a delayed diagnosis of more than two years in over 60 percent of the cases. Again, the reasons for this are still not understood, but female biology could be playing a role.

You'll recall Dr. Miller's story from the first chapter. He's the Mayo Clinic–trained rheumatologist whose daughter-in-law developed ALS in her forties after doctors missed her underlying infection for far too long. Dr. Miller now questions the whole concept of autoimmune disease. According to him, "The body is not fighting itself — the body is fighting an infection. 'Autoimmune' is a cop-out."

THE HAZARDS OF UNDERLYING INFECTION

The following is a partial list of conditions often linked to — and caused by — Lyme, *Bartonella*, and other frequently associated infections:

- Fibromyalgia
- Chronic fatigue syndrome
- Multiple sclerosis
- Rheumatoid arthritis
- Spondyloarthropathy — psoriatic arthritis, spondylitis
- Psoriasis
- Lupus
- Mixed connective tissue disease
- Migraines
- Inflammatory bowel disease i.e., Crohn's and ulcerative colitis
- Irritable bowel syndrome (IBS)
- Interstitial cystitis, bladder symptoms
- Psychiatric illness (e.g., depression, anxiety, OCD, bipolar disorder, and psychosis)
- Dilated cardiomyopathy

▪ Neurodegenerative diseases including ALS (Lou Gehrig's disease), Alzheimer's disease, Parkinson's disease, and Lewy body disease*

If you suffer from any of the above, you will probably do anything to find relief. These illnesses can mean lifelong disability and even premature death. To gain an understanding of how these ailments can be rooted in Lyme+, it helps to see the complexity of a few serious conditions — some neurodegenerative, others autoimmune — that are often rooted in an infection.

THE ALS AND LYME+ CONNECTION

ALS has historically been an almost always fatal illness characterized by progressive motor neuron disease, leading to paralysis throughout the body, including the muscles that control breathing. Although there is considerable published medical data linking Lyme+ to ALS, it appears that there are many pieces missing from this puzzle because, although a portion of ALS patients improve greatly with antibiotic therapy, ALS is among the less responsive of the diseases linked to Lyme+. The question that naturally follows: Is ALS at the top of a large multifactorial pyramid with probably several contributing causes at the base of the pyramid? Is it Lyme that's causative? Is it another associated Lyme+ infection like *Brucella*, *Bartonella*, or mycoplasma? Is it another infection entirely, like HERV-K (a retrovirus)[1] or enterovirus (both of which have been linked to ALS and for which entirely different treatments would be necessary)?[2] Or is it something else entirely? For example, a history of toxic exposure to pesticides[3], to formaldehyde[4], and to the toxin BMAA (beta-methylamino-L-alanine), which occurs from exposure to blue-

---

* In my (Dr. Phillips') experience, these illnesses do not respond well to treatment in most cases; only about 15 percent of people improve a lot. By the time someone is suffering from a serious neurodegenerative disease brought on by an underlying infection or multiple infections, a large part of the damage has been done.

green algae (which are actually cyanobacteria, not true algae), have both been implicated in ALS.[5] In an interesting study, the progression of ALS was slowed by treatment with L-serine, an amino acid that nullifies the toxic effect of BMAA.[6] We could go down a number of lines of research into the cause(s) of ALS, but there's no single answer in many cases. However, since a portion of ALS patients respond well to antibiotics, it's prudent to explore its relationship to Lyme+ in depth.

In one of the oft-cited cases documenting the Lyme–ALS connection, a patient with a motor neuron disease who was initially thought to have ALS improved on antibiotics to the point that her diagnosis had to be changed.[7] And in a larger study from *JAMA*, ALS patients were almost five times more likely to test positive for Lyme than healthy controls.[8] When these patients were treated with antibiotics, one-third improved, one-third didn't change, and one-third got markedly worse and didn't improve. The fact that a course of antibiotic therapy was impactful in two-thirds of the cases — those that improved and those that worsened — is noteworthy, even in the unfortunate cases where the patients declined. But how do we explain this pronounced worsening? Was it a Herxheimer reaction due to bacteria shedding toxins to which the body responds? And if so, why didn't the patients eventually improve? What if some of the ALS cases were caused by Lyme, some were caused by *Bartonella*, and some were caused by mixed or other infections? (*Brucella*, the close cousin to *Bartonella*, has been published to be capable of causing ALS.[9] Although *Bartonella* has not yet been published as a cause of motor neuron disease, keep in mind that it's only been taken seriously for the past decade and there's still a dearth of research on the topic. Typically whatever *Brucella* can do, *Bartonella* can too, so we remain suspicious.)

Only physicians who are very experienced in the treatment of ALS patients with antibiotics should be handling such cases, due to the already mentioned potential for marked worsening in some patients upon starting antibiotics which may not be followed by improvement. The answers to these questions from a microbial perspective are complex, largely because there are so many different strains and species of these organisms, with different patterns of antibiotic sensitivity, resistance, and persistence. As a reminder, resistance is the ability of an organism to grow in the face of an antibiotic, whereas persistence refers to its ability to enter a less metabolically active state while under attack from antibiotics, only to re-emerge when the coast is clear. For example, *Borrelia burgdorferi* tends to be more antibiotic-sensitive than *Bartonella*, but it has a high rate of persistence. And for *Borrelia burgdorferi*, there's a vault of data documenting its persistence despite even long-term antibiotic therapy. On the other hand, *Bartonella* infections, just like *Brucella*, can frequently be difficult to control with antibiotics due to the high level of resistance inherent to the class of bacteria. Moreover, adding to the complexity are an individual's unique vulnerabilities due to genetic forces that can come into play, such as DNA variants that increase or decrease one's risk for developing an ailment like ALS.

Consider the extraordinary case of the respected oncologist/hematologist Dr. David Martz, who in 2003, after thirty years of practicing medicine in Colorado Springs, had sudden onset of a litany of debilitating symptoms like body-wide pain, progressive muscle weakness, and extreme fatigue. He deteriorated rapidly, leading to a devastating ALS diagnosis, with two years to live. He was forced to close his practice and was told to get his affairs in order to prepare for his demise.

Dr. Martz would not accept this death sentence, and in his research for underlying causes of ALS, he discovered that Lyme could be at its root. Though he tested negative for Lyme several times, he decided to try a course of antibiotics anyway with the help of a Lyme disease specialist who prescribed the medication, which caused his next Lyme test to turn positive. (In an ironic twist, taking antimicrobials can provoke the conversion from a negative to a positive antibody test. It's thought that the mechanism is due to killing some microbes, thus making dead fragments from the organisms more visible to the immune system with the creation of new antibodies and/or freeing up some pre-formed antibodies that were linked to the microbes so those antibodies can be picked up on the tests. It's a phenomenon that doesn't just happen with Lyme, but is common to many of the Lyme+ infections.)

Dr. Martz got markedly better on both IV antibiotics and oral antimicrobials; by the end of 2004 he had fully regained his health and the doctor who had diagnosed him with ALS said the condition was gone. He remains well today, sixteen years after being told he was going to die.

Another Lyme-induced ALS case that's made headlines is that of Jim Young of Raleigh, North Carolina, an executive at a computer company. Young got a tick bite while golfing in 2007, accompanied by a rash that was "not a bull's-eye," according to his wife, Dr. Erica Kosal, a biologist and professor at North Carolina State University. That led her to believe "it can't be Lyme, and that was that."

Young soon began getting severe headaches, neck pain, fatigue, and constant flu-like symptoms. Doctors prescribed two weeks of antibiotics, but when his symptoms worsened to include muscle weakness, they diagnosed him with ALS.

Young and Kosal were convinced that Lyme was the driving force behind his ALS and continued pressing for answers. Young was eventually diagnosed with chronic Lyme, and although he appeared to be responding to treatment at certain points throughout his seven-year battle, it was too late to turn back the clock. On June 27, 2014, at the age of fifty-six, Jim Young passed away. Kosal laments, "If only we knew any rash is bad news.'"

Advanced cases of ALS, at least in our experience, tend to be more difficult to treat than many other illnesses linked to Lyme+. Clearly there are pieces to this puzzle that remain to be figured out.

THE MS AND LYME CONNECTION

Lyme can be clinically indistinguishable from multiple sclerosis,* a

---

* For an in-depth exploration of the relationship between MS and Lyme, as well as other complications that include lymphomas, chronic fatigue, and autoimmune disease, we recommend Bonnie Bennett's *Tick Bites and MS*. The book chronicles her fight to find the cause of her husband's malaria-like illness that began in 1982. He had tick-borne relapsing fever caused by *Borrelia hermsii*. Bonnie became a citizen scientist and spent four decades entrenched in the research to understand the many different species and strains of *Borrelia* and its wide scope of animal host/reservoirs, such

fact that has been documented for decades.[10] Before the 1950s, spirochetes were visualized in the brains of MS patients and found from their spinal fluid. As documented in the *Official Journal of the California Medical Association* by a group of Stanford-based researchers, they named these organisms *Spirochaeta myelophthora*. After that, a series of inoculation studies demonstrated that the tissue from the central nervous system of MS patients could be contagious.[11] When lab animals were injected with this tissue, they became infected—their immune systems became inflamed and neurologic illness followed, sometimes resulting in paralysis and death. In a 2001 study done in Norway, when researchers looked for infectious agents in the cerebrospinal fluid of MS patients, they found *B. burgdorferi* cysts in all of them, but not in healthy controls, with the exception of one who had a prior history of Lyme.[12]

Conventional wisdom says many of the ailments listed on page 110 are autoimmune diseases, meaning they result from the body's natural defense system attacking healthy tissues. Or, in the case of chronic migraines or psychiatric illness, they are brought on by something else not working right in the body's physiology, such as chemical or hormonal imbalances. One thing all of these conditions share is inflammation, which is now known to be at the heart of virtually all manner of chronic disease, disorder, and dysfunction. Classically, inflammation has always had its roots in infection, so why did we stray from this time-proven path of scientific inquiry? How can Lyme and other vector-borne pathogens lead to these disorders?

Once you label me, you negate me.

—*Søren Kierkegaard*

---

as chipmunks and squirrels in Ponderosa forest habitats, that most certainly are not confined to the deer-tick areas mapped out for "Lyme disease." She describes the later manifestations and persistent disease complications of tick-borne relapsing fever and connects the dots from *Borrelia* and its related tick-vectored disease agents to many cases of multiple sclerosis. She had many communications with the man who identified *Borrelia* to begin with: Willy Burgdorfer.

THE FACTS OF AUTOIMMUNITY

The prevailing wisdom on the street about autoimmune disease is often along the lines of: "autoimmune diseases are genetic"; "autoimmune diseases have no known cause"; "autoimmune diseases have no cure—the best you can do is manage symptoms." These statements are far from true. While there are some underlying genetics involved that may make one vulnerable, DNA doesn't tell the whole story. And neither does the notion that autoimmunity is *idiopathic*, meaning that it arises spontaneously or that the cause is unknown.

What is the definition of autoimmunity? Autoimmune disorders are purported to occur when the body's immune system, which normally helps protect you from infections, instead turns against your organs and tissues. In MS, for example, the immune system causes inflammation that damages myelin—the insulating covers of nerve cells in the brain and spinal cord. The nerve fibers and the specialized cells that make myelin are also damaged or even destroyed. This disrupts the messaging within the central nervous system, leading to a number of effects, from problems with vision, balance, and muscle control to basic body functions. Contrary to what you might think, or what the term "autoimmunity" connotes, MS can be an infection-related condition that affects the immune system. The link between MS and several germs that infect the central nervous system, including viruses and bacteria, has long been studied.[13] Among the culprits suspected in studies: human herpes virus 6 (HHV6), Epstein-Barr virus (EBV), mycoplasma, *Chlamydia pneumoniae*, and of course *Borrelia burgdorferi* (Lyme), as we have already noted.

Not everyone infected with these germs will develop MS, but in some people there is underlying genetic or epigenetic susceptibility due to a variety of factors. ("Epigenetic" refers to biological mechanisms that switch genes on and off.) Think of it this way. Everyone has symptoms that are a little bit different. There are common denominators, but how Lyme+ affects any given person depends in part on their vulnerabilities and strengths, both inborn and at the time of infection. In some people, one gene will make them more susceptible to one symptom, while others will be susceptible to other symptoms. If you got bitten on the neck you may have different symptoms than if you were bitten on the toe. And it also depends on what other associated infections are involved, how long they have been able to inflict damage on the body before diagnosis, and how much stress you're under. Even low vitamin D has been implicated in immune dysfunction, autoimmunity, and MS, so it's important to have that checked. As you can see, there are quite a few variables in the equation, which is why no two patients are alike. As we grow older, our overall infectious burdens increase due to cumulative exposures over time, and as we said previously, you may never know how a certain infection you contract will affect you in the months or years to come. Multiple forces are likely interacting, from the genetically programmed strength of your immune system to non-genetic environmental factors that can change how your DNA behaves and expresses itself.

Even though genes encoded by DNA are essentially static (with the exception of mutations), the behavior of those genes can be highly dynamic in response to environmental influences. This field of study, called epigenetics, is now a popular area of research. Epigenetics, defined more technically, is the study of sections of DNA (called "marks" or "tags") that have been influenced by the environment, so they instruct your genes when and how strongly to express themselves. These epigenetic marks trigger small changes to DNA or its associated proteins that change the level of gene expression, thereby controlling not only your health and longevity, but also potentially how you pass your genes on to future generations. Another way of picturing this phenomenon is to view the epigenetic tags as gatekeepers, blocking or allowing access to a gene's "on" switch. The expression of your DNA today can have effects that are passed on to your offspring, affecting how their genes behave and whether or not *their* children will face a higher risk of certain diseases and disorders. But, by the same token, these marks can be changed to read differently, making it fully possible to *reverse* the process and lower one's vulnerability to these same diseases. For example, researchers have found that many origins of leukemia, a type of blood cancer, lie in mutations in the enzymes that add or remove these chemical tags on DNA.[14] Now scientists can adjust the enzymes that add or remove the chemical tags, thus restoring the gene's normal role and treating the cancer. This revolutionary finding is paving the way for new cancer treatments; manipulating epigenetics with drugs will likely have a role in the treatment of other types of cancers.

Epigenetic forces affect us from our days in utero until the day we die. We inherit epigenetic changes and accumulate them over time throughout our lives. There are likely many windows during our lifetime when we are sensitive to environmental impacts such as infections that can change our biology and have major effects, including an autoimmune disorder.

Rheumatoid arthritis (RA), for example, was originally believed to be caused by an infection.[15] Retroviruses, parvovirus B19, rubella, Epstein-Barr, and other herpes viruses have all been studied as potential causes of RA.[16] But the development of the steroid drug cortisone in the late 1940s, which had such an immediate suppressive effect, temporarily covering up painful inflammatory symptoms, led to a new assumption: that rheumatic disease was autoimmune and tended to run in families. By the time the side effects and dependency created by the overuse of cortisone became evident and its promise of a "cure" was dispelled, a new medical paradigm and approach to treatment had become firmly established: treat the symptoms, stop looking for a cause, never find a cure. Research into infectious causes for rheumatic diseases was thus sidelined as financial market forces began to drive the creation of lucrative immunosuppressants that patients would take for the rest of their lives, and doctors followed along.

Today, we can say the same for the slew of autoimmune diseases for which strong steroids and immunosuppressants are prescribed. As we've been reiterating, these drugs mask symptoms rather than treat root cause, at great risk to patients, at great financial cost to our healthcare system, and at great profit for Big Pharma. As previously mentioned, there have been about a dozen randomized controlled trials comparing antibiotics to placebo, demonstrating benefits from antibiotics but not placebo in RA patients. And some of these studies used antibiotics that were devoid of anti-inflammatory effects. What's more, studies show benefits from antibiotics in RA patients, over and above the typical drugs prescribed, namely steroids and the chemotherapy drug methotrexate, which we described earlier.

We are often asked how this is possible. It helps to understand that medical doctors, including those in the field of rheumatology, adhere to standards of care that are created by their respective medical societies. These standards rely on evidence-based medicine and the conclusions drawn from large-scale clinical trials of various treatments. And therein lies the rub. Even though many clinical trials designed to test the efficacy of antibiotic treatment for autoimmune diseases have demonstrated efficacy, there is no profit to be made from studying cheap, generic antibiotics that are already approved by the FDA. So it's extremely unlikely that expensive, large-scale clinical trials will ever be funded by pharmaceutical companies in order to get a second FDA indication for a drug that won't make them any money. It's also difficult to design an optimum clinical trial because of the differences from patient to patient due to the various strains and species of infection, as well as the genetics and epigenetics of the patients themselves. Again, it helps to turn to cancer for a useful analogy. For example, scientists used to think that breast cancer was just "breast cancer," the same in every patient, end of story. Now we know that there are all different sorts of breast cancers, which respond to therapies far better when you individualize the care so that it's specific to each patient's type of breast cancer. The same is true for most types of cancer, for there are innumerable molecular pathways that can all result in "cancer"; sequencing tumors to figure out which drugs, for example, will target that particular tumor has revolutionized cancer therapy today. This information was gleaned only through an enormous amount of research funding, but such funding doesn't exist for these vector-borne infections. The lack of funding, in and of itself, is a scandalous transgression.

For another powerful example, let's turn to the infection theory of Alzheimer's, which was only recently established and is receiving much-deserved attention in neurological circles for the right reasons: evidence is mounting that it's not just bad genes combined with old age. In 1987, Drs. Alan MacDonald and Joseph Miranda published a study in *Human Pathology* showing that the plaques found in the brains of Alzheimer's patients were infected with *Borrelia burgdorferi*.[17] Sadly, it took nearly thirty years for modern science to catch up to this observation.[18] Well-designed research by Dr. Rudolph Tanzi and the late Dr. Robert Moir at Harvard, and Dr. Judith Miklossy at the International Alzheimer Research Center in Switzerland, had also found that Alzheimer's-riddled brains are frequently suffused with pathogens, *Borrelia burgdorferi* among them. Amyloid, the aberrant protein in a diseased Alzheimer's brain, has now been documented to be the brain's *response* to an infection, with those hallmark tangles and plaques as the end result.

Tanzi's lab is now leading the Brain Microbiome Project to learn what microbes can be found in the brain and decipher which types can be harmful. In a 2010 study, the duo proved that amyloid is in fact an antimicrobial peptide — basically, a protein that the immune system creates to physically trap a germ.[19] The microbe, like a fly in a spider web, becomes trapped in the cage. The cage is a plaque that is the hallmark of Alzheimer's. All the while, the brain is under siege by inflammation that then kills more nerve cells and inflicts more damage, laying the groundwork for future dementia.

In 2017, Gina Kolata finally wrote about the infection theory of Alzheimer's disease for the *New York Times*, and it is now among the intriguing, well-supported, yet still hotly debated biological paths to the dreaded disease in people who, by genetics and/or environment, are susceptible.[20] Although the infection theory has been around for a century (even Dr. Alois Alzheimer, the doctor to first describe the disease in a patient, noted a possible connection between dementia and tuberculosis), it was hard for scientists to get their research published in medical literature to support the idea. Finally, in 2016, sending a clear message, thirty-two researchers from universities around the world signed an editorial in the *Journal of Alzheimer's Disease* calling for "further research on the role of infectious agents in [Alzheimer's] causation."[21] This is not to say that all cases of Alzheimer's are caused by Lyme disease. It does imply that there may be more than one pathway to the degenerative illness, with brain infection being a common culprit.

Alzheimer's is not the only game in town. In the case of Parkinson's, the aberrant protein is called alpha-synuclein. And it turns out that alpha-synuclein also plays the role of antimicrobial peptide, leading to the natural conclusion that Parkinson's may also be an end result of a brain infection.[22] For ALS the protein is called TDP-43, and although the data doesn't yet appear to show clearly that it's an antimicrobial peptide itself, it has been demonstrated that nerve cell expression of TDP-43 induces antimicrobial peptide gene expression in fruit flies.[23] The sum of this evidence implies that the major neurodegenerative illnesses may have their roots in infection and have overlapping themes. We mentioned before that ALS patients can be challenging to treat with antimicrobials, as only a portion respond to current therapy in my (Dr. Phillips') experience. The same can be said for Alzheimer's and Parkinson's; pieces of the puzzle are missing for all three. Perhaps it's analogous to tertiary (late stage) syphilis, where treatment can stop progression but doesn't reverse the damage that's done, which seemed to have been the case with Miller's daughter-in-law. If you remember, he's the Mayo Clinic–trained rheumatologist who, after a lifetime of practicing medicine according to the status quo, ultimately came to his dogma-challenging epiphany that vector-borne illnesses can cause a broad swath of rheumatologic and neurologic disorders.

At present, Alzheimer's, Parkinson's, and ALS are not considered autoimmune disorders. They are considered neurodegenerative. The next question then becomes: How can invading germs flip the "switch" on the body's immune system and cause what are commonly described as autoimmune disorders, like lupus or RA? There are two potential ways: antibodies produced in response to the infections may also attack normal cells because they resemble the invader that caused the infection, or the infection itself may actually damage the immune system, leading to symptoms of autoimmune disorders, which can be painful, confusing, and migratory. You'll recall that the outer coat of the Lyme bacteria is similar to tissue found in our nervous system. When the immune system rallies to attack the bacteria, it can mistakenly attack nerve tissue as well, causing secondary autoimmunity. The bacteria that were not eliminated via antibiotics "confuse" the immune system, causing symptoms in many systems of the body. The word *primary* in medical language means "without known cause," a synonym to "idiopathic." Every *primary autoimmune condition* is just a secondary one whose cause has yet to be determined. If a treatable cause is not determined, chronic symptoms thereafter are usually misattributed to an autoimmune disease. And the same inflammatory response caused by these infections can also trigger one of our most debilitating illnesses on the planet today: mental illness. The data is clear that much of what is called autoimmunity is actually an infection waiting to be identified, and that symptoms will dissipate when infections are treated. If we can understand how an infection can lead to neurodegenerative illness, such as Alzheimer's and Parkinson's, countless lives may be saved through prevention and proper treatment.

Can Lyme+ be linked to certain cancers? Throughout the years, many infectious agents have been found to cause cancer. Who would have thought thirty years ago that *H. pylori* was a causative agent for stomach cancer? Or that HPV, the virus that causes warts, can cause cervical and head and neck cancers? Or that Epstein-Barr can cause lymphoma, hepatitis B and C can cause liver cancer, or the parasite schistosoma can cause bladder cancer? So it is not far-fetched to say that a bacterium that causes inflammation can create the perfect storm for developing a tumor. There's already published research linking Lyme to a type of lymphoma, and research is beginning to emerge that in fact implicates *Bartonella* in facilitating the development of some cancers.

THE MISEDUCATION OF THE
FRIENDLY MICROBIOME

We should pause here to define the human microbiome in more detail. We've already mentioned how scientists are beginning to map out the brain's biome in order to understand complex neurological diseases like Alzheimer's. You've probably heard about the microbiome mostly in terms of your gut and the intestinal microbes that aid in your digestion, metabolism, and immune system. The microbiome actually refers more broadly to the genetic material of all the microbes — bacteria, fungi, protozoa, and viruses — that live on and inside the human body. It is currently thought that the number of genes in all the microbes in one person's microbiome is two hundred times the number of genes in the human genome. This area is currently under study around the world and goes far beyond the gut's and brain's microbiomes. There are biomes in placentas, breast milk, bladders, lungs, genitals, skin, and even tumors and blood. I (Dr. Phillips) once grew non-Lyme spirochetes, confirmed by electron microscopy and PCR, from the blood of three healthy beluga whales. This shows that biomes not only exist in other species, but quite likely in all of them. After all, bacteria were among the first living creatures on this planet, so it makes sense that they learned to take up residence in and on us for their own survival.

Amy Proal, PhD, is a microbiologist with a specialty in the role of infectious agents in chronic diseases. Since 2005, she has been studying chronic inflammatory diseases rooted in infectious agents. She has lectured at numerous international conferences and the NIH. Dr. Proal set us straight on the definition of microbiome and its relationship with human health and disease. When we asked her about the denial of chronic Lyme in particular, she put it bluntly: "That Lyme isn't being primarily studied as chronic is one of the most ridiculous things I've ever heard."

Although the microbiome is often couched in terms of "friendly" versus "unfriendly" bacteria, Dr. Proal doesn't like to use those terms. According to her, the notion that the microbiome is "good" misrepresents the nature of it. These microbes just want to survive, not necessarily "help" us. She uses the term "pathobiont," which refers to any potentially disease-causing organism that, under normal conditions, lives as a non-harming symbiont. "Almost all organisms in the human body can act as commensals (be tolerated) but can also change their gene expression under different circumstances or environments to begin acting in ways that promote *their* survival over ours," she states. She also debunks the idea that antibiotics are completely to blame for the current superbug crisis, and that we should subsequently decrease antibiotic use in the treatment of chronic disease. "Antibiotics are some of the best tools we have to keep pathobionts and pathogens in check in patients with these conditions. Immunosuppression is actually the biggest driver of superbug resistance," she told us. Indeed, Proal regards immunosuppressants as one of the biggest mistakes in medicine. "Most of what we call autoimmunity is the immune system trying to target persistent organisms. Autoimmunity is a theory. Scientists had to come up with a way to explain why there were signs of antibodies under 'sterile' conditions. We've taken an entire generation of patients and lumped them into one group, creating a pharmaceutical industry that shuts down their immune systems. Put simply, we've created an industry around the wrong paradigm."

She uses influenza as an illustrative example. Flu symptoms result from a reactive immune system. If you have the flu, you can take drugs to reduce part of that inflammatory response and you'll feel better. But the drug is doing nothing to the virus. Similarly, giving immunosuppressive drugs will temper the battle between the germ and immune system but the drugs are not getting to the root cause.

Dr. Proal is not alone in thinking that microbes play a much larger role in chronic diseases than what's acknowledged—or studied. We need only look at evolutionary biology to understand the logic that chronic disease almost always involves microbes. And it may even help us understand how certain diseases run in families. Historically, science has routinely attributed inherited risk factors for disease mostly to genetics. But what if inherited organisms are also to blame? Paul W. Ewald is an evolutionary biologist, specializing in the evolution of infectious disease. He received his Ph.D. in zoology from the University of Washington, with specialization in ecology and evolution. He is currently director of the program in evolutionary medicine in the Biology

Department of the University of Louisville. Dr. Ewald agrees that microbial agents—bacteria, viruses, fungi, protozoa—are overlooked as causative agents in human disease.

Evolutionary biologists like Dr. Ewald understand that if a DNA sequence that codes for a gene were to code for a severe disease that manifests early in life before childbearing age, it would slowly get weeded out of the population, particularly since people who are sick are much less likely to reproduce. It might not be entirely selected out of the population, but the prevalence would be low. An example that's often used to explain this phenomenon is schizophrenia. A person's chances of getting schizophrenia are 1 in 100. The reality is that faulty genes cannot maintain this frequency. If schizophrenia were a genetic disease, then according to the rules of mathematics, it would only occur in about 1 in every 10,000 people; the current frequency of the disease is just far too high to be explained genetically, and also appears to be *increasing*—which is another clue.[24]

Which bring us to the facts of certain diseases "running in families." The fact that illnesses tend to run in families does not mean that only faulty genes are at work. Family members could be passing each other pathogens. If one member of a twin pair has schizophrenia, there is a 35 to 60 percent chance that the other member of the twin pair will have it. But this may reflect both genetic and environmental factors (including infections), as the twins were exposed to the same environments in the womb.

Dr. Ewald points out that pathogens also have the ability to evolve and adapt at rapid rates, meaning that even if the host acquires a defense against them they can often find a way around it. As previously mentioned, genetic disease would gradually be weeded out of the population. But as soon as you hypothesize that a disease has an infectious origin, and that the pathogens causing it can adapt and evolve, it is possible to explain how diseases can be perpetuated indefinitely in quite severe forms.

Although this new perspective on the origins of disease may sound radical, the idea that microbes could be a root cause of ailments not

historically considered infectious is not a new concept. Bennett Lorber
is the retired chief of Temple University's School of Medicine. In 1996
he published a paper in the prestigious *Annals of Internal Medicine*
that had a provocative headline: "Are All Diseases Infectious?"[25] In it,
he argues that pathogens cause many diseases that we never previously
attributed to germs. He writes: "Although we have been flooded with
interesting and sometimes dramatic reports of emerging infectious
diseases and antimicrobial-resistant bacteria, the media have largely
ignored a quieter revolution that has been taking place in our understanding of human microorganism interactions: the discovery that
transmissible agents are responsible for diseases that were never suspected of being infectious in origin. Examples include ulcers, neurodegenerative diseases, vasculitis, inflammatory disease, and cancer. In
some instances, the pathogen is truly causal."

Some of the historical notes he cites leave us angry for what
should have been. In 1947, for example, it was observed that RA patients who were treated with a tetracycline experienced relief from
their illness. This was presented at the Seventh International Congress on Rheumatic Diseases in 1949, but fell on deaf ears because
the symptom-suppressive effects of cortisone in the treatment of arthritis were introduced at the same meeting. We were so close to going down a different path, but it would take nearly fifty years for the
salutary effects of antibiotics on rheumatoid arthritis to be considered.[26] Other diseases he links to microbial origins include coronary
artery disease, acute renal failure, inflammatory bowel disease, and
diabetes.

The Mysterious Power of Curcumin

Curcumin is a natural substance that is extracted from the
curry spice turmeric, which is a member of the ginger family.
It has long been shown that in populations where this spice is
frequently used in cooking (e.g., India), incidence of Alzheimer's

and other dementias is low. In mouse studies, curcumin has been shown to lower levels of the characteristic plaques and tangles of Alzheimer's and improve disease-like symptoms.[27] In addition to the substance's anti-inflammatory and antioxidant powers, it also has antimicrobial actions that could have a therapeutic role. Here's what we know.

As previously mentioned, herpes simplex virus type 1 (HSV-1) DNA is more frequently found in the aged brains of people with Alzheimer's disease. Studies show that reactivation of HSV-1 is a big risk factor for the development of Alzheimer's; patients with HSV infections may have a 2.56-fold increased risk of developing dementia. And studies have demonstrated a reduced risk of developing dementia in HSV-1-positive patients who are treated with anti-HSV-1 medications.[28] The virus can cause increased formation and accumulation of amyloid-beta and abnormal tau protein (tau proteins are other brain structures implicated in the disease; they can become tangled and damage brain cells). Where does curcumin come in? It blocks the expression of HSV-1 genes, thereby hampering the virus's destructive paths in the brain. In Chapter 8 we'll list curcumin as a potential therapeutic supplement to take. The key is finding one that's easily absorbed, and for that we have a recommendation. In the future, we may soon see it also in an inhalable form that travels easily from your nose to the brain.[29]

THE LINK TO MENTAL ILLNESS

I (Dr. Phillips) once had a case where a woman brought in her husband for evaluation of mental status changes over a period of a few months, which began after the patient had been diagnosed with Lyme by his previous physician and was unsuccessfully treated with doxycycline. Upon examination, the patient behaved as if he were in slow motion, but wasn't violent or agitated. His clinical and lab findings were consistent with Lyme, and I treated him with tetracycline. About one week into treatment, he suddenly developed severe agitation. He began kicking and punching holes in the walls of his house, the police were called to restrain him, and he was admitted to a local psychiatric hospital. When I spoke to the admitting psychiatrist, I was pleasantly shocked to hear him say, "I think your patient is having a neuropsychiatric Herxheimer reaction." I concurred. We agreed to continue antibiotic treatment while the patient was hospitalized, and his psychiatric symptoms lessened in about another week. A month later, the patient returned to see me, back to his old self. He said that he felt like it had all been a bad dream. This fortunate man had no further complications.

In another case, a young woman without any history of an eating disorder developed anorexia in her mid-twenties, losing thirty pounds. Upon evaluation, I noted the typical multi-system clinical features for Lyme, along with lab results that supported a Lyme diagnosis. I treated her with several courses of pulsed antibiotics for nine months. Although there were significant Herxheimers, they were mostly physical rather than psychiatric, and her food obsessions gradually cleared during treatment. Midway through her treatment, her anorexia had largely vanished and she gained back the weight she had lost. She eloquently described how her food obsessions dissipated during antibiotic therapy.

The author, artist, and designer Ally Hilfiger suffered through twelve years of torture caused by a tick bite she got when she was seven years old. She saw almost a dozen doctors, who diagnosed her with everything from RA to MS. She spent years deteriorating until she was committed to a psychiatric hospital at age nineteen. She recalls, "I was having terrible panic attacks, major nausea attacks, and my brain started to shut down. I was crying, 'My body is sick, there are bugs inside of me, I need help! Do something!'" Finally, four months into her hospital stay, a savvy psychiatrist recognized she might have Lyme and sent her to be evaluated by me. Blood tests and clinical evaluation revealed that she had Lyme and babesiosis. Ally began long-term antibiotics and got well, but only after several years on treatment.

These three patients are dramatically different but also similar, in that each reflects serious psychiatric manifestations of Lyme disease. This phenomenon has been well documented in the literature. In 1994, no less an authority than the *American Journal of Psychiatry* published a seminal paper by two Columbia University Medical Center doctors declaring Lyme disease a neuropsychiatric illness.[30] They wrote that up to 40 percent of patients with Lyme develop neurologic symptoms within the first few weeks of infection, and that the broad range of psychiatric reactions associated with Lyme disease includes paranoia, dementia, schizophrenia, bipolar disorder, panic attacks, major depression, anorexia nervosa, and obsessive-compulsive disorder. Depression in particular has been documented to occur in up to 66 percent of patients. And the way the Lyme bacterium behaves in the body explains why the resulting disease can wax and wane, and why it can be so stubborn, resistant, and unresponsive to treatment.

Shamefully, complex and poorly understood diseases, many stemming from infections like Lyme, *Bartonella*, and others, are often defaulted to a psychological cause when an obvious physical cause isn't readily apparent. Tuberculosis, hypertension, and stomach ulcers were once considered to be stress-induced. This unfortunate presumption is rampant and damaging. Patients with real, albeit confusing, symptoms are frequently cast off by the medical community — and, largely as a result of the medical community's dismissal, even their loved ones do the same, because on some level they think the doctors must be right, which inflicts emotional trauma on top of pain.

Part of the problem lies in their training. Doctors are taught to follow one-size-fits-all guidelines, which allows them to squeeze lots of patients into their daily schedule. But good medicine involves problem solving, and that takes time. This is especially true for specialists, who rarely think outside the boxes within their fields. As stated by Dr. Ramzi Asfour, board certified in infectious diseases and internal medicine, and Assistant Clinical Professor of Medicine at UCSF, "You have to address the nervous system. Unfortunately, infectious disease doctors don't want to deal with that."

The presence of a psychiatric diagnosis does not eliminate the possibility of a physical cause of the psychiatric condition. Many patients are given a psychiatric diagnosis as a result of an inadequate medical workup. Jill Buchwald, PhD, has been a clinical psychologist for over two decades and served as Assistant Professor of Psychiatry at The Payne Whitney Clinic at New York Presbyterian Hospital and Associate Director of the Cornell Cognitive Therapy Clinic. "I've been astounded by patients I've known for years who have only gotten so far with meds and therapy but who've ultimately been diagnosed with a tick-borne disease and gotten better with antibiotics in an unprecedented way," she told us. "In training, you don't learn about the profound connection between psych symptoms and infections, and that's a huge loss for patients. It's totally wrong that clinicians are not only not taught, but are steered away from looking at cause. In my most treatment-refractory patients with depression and anxiety, I am finding that so many of them actually have underlying infections. And when treated properly, I have seen them respond in miraculous ways." She now feels it's her duty as a mental-health professional and human being to make this known. According to her: "A ridiculous number of people with psychiatric illnesses actually don't need psych meds. They need antibiotics."

We're not happy to report that many doctors generally lack even a cursory insight into what Lyme+ can do to the body and brain. Countless patients come to us after being told that their illness is "all in their head," that Lyme is a "trendy disease," that they're "just depressed," are "going through a midlife crisis," they have "sickness syndrome" (meaning they like being sick so they pretend to stay that way), or worse, in the case of parents with chronically ill children, that they have "Munchausen syndrome by proxy," which, you'll recall, is when a parent or caregiver fabricates or exaggerates a child's illness. Our poll of over 1,100 Lyme patients revealed that 79 percent were first diagnosed with a psychiatric illness!

Dr. Bob Bransfield is a well-published psychiatrist and Clinical Associate Professor at Rutgers' Robert Wood Johnson Medical School, widely recognized as being at the forefront of treating patients with the neuropsychiatric symptoms of tick-borne illness. In a 2017 review paper, he wrote about the link between suicide and Lyme+, attributing more than a thousand suicides a year in the U.S. to Lyme and its associated diseases. But this is not hot-off-the-press news. In the 1994 review paper for the *American Journal of Psychiatry* that we mentioned above, co-author Dr. Brian Fallon, who is the director of the Lyme and Tick-Borne Diseases Research Center at Columbia University Irving Medical Center, documented very significant neuropsychiatric features of the illness.[31]

Bransfield believes there's a lot of misunderstanding when it comes to neuropsychiatric Lyme, especially in regard to those who deny or dismiss the strong connection between mental illness and underlying infection. "You don't always get psychiatric symptoms immediately after infection. There can be a sequence of how these symptoms present," he says. "The cognitive and tic disorders come sooner, but the psychiatric — the depression, anxiety, mood changes, panic attacks — a lot of that can emerge farther down the road post-infection. And at that point, people aren't always connecting the dots . . . People like hard-line IDSA folks think that psychiatric symptoms come out of nowhere from a vacuum. They don't see the connection. It's a very clear connection: A lot of infections increase the risk for psychiatric illness. And there's very little training in this area." Again, it's like the German physicist Max Planck's famous quote: "Science advances one funeral at a time."

Unfortunately, there's much confusion over what mental symptoms can mean. According to Bransfield, if you have mental symptoms from an infection, then it's assumed you have an infection within the central nervous system. But that's not always the case. You can have infection within the body *provoking the immune system*, with the results of the infection (e.g., antibodies, inflammatory agents) crossing the blood-brain barrier and causing symptoms. This is not a trivial point. It has great importance because psychiatric patients whose illness is caused by underlying Lyme, *Bartonella*, or others can be inappropriately relegated to a "primary psychiatric" group, meaning that there is no infectious cause of their illness, purely on the basis of a normal spinal tap. As previously highlighted, the interaction can be in the brain, even with normal-appearing spinal fluid.

The flawed diagnostic testing for Lyme+ makes it easier for some doctors to ignore the ramifications of a potential infectious cause of psychiatric disease. "You're not going to convince people who have been so invested in hanging on to a 1970s definition of Lyme disease,"

Bransfield states. "To a rheumatologist, everything can be a rheuma-tologic disease." Undoubtedly, the silos in medicine are causing much suffering; it can be hard to see outside your own box. "Money, ego, and power are part of it," Dr. Bransfield states. "But it's also that they just don't understand. And they've dug themselves into a corner so much that they created this whole idea of 'post-treatment Lyme disease syndrome': That's a back door that lets you get out of the corner you've put yourself into. They are not graciously taking it. It's an outrageous position to say there's no such thing as chronic Lyme. Totally outra-geous. They've taken that position and are locked into it. And then when you show evidence to the contrary, instead of trying to under-stand it — instead of trying to understand the evidence that conflicts with their belief system — there's a tendency to try to demean instead. It forces them to defend. It's a rare person who can say 'I was wrong, and let me see things in a different light than I used to.'"

As noted, the psychiatric symptoms sometimes don't develop right away. They can emerge years or decades after infection. "One of the greatest disservices is this perception of the two-tier testing," states Dr. Bransfield. "It was never standardized for late-stage disease. So it might be useful a few months after infection, but if it's ten or twenty years ago that you were infected, it's not reliable. Yet that's when the psychiatric symptoms can surface. And you're using an immune-based testing for an organism that suppresses and evades the immune system. It's ab-surd . . . If you look at standard of care in medicine, it's the same no matter what the disease: you do a thorough exam, you take a thorough history, you use clinical judgment, and you individualize your think-ing and your treatment plan. And we do that in every disease that ex-ists except Lyme disease. Why should Lyme be an exception?"

We should point out that depression is no longer considered just a "chemical imbalance in the brain." Quite to the contrary, the in-flammation model of depression is quickly taking hold.[32] That's right: Depression is now considered an inflammatory disorder. Cytokines, which are chemical messengers that cause inflammation, along with markers like C-reactive protein which tell us that inflammation is oc-curring in the body — the same things we see elevated in heart disease

— are often elevated in depression, especially in the forms that are resistant to antidepressants.[33]

This is not new information; two decades of scientific literature describe the role of inflammation in mental illness, from depression to schizophrenia.[34] The field of psychiatry has known about the immune system's part in the onset of depression for a long time, but only recently have we begun to understand the connection, thanks to better technology and longitudinal studies. Higher levels of inflammation are associated with a higher risk of developing depression. Infection is an underlying cause of inflammation, and the higher the levels of inflammatory markers, the worse the depression. This places depression right in line with other inflammatory disorders such as Parkinson's disease, multiple sclerosis, and Alzheimer's disease. In spite of the long-documented infectious link to mental illness, the field of psychiatry is still largely in the dark ages, using long-term psychiatric medications that often don't work well, don't cure, and in most cases don't address the root cause.

MTHFR Gene Variant

You may have heard about these genes that are now mentioned in psychiatric circles. There are at least two genes that encode for the enzyme methylenetetrahydrofolate reductase, or MTHFR for short. These are frequently mutated in the population, and cause varying levels of metabolic disruption depending on how many copies of each mutated gene are present. Mutations of these genes contribute to increased levels of homocysteine, an amino acid, which is recognized to be a significant risk for vascular disease, dementia, psychiatric illness, and certain cancers.

The American College of Obstetricians and Gynecologists, College of American Pathologists, American College of Medical Genetics, and American Heart Association do not recommend testing for MTHFR.[35] Likewise, most medical societies do not recommend routine screening for homocysteine levels. I (Dr. Phillips) have been very surprised by this, given the following:

Studies show that certain B-vitamin supplementation resulting in lowered homocysteine reduces the risk of stroke,[36] which is confirmed by a metanalysis of many studies.[37] Homocysteine reduction by vitamin supplementation also reduces retinal atherosclerosis[38] in diabetic patients with high blood pressure, as well as brain shrinkage[39] and cognitive decline[40] in patients with early dementia. Other studies also demonstrate a significant treatment benefit to psychiatric symptoms in patients with depression[41] and eating disorders.[42]

Although studies of homocysteine reduction by vitamin supplementation demonstrate a reduced rate of recurrent blockage of the coronary arteries[43] after balloon angioplasty, a procedure to open clogged arteries, most studies do not demonstrate a reduction of overall heart disease[44] that meets statistical significance. This may be because the B-vitamin regimens used in those studies were sub-optimal, as homocysteine levels were frequently only modestly reduced. I offer my patients with elevated homocysteine vitamin therapy to lower it. For most patients, methylfolate and methylcobalamin will markedly lower homocysteine. For some patients, additional therapy is required, such as vitamin B6, but it can cause heartburn in some patients, and if taken in excess, can damage nerves. Thus, it's always best to follow up with your doctor before starting any supplements.

THE INFECTION THEORY OF AUTISM

There is one more angle in the conversation related to brain function that we'd like to discuss: the development of autism. We realize this is a hot-button topic in medical circles today, with so many competing theories and ideas on the matter, but most experts agree that autism spectrum disorder (ASD) has both genetic and environmental origins. A number of risk factors are being studied, including genetic, infectious, metabolic, nutritional, and environmental, but less than 10 to

12 percent of cases have specific, identifiable causes. The million-dollar question is how big a role infections may play in the growing number of cases. One in forty-five children aged three to seventeen — more than a million children in the U.S. — have been diagnosed with ASD, a neurologic disorder that usually appears by age three and affects the development of social and communication skills. Studies suggest that ASD is still significantly underdiagnosed and increasing, especially among females.[45] Symptoms can range from relatively mild, such as social awkwardness, to profoundly severe, and include developmental disabilities, debilitating repetitive behaviors, and an inability to communicate. It can result from a variety of different pathways, each one unique to the individual. One root cause may stem from infection.

The pediatricians and psychiatrists we spoke with share a collective wealth of experience in seeing children with autism, some cases of which come on suddenly with an infection like Lyme or *Bartonella*, after the child has been developing normally since birth. This is known as retrograde autism, and while it mystifies doctors, we think the science will eventually show that underlying infections from Lyme+ could very well be a cause — and that it can happen in utero via the mother as the fetus develops, later when the child is a toddler, or perhaps older but when the brain is still "under construction" and vulnerable. The human brain is not fully mature until about the age of twenty-five. It is the organ that takes the longest to fully develop. This may explain why Lyme+ infections can present so differently in children and adolescents than in adults, especially with regard to brain-related, neurologic effects such as problems with learning, behavior, anxiety, depression, and, yes, sudden autistic presentations, which can occur after immunologic triggers.

The medical literature is already filling up with risk factors for autism that have everything to do with infections. In 2017, for example, a study overseen by Dr. Ian Lipkin, an epidemiologist and infectious disease expert at Columbia, showed that infections during pregnancy may cause some cases of autism.[46] And once again, similar to the cause-and-effect of other infections, it's believed that the immune system's response via inflammation damages the brain of a developing fetus, resulting in the brain disorder. This particular study found that women who had active genital herpes infections early in pregnancy were twice as likely to have a child with autism than women who did not. A range of infections are already known to cause birth defects and impact a baby's brain — viruses like Zika, cytomegalovirus, herpes simplex 1 and 2, and rubella, as well as infections like syphilis. So why not other germs in the Lyme+ family, too? We know that congenital Lyme, *Bartonella*, *Brucella*, and *Babesia*, among others, exist and can cause everything from devastating birth defects to stillbirths, so it's not a stretch to also posit that a developing fetus can be gravely impacted, not just by an invading pathogen crossing the placenta and then the growing baby's blood-brain barrier, but also by an injurious immune response arising from the mother's infection and resulting in inflammation of the baby's brain.

This study comes on the heels of others demonstrating a wide range of different types of infections triggering brain disorders like autism in vulnerable kids. A 2013 study at UC Davis found that women who had the flu while pregnant were twice as likely to have a child later diagnosed with autism.[47] Those who had a fever lasting a week or longer — perhaps caused by the flu virus or maybe by something else — were three times as likely to have an autistic child. And our friend Dr. Bob Bransfield published his findings in 2014 that there's a high rate of Lyme in children with autism, many of whom went undiagnosed for a long time.[48]

Dr. Amy Proal offered her thoughts on this topic. Although she sees a combination of genetic and environmental forces at work in the development of autism, she sees evidence that pathogens are a driving force in this brain disorder. She sees many root-cause connections among autism and conditions like Alzheimer's, RA, and even cancer. "There are common underlying mechanisms in all of these conditions," she says. "They run in trends of environment acting on the genome — trends like persistent infections and chemical exposures. The symptoms you get just depend on the set of unique organisms you end up sustaining and how other environmental variables allow such organisms to survive and persist. You become the sum of your infectious and environmental history."

Her answer as to why autism tends to run in families and is more prevalent in the children of older parents echoes what Bennet Lorber and Paul Ewald have articulated: Because it runs in families doesn't mean it's explained by the human genome alone. Although people on the spectrum tend to reproduce later in life, which supports the genetic theory of autism, it can also be explained by inherited communities of pathogens that accumulate as we age and then are passed on. The longer you live, the more the environment affects you from both an epigenetic and infectious burden perspective.

PART II

The Remedy

CHAPTER 6

The Difficulty in Diagnosis

If you listen long enough, the patient will give you the diagnosis.

—*Sir William Osler*

F YOU KEEP telling people that their debilitating symptoms are medically unexplainable and psychosomatic, many begin to believe it and give up. The ones who won't be deterred will endure just about anything for a diagnosis and cure. And with Lyme, as well as many of the infections included in Lyme+, there is no part of the body that they can't infect, including the brain, as we've just described in the previous chapter. This should not come as a shock to anyone because we already know that psychiatric and neurological illnesses can be caused by other similar infections, like syphilis and leptospirosis, both of which are closely related to Lyme, and brucellosis, which is closely related to *Bartonella*. And it's not limited to those. Psychiatric symptoms can also be caused by a host of other infections, including tuberculosis, as well as lesser-known infections included in Lyme+, such as *Coxiella* (another bacterial infection) and *Toxocara*, neurocysticersosis, and schistosomiasis (parasitic infections). Most doctors today, including infectious disease doctors, will never have seen many of these diagnoses in patients. They are not thinking about or looking for them.

You can't refute solid data. In Part 1, we explained that many of the infections in Lyme+ can evade most, if not all, of the major antimicrobial classes of drugs, persist, and cause serious health problems throughout the body—from joints to the brain. Now, in Part 2, we offer solutions to getting the right treatment and finding a path to healing. We'll start with a question often asked: Why no vaccine?

A FAILED VACCINE

Vaccines have a long and colorful history. They have eradicated many ills that used to debilitate, disfigure, or kill entire swaths of populations. The first vaccine was for smallpox, a common epidemic prior to the eighteenth century. In the late 1700s, a small-town doctor, Edward Jenner, noted that farmers and milkmaids exposed to cowpox, which was common among cattle at the time, never seemed to suffer from smallpox during its frequent outbreaks. They would have a brief bout with the illness, which was less serious and less deadly than smallpox, but retained their beautiful complexions. Others, who suffered immensely from the disease, would either die from it or be left with severely scarred skin. For Jenner, this was a huge clue. He began looking into whether or not these workers were being naturally vaccinated by exposure to the cowpox virus. Perhaps the cowpox virus conferred protection against the related smallpox virus. (Interesting trivia tidbit: the word vaccine comes from the Latin word *vacca*, which means "cow."*)

In 1796, Jenner met a young dairymaid named Sarah Nelms who had cowpox lesions on her hands. He carefully extracted material from her lesions and injected it into an eight-year-old boy, James Phipps, who was the son of a gardener. This was before the days of informed

---

* Although the Oxford English Dictionary credits the French for coining the term "vaccine" in 1800 and "vaccination" in 1803, the term was used as an adjective by Edward Jenner in 1799, and his friend Richard Dunning introduced the term "vaccination" in 1800.

consent, not to mention parental involvement in such consent, but it also speaks to the long tradition of medical researchers experimenting on the poor. Phipps developed fevers, chills, and loss of appetite about a week later, but recovered thereafter. The real experiment came two months later, when Jenner injected Phipps with smallpox material. As he predicted, the boy stayed well, leading Jenner to conclude that Phipps was protected from the deadly smallpox. The boy was now "immune" to the disease. Better yet, two other children who shared a bed with Phipps did not catch smallpox from him either, further strengthening his evidence. His report of the events called for more vaccinations, and elicited skepticism. Jenner was not discouraged. He documented more vaccinations throughout the next year. By 1800 Jenner's work had been published in all the major European languages and had reached Benjamin Waterhouse in the U.S., a respected physician and a cofounder of the Harvard Medical School. The rest, as they say, is history. Other vaccines for many other diseases would follow.

After decades of continuous worldwide vaccination and improvements in public sanitation and hygiene, in 1972 smallpox was declared eradicated in the United States; in 1977 a single case of smallpox occurred in Somalia, the very last one. By 1980, the WHO considered smallpox to be eliminated worldwide.

All vaccines work the same way: they prime the immune system to recognize and attack a particular pathogen, or in the case of a toxoid vaccine, a pathogen's toxin, if it shows up in the body in the future. This can be done in four main ways: inactivated vaccines, live attenuated vaccines, toxoids, and subunit/conjugates. Inactivated vaccines do not contain live viruses or bacteria, but either whole killed germs or simply parts of these organisms. (The development of a vaccine against parasites continues to be elusive—deeply troubling, given the breadth of their presence and toll that they take on our global health.) These microbial parts are either DNA, protein, or specific molecules on the germ's surface. They allow your immune system to identify this as the enemy and obtain advance notice if that virus or bacterium were to invade. Immune system cells then have memory to be able to recognize the organism when they next encounter it, in order to produce antibodies to fight it. The immune cells remain circulating in your blood on guard, ready to stop an infection in its tracks if your body is later exposed to the real thing. However, these antibodies often don't remain for your whole lifetime or aren't strong enough to protect you after just one shot, which is why booster immunizations are recommended, for example for whooping cough or rabies.

The smallpox vaccine was a live attenuated vaccine, but it was given in much smaller concentrations than the original, Jenner-like smallpox vaccine. These types of vaccines often confer lifelong immunity after one or two doses. But people with compromised immune systems are usually not able to receive these. Examples of live attenuated vaccines include the measles vaccine, the rotavirus vaccine, and the yellow fever vaccine. There's a vaccine for tuberculosis that's given in several countries around the world, known as BCG, which is also a live bacterial vaccine, but the CDC recommends that it should not be given to those with weakened immune systems.

A toxoid is a form of vaccine that is an inactivated bacterial toxin. Examples of these include toxoids against diphtheria and tetanus. These types of vaccines enable the body to render the real toxin harmless if it were to show up in the future. Tetanus is exceedingly rare today (fewer than thirty cases per year occur in the United States) and most doctors have never seen a case. Tetanus is not like other infections that can spread between people. It's a spore-forming soil bacterium and is transmitted by entering an open wound. Its spore can survive on surfaces, like a rusted nail, for long periods, only to start replicating in the unsuspecting person who steps on the nail. The spore produces a toxin that causes powerful and life-threatening muscle contractions, unless of course the person has been vaccinated.

Like inactivated whole-cell vaccines, subunit/conjugate vaccines don't contain live components of a pathogen, but rather small fragments of its outer surface protein, which stimulates a protective immune response. Some examples of subunit/conjugate vaccines are those for influenza, hepatitis B, HPV, and some for shingles.

At a time when many infectious diseases have been brought or kept under control with global vaccination efforts, one has to wonder why it has taken so long to develop a vaccine for Lyme+. There are several reasons for this. Lyme is the only one in the family that has gotten any significant attention by the medical community, and that attention has been fraught with controversy. *Bartonella* is an emerging infectious disease that has only been recognized in earnest since the 1990s. Before that, only two species were known—one that was restricted to the high Andes Mountains and caused Carrión's disease, and the other that caused trench fever. Over the past twenty years or so, about forty-five more species of this bacterium have been discovered. In sum, we're dealing with a tribe of infections, all of which are poorly understood, and all of which have been mismanaged by the medical community.

Moreover, these are complex germs that behave in crafty ways in the body. A good analogy is to consider the human immunodeficiency virus, or HIV, for which we still do not have a vaccine after decades of research. Not only are there many different types, subtypes, and strains of HIV, each genetically distinct, but the virus also mutates frequently. These characteristics make the prospect of a vaccine practically impossible — there are too many rapidly moving targets. The Lyme+ family of infections suffers from similar complications. It's like trying to shoot a gun at a swarm of flies.

Not that vaccines for Lyme haven't been developed and tried. SmithKline Beecham (now GlaxoSmithKline) developed the first and only licensed vaccine against Lyme disease. It was called LYMERix and it was rolled out in 1998. Given in a three-dose series, the vaccine had an unusual method of action: it stimulated antibodies that attacked the Lyme bacteria in the tick's gut as it fed on the human host — before the bacteria were able to enter the body. More specifically, it was a recombinant vaccine containing an outer surface protein (OspA) from *Borrelia burgdorferi*, the Lyme bacterium. A recombinant vaccine is one that's been engineered using recombinant DNA technology, which means inserting DNA into a bacterium. The bacterium then produces a specific antigen, in this case the surface protein from *Borrelia*, which is then purified and used as the vaccine.

Before licensure by the FDA, 6,478 people received a total of 18,047 doses of the vaccine during clinical testing. It was reported to be about 78 percent effective in protecting against Lyme after all three doses of the vaccine had been given (note that what constitutes efficacy is subject to interpretation, since we're talking about *Borrelia burgdorferi* only — not any of the myriad other virulent infections included in the Lyme+ family such as *Rickettsia, Ehrlichia, Anaplasma, Bartonella, F. tularensis, Coxiella*, the Powassan virus, and *Babesia*, just to name a few).[1] Between the time of its licensure in 1998 and July 31, 2000, about 1.5 million doses of the vaccine were distributed. It was intended for use in individuals between fifteen and seventy years old living or working in areas with high rates of Lyme disease.

By 2002, SmithKline Beecham had withdrawn LYMERix from the market. Reports of sobering side effects were accumulating, some of which were serious — resulting in life-threatening illnesses, long hospital stays, or severe disability. The vaccine was followed by crippling arthritis in some and neurologic disorders, including cognitive issues, in others.[2] It was a cruel twist of irony, given that Lyme itself can cause all of those conditions. But people couldn't get an active Lyme infection from the Lyme vaccine, as it contained no live bacteria. That's true, but it's also true, and indeed well known among Lyme researchers, that asymptomatic or minimally symptomatic Lyme infection is common. What if Lyme was widespread in the general population but the narrow CDC surveillance laboratory criteria adopted by IDSA for its diagnosis missed a large proportion of those infected? Well, it turns out that Lyme *is* common in the population — 11 percent of healthy people without symptoms turned antibody-positive by the CDC criteria. Although it wasn't admitted by the CDC at the time the vaccine was released, in 2013 the CDC admitted that the true number of Lyme cases is approximately ten times higher than the number reported to them.[3] This means that the true infection rates with Lyme are alarmingly high. So what happens if the Lyme vaccine is given to a patient with asymptomatic Lyme infection? Since the symptoms of Lyme are caused largely by the immune system going after the bacteria, can vaccinating someone with hidden, undiagnosed Lyme turn that asymptomatic infection into a symptomatic one?

During a heated meeting with the FDA, Donald H. Marks, MD, PhD eviscerated LYMERix and its makers. Dr. Marks was the director of the Lyme vaccine program for the pharmaceutical giant Aventis Pasteur, previously called Connaught, and had been brought in as a consultant to independently review the reported adverse events of LYMERix. He accused SmithKline Beecham of using "confusing" language to mislead physicians administering the vaccine. His strong words:

"SKB (Glaxo) has acted in an unreasonable manner by marketing LYMERix without adequate warnings about the risks of severe rheumatologic, neurologic, autoimmune and other adverse events, and by failing to caution and educate physicians about these dangers.

"In my opinion," he told FDA officials, "there is sufficient evidence that LYMERix is causally related to severe rheumatologic, neurologic, autoimmune, and other adverse events in some individuals. This evidence is such as to warrant a significantly heightened degree of warnings and possible limitations or removal from marketing of LYMERix."[4]

With that, LYMERix was hastily pulled from the market, though the official PR story from its maker was that it was yanked due to lack of demand. Many individual lawsuits followed, as well as a class-action lawsuit from vaccine recipients who became ill after vaccination.[5] We continue to hear from patients who say they have still not recovered from their LYMERix injuries.

Vaccines are enormously expensive to develop, often costing more than $1 billion, as was the case with the rotavirus vaccine — a vaccine for a condition whose seriousness doesn't compare to what Lyme+ can do. Federal institutions and global organizations have already spent more than $9 billion trying to develop an HIV vaccine. At this expense, it is hardly believable that a drug company would pull an approved vaccine due to a relative "lack of demand."

Today drug companies are trying to develop vaccines for zoonotic infections, among them some that target multiple tick-borne pathogens and some that target tick saliva, but this area of medicine continues to be fraught with challenges. Lyme+ presents unique difficulties that make developing a vaccine a very onerous, if not impossible, task.

(The same is true of malaria, which has its own unique complexities and no commercially available vaccine despite more than fifty years of trying.) There needs to be a major leap in vaccine technology and a cleanup of the industry; otherwise, it's an enormous waste of resources. with so many different strains of Lyme and with so many other pathogens that can be transmitted with Lyme, or on their own, there may never be a single vaccine to cover this extensive territory. And a "Lyme vaccine" could give people a false sense of security since it will not prevent any of those other infections from taking hold. The hurdles are formidable, just like those for testing and diagnosing.

THE SCIENCE OF IMPERFECT DIAGNOSTICS

If you become diabetic, a fasting blood sugar test will tell you that. If you get strep throat, a culture will identify the bad bacteria. If you become infected with HIV, there's a test to detect both HIV antibodies and antigens (pieces of the virus). These areas of medicine are black and white. When it comes to Lyme, *Bartonella*, and related infections, it's anything but.

Diagnosing Lyme+ requires an exhaustive exploration into a person's history and symptoms, as well as a good physical examination and thorough laboratory testing. As we have seen, most Lyme patients never see the stereotypical "bull's-eye" rash and never recall getting a tick bite. And chances are very good that your primary care doctor hasn't checked you for any of the less well-known infections in Lyme+. To make matters worse, signs and symptoms of these diseases can emerge a long time after the initial infection, making an accurate clinical diagnosis harder because the trail has grown cold.

Serologies (blood antibody tests) are the most commonly performed diagnostics for Lyme+ infections. Contrary to what you might assume, these tests do not identify the presence or absence of the microbes, but rather detect the presence of an antibody response caused by exposure to the pathogen. Lyme is particularly controversial in this regard. Here's the shocker: Of the dozens of Lyme serologies available in the U.S., none are FDA-approved and none has been shown to be the best one. A minority are FDA-*cleared*, which means that they perform at least as well as similar tests already in use, but that does not mean they have been clinically validated in studies. So when your doctor recommends "only FDA-approved Lyme testing," you now know why that statement doesn't make sense.

Keep in mind that the reliability of diagnostic testing in general, no matter what kind of diagnostics we're talking about, is a function of three important scientific concepts: sensitivity, specificity, and reproducibility. *Sensitivity* is a test's ability to detect disease when it is present, and *specificity* is a test's ability to not detect disease when it is absent. *Reproducibility* is the ability of a test to give the same result for a specimen on repeat testing. Highly accurate tests generate few false negatives and few false positives. Unfortunately, Lyme serology produces a great many false negatives and some false positives. Additionally, researchers have repeatedly demonstrated that results and interpretation of both ELISA and Western blot tests (more on these shortly) for Lyme vary from lab to lab.[6] Translation: they're not reliable.

Apart from Lyme, why can't we easily detect many other active Lyme+ infections? Many of these infections are caused by fastidious organisms, which means that they have complex growth requirements and are difficult to culture from infected patients. Non-fastidious infections, on the other hand, such as those caused by bacteria like *E. coli* and *Streptococcus*, can be detected by culture or PCR analysis (polymerase chain reaction, a method for amplifying target DNA). Trying to grow many of the Lyme+ microbes out of infected tissue or detect their DNA in blood, joint fluid, or even cerebrospinal fluid is incredibly hard. In fact, so-called direct-detection tests (i.e., culture, PCR) for *B. burgdorferi* (along with others in the Lyme+ family) have historically performed poorly—so much so in the case of Lyme culture that these tests are not available through chain or hospital labs. Although there have been some labs trying to offer an innovative Lyme culture test, they have been met with great controversy. PCR testing is getting better with new technologies to sequence not just different strains and species of *Borrelia* but also associated infections, like *Bartonella, Brucella, Babesia, Rickettsia, Francisella, Coxiella,* and many others.

Indirect testing seeks to find signs of the body's response to an infection rather than the infection itself, which makes this whole business suspect, given the sneaky behavior of these organisms. False negatives (not false positives) are a major problem in Lyme and *Bartonella* diagnostics, and a significant issue for other stealthy Lyme+ infections, including brucellosis,[7] tularemia,[8] babesiosis,[9] *Coxiella,*[10] *Toxocara,*[11] and *Strongyloides.*[12] However, Lyme is still the illness that gets most of the attention, so we'll focus on that in the following paragraphs.

It's often said that when antibody testing is done too early in Lyme infection, false negatives may result, but this is a common scenario at any stage of infection. What's more, it has been shown that after a Lyme antibody response develops, it can wane or persist regardless of disease status.[13] In one oft-cited study of primates infected with *B. burgdorferi,* some untreated animals had antibodies develop and then disappear over time, despite persistence of infection.[14] The same disappearance of antibodies despite continued infection has been published for humans.[15] Worse, many Lyme patients fail to develop antibody responses to this infection at all and studies show that these patients tend to be sicker than those who develop positive tests.[16] Equally troubling, false-negative antibody tests also occur with *Bartonella* infection, even in severe disease resulting in fatality.[17]

Differences in how a test performs are affected not only by the timing of the testing (how soon after initial infection) but also by the symptoms being evaluated. The most commonly available Lyme serologies, for example, have been found to perform better in cases of arthritis but poorly in neurologic presentations. Note that even when the tests perform better, cases will be missed if doctors rely solely on test results. This is why a clinical diagnosis made by a physician, based upon signs and symptoms and ruling out other illnesses, is crucial. You cannot rely solely on test results because, unlike other areas of medicine, Lyme and *Bartonella* testing is not reliable, and testing for the other infections in Lyme+ is almost as bad.

TWO-TIER TESTING FOR LYME

There are two commonly performed blood tests for Lyme, which, if executed according to the CDC surveillance criteria — a protocol we don't agree with for diagnosis — go in sequence. The first test is called an ELISA, and if that comes back positive, then another test called the Western blot is ordered. Unfortunately, many Lyme cases are not picked up by the ELISA. If the ELISA comes back negative in a Lyme patient, he or she will probably not get the second test — the Western blot — and will go on to suffer from the missed diagnosis.

ELISA stands for enzyme-linked immunosorbent assay. This test measures certain antibodies in the blood — IgM, IgG, or a combination of IgM and IgG antibodies — that are indicators of exposure to an infection. The sensitivity of this test for Lyme varies depending on where the patient is in the course of the disease (early, late) and how it is manifesting in the body. In the early stages of the infection, for instance, this test returns lots of false negatives because the body has yet to produce those antibodies. It takes time — weeks, often — for the body's immune system to get the message that it's been infected by an invader. But when there's a positive result in a Lyme ELISA test, chances are it's a true positive for either Lyme or something similar. Although it's possible for the ELISA to be false-positive, this can be because it is detecting other closely related infections such as syphilis, leptospirosis, relapsing fever spirochetes, or other *Borreliae*, such as *Borrelia miyamotoi*. Negative Lyme ELISA test results, on the other hand, are not as dependable. By some estimates, the Lyme ELISA can be falsely negative nearly 50 percent of the time.[18] And it's rarely of use for late-stage, chronic Lyme if the person does not have typical Lyme arthritis. It has been shown that in people who have Lyme arthritis, chances are good that an ELISA test will give a positive result. But those who have other manifestations of the disease, such as neurological issues or symptoms of fibromyalgia or chronic fatigue syndrome, are less likely to have a positive ELISA.

The *Western blot* is a test widely used in molecular biology to detect specific proteins in a sample of tissue or body fluid. The procedure was named for its similarity to an earlier method known as the Southern blot, and the word "blot" refers to how the test results are developed like a photograph on a film and interpreted: the scientist looks for dark spots or "bands" on a special film that correlates with the identity of specific proteins. Like the ELISA, the Western blot measures the presence of antibodies that form in the body upon infection. In particular, the Western blot tries to find reactivity against a group of different proteins found on the Lyme bacteria which corresponds to the particular bands that are demonstrated in the test. These bands all have numbers (e.g., "band 31") and some are more strongly associated with the presence of a Lyme infection. The problem is that there's no universal acceptance in the medical community about which bands equal a positive Lyme infection. The CDC's list of bands is not comprehensive enough, and remember that strict adherence to their reporting criteria fails to capture 90 percent of Lyme cases, by the CDC's own admission; ILADS recommends looking for a broader range of Lyme-centric bands.

Some of the most compelling bands supporting a history of Lyme infection are numbers 23, 31, 34, 39, and 93. This means that a Western blot that comes back with these bands showing up is consistent with a Lyme infection. Unfortunately, the debate over which antibody reactions to include in establishing criteria for a positive Lyme Western blot continues to rage on. Most of the largest commercial labs omit not only band 31 but 34 as well, leading to many false-negative results in infected people. We are strongly in favor of labs including those bands.

The above-mentioned tests are the most commonly used for Lyme specifically. Different tests need to be administered for other infections that can ride along with it, or be transmitted on their own, such as *Babesia*, *Ehrlichia*, *Anaplasma*, and *Bartonella*. And then there are the other less commonly discussed infections, including Q fever from *Coxiella*, brucellosis from *Brucella*,[19] tularemia from *Francisella tula-*

rensis, and spotted and typhus fevers from *Rickettsiae*, to name a few. All of these can be transmitted via tick and other vectors, and some by other means as well (i.e., airborne transmission for *Coxiella* and ingestion of contaminated dairy for *Brucella*). There are also other stealthy infections that contribute to chronic illness around the world, such as TB, Whipple's disease, *Toxocara*, filaria, *Strongyloides*, schistosoma, trichinella, cysterercus, echinococcus, leishmaniasis, and entamoeba, the first two of which are bacterial and the rest of which are parasitic. Symptoms of chronic Lyme+ warrant a high degree of suspicion for an infection with at least one species of *Borrelia* and up to several other microbes—and testing has to be rigorous in order to investigate this.

When testing for Lyme+, I (Dr. Phillips) order both the Lyme ELISA and Western blot tests sent to Stony Brook University, requesting "all bands reported" (which means that even Lyme-specific bands that aren't on the restrictive CDC list can be reported). Note that widely available tests are based on a single *B. burgdorferi* strain, which increases the risk of false-negative results since many people are infected with other Lyme strains.[20] Doctors tend to lean too heavily on testing and don't realize how flawed it is. We can't stress it enough: The diagnosis of Lyme+ should be made *clinically*, based upon signs and symptoms, with antibody tests playing a supportive but not linchpin role. A negative test does not necessarily rule out a diagnosis of Lyme+.

- I send the blood to more than one lab since results can vary. I prefer to use Stony Brook University's lab. In my opinion, they have about as sensitive a test as anyone out there, they take most insurance, and they report all bands (though doctors still must specify "all bands" when filling out the requisition). Even if you live in other parts of the country, you can still send your blood to Stony Brook.
- I test for almost all of the other infections in the Lyme+ family at the major chain labs, such as Bioreference, Quest, LabCorp, or whichever lab takes my patient's insurance. I do this for two reasons: 1) to save my patients money at a fully covered lab because otherwise these tests would run into the thousands; and

2) because I think that the sensitivity of testing is decent for these other infections included in Lyme+. (We can always do more expensive send-out labs later if need be.) The other test that I feel is prone to false-negative results and requires a send-out from the start is *Bartonella*. I prefer North Carolina's Galaxy Diagnostics *Bartonella* IFA (immunofluorescence assays). The research team at Galaxy is composed of leaders in the field and I've observed that their test has superior sensitivity compared to most tests on the market. Other options include *Bartonella* antibody tests at Medical Diagnostic Laboratories and Focus Labs.

■ As a general rule, it's always a good idea to get a copy of all your test results and medical records. You may have been told by your doctor that you've tested negative, but the actual results in your medical record may indicate otherwise. If we had a nickel for every time we hear of a patient developing chronic illness because of delayed diagnosis and treatment, due simply to reading a Lyme Western blot with three or four bands as "negative" because it failed to meet the CDC criteria, or even worse, ignoring a frankly positive test (which happens a lot!), we're talking a ton of nickels.

Dr. Christienne Coates is an ophthalmologist who commonly sees manifestations of Lyme in her patients' eyes. She also has a daughter who was initially diagnosed with an autoimmune disease and had to drop out of college before finding proper treatment for her Lyme and *Bartonella*. "It's unfortunate that Lyme patients can't always easily get the care that they need," she says. "Doctors don't always have time to reflect when they are seeing patients all day. It's going to take awareness and public outcry for things to change. People don't realize that Lyme is a clinical diagnosis—you have to sit, listen, and draw things out of your patients because the testing is so poor." Her daughter saw a few doctors before coming to me (Dr. Phillips), but unfortunately, none of them offered a Lyme diagnosis. The general message was: "Whether she takes antibiotics or not, the results will be the same." Little did they know that the results would not be the same. She came to me and I had the privilege of helping her back to good health.

Dr. Charlotte Mao, the pediatric infectious disease expert you met in the previous part, puts it bluntly: "Trust your instincts, ask questions, and don't believe what you're presented with if you don't agree. You have to be your own best advocate and educate yourself widely and deeply until medicine catches up with you."

RULING OUT OTHER CONDITIONS

It's important to rule out other conditions either not related, or less directly related, to a Lyme+ infection but that could be creating, or contributing to, Lyme+-like symptoms. These include, but are not limited to:

- cancer, including solid tumors as well as lymphomas (cancers of the lymph system) and leukemias (blood cancers)
- HIV
- chronic hepatitis B or C
- tuberculosis
- Whipple's disease
- parasitic infections (we include these as Lyme+ but they can cause symptoms on their own as well as exacerbate Lyme)
- heart disease
- cerebrovascular disease
- sleep apnea
- anemia
- thyroid disorders
- parathyroid disorders
- vitamin B_1, B_6, or B_{12} deficiency
- heavy metal poisoning
- age-related degenerative joint and spine disease
- vitamin D deficiency

As we've been underscoring throughout the book, people with Lyme+ are up against an enormously fierce set of challenges. First, there's the stigma associated with Lyme and the intense controversy that swirls around its diagnosis and treatment. And then there's the

question of who's qualified to treat it, since medical providers are notoriously polarized. If you are lucky enough to get over the diagnostic
hurdles, the struggle to get insurance companies to cover long-term
treatment, and sometimes *any* treatment, awaits. Virtually everyone
we know who is dealing with these pernicious infections has encountered unacceptable roadblocks from the beginning, leaving them feeling desperate and demoralized.

Keep in mind that doctors are also in a bind. They may earnestly
want to help by prescribing longer-term antimicrobials, but legiti-
mately fear risking their licenses if they choose to treat outside IDSA's
erroneous and outdated guidelines. In an ongoing antitrust lawsuit
against several major health insurers, brought by twenty-eight chronic
Lyme+ patients who claim they're being wrongfully denied long-term
care, costing them hundreds of thousands of dollars in treatment, it
was revealed that doctors who defied the IDSA Guidelines were targeted by insurers. The complaint states: "As a result of their speaking
out, from 1997 to 2000, more than 50 physicians in New York, New
Jersey, Connecticut, Michigan, Oregon, Rhode Island and Texas were
investigated, disciplined or had had their licenses removed. Many of
these doctors were reported to their medical boards by the insurance
defendants."[21] Should an insurance company have the right to report a
doctor simply for prescribing medications that the insurance company
doesn't want to cover? Isn't that a conflict of interest?

Medical uncertainties surrounding vector-borne diseases lead
some doctors to take a hands-off approach, failing to coordinate with
a Lyme+-treating colleague. They are often just as perplexed by the
mysteries of Lyme+ as their patients. Hence patients experience misdiagnoses, their symptoms often erroneously attributed to an "autoimmune" or psychiatric condition. As described in Part 1, Lyme+ is said
to "mimic" (though we prefer the more accurate word "cause") a range
of other conditions. Doctors who are unfamiliar with vector-borne
illnesses can be short-sighted and tend to focus narrowly on a single
symptom. If you complain of arthritis in your hands and hips, for example, your doctor probably won't consider an underlying infection

as cause. If your primary care physician is offering treatment to palliate chronic symptoms that could be attributed to Lyme+ but they're not evaluating for these infections fully, you're not getting at the root of the problem.

A good first step may be to consult a physician trained by ILADS. Otherwise, Lyme+ may not be properly evaluated, which can lead to years or decades on the medical merry-go-round. To find a provider, ILADS has a provider search on their website (www.ilads.org). A next step would be to read reviews and look at the doctors on YouTube, if possible, as sometimes their lectures have made their way to the internet, to get a sense of who's the best fit. Watching a video of a physician speaking is going to tell you much more than reading something he or she has written. Facebook groups and message boards can also provide invaluable resources and support.

Doctors will differ on their approach to treatment due to all the controversies, variables, misconceptions, biases, and unknowns. Don't hesitate to get second (even third) opinions. In the next chapter, I (Dr. Phillips) will give you insights into how I treat my patients. By no means is it the only road to recovery, but by building on what works and discarding what's a waste of time, it provides a path toward getting better. I hope that my experience provides context to this puzzle, helping both physicians and patients appreciate the complexity of these diseases.

Dr. Z, who prefers to remain anonymous, is a post-doctorate medical fellow in infectious disease at a top-tier, prestigious university who can't talk about Lyme with her attendings because she hears them bash chronic Lyme patients and Lyme doctors almost daily. Consequently, she hasn't told any of her colleagues about her own complex health issues. As a young teenager, she was given five years to live after being diagnosed with scleroderma, a serious autoimmune disease that attacks the skin and connective tissue and can be fatal. Her life was saved by getting properly treated with five years of antibiotics for her underlying infection. She's now healthy and whole. But still, she regularly hears chronic Lyme patients being ridiculed and demeaned by the attendings under whom she trains, her academic superiors to whom she can't talk back. "These people are my mentors," she says. "I almost wish I didn't know their opinion. I feel like I'm living in an 'alternate universe.' My experience was part of my inspiration to go into medicine."

Although she now enjoys good health, tragically, she can't share her learned lessons with others currently struggling with her former illness. She feels so constrained by a broken and intimidating medical education hierarchy that she's not been able to tell her story and share her wisdom with critically ill scleroderma patients on whom she's consulted, and has had to watch some of them die.

WHAT'S CAUSING YOUR SYMPTOMS?

Whether they be sudden and intense, or chronic and smoldering, experiencing many strange symptoms is frightening. Don't be afraid to ask WHY?! Don't be afraid to demand answers that make sense to you! Don't be afraid to move on when you're not being heard or believed or respected! Many doctors have a reflexive, automatic "it's-not-Lyme-but-I-don't-know-what-it-is" response. We've heard it a lot and it was said to us, too, as patients. In cases of unexplained chronic illness, raising the possibility of an underlying infection as cause, even if the doctor thinks it's anything but that, can be the golden ticket.

It's a logical question: What could cause, say, a healthy twenty-five-year-old individual from New Hampshire to get multiple sclerosis or rheumatoid arthritis or psychosis or all three? It's a crucial question that usually goes unasked by mainstream medicine. Bodies do not just start attacking themselves for no reason. The human body is incredibly well designed after millions of years of evolution. It has backup systems and redundancies, like any highly engineered piece of machinery. It does not easily or suddenly break on its own. Often, the reason is an underlying, common infection. If any doctor is dismissive and refuses to consider Lyme and other vector-borne pathogens as a possible cause for a multi-symptom illness, it's reasonable to move on to another doctor. A doctor should never bully or intimidate, and you should not feel compelled to stay. Doctor-patient relationships are partnerships. We all need free-thinking physicians who will be partners in our health-care, so why waste time on those who aren't? We recommend that you bring someone with you — a friend or family member — who can advocate, ask questions, and take notes. Do not be afraid to challenge doctors, to engage them, to bring them studies, to show them cases similar to yours in the published literature. Seek out similar accounts too, on blogs and news sites. There are great resources within the Lyme+ community, which is growing online every day (you can start on our websites — StevenPhillipsMD.com and TheChronicBook.com — and follow the links to other sites we trust).

We both know what it's like to be ignored and rejected by the system. At one point, when first diagnosed with Lyme in med school and about twenty years before getting the *Bartonella* that nearly killed me (Dr. Phillips), I was seen by an infectious-disease physician who later went on to become an author of the much-contested IDSA Lyme treatment guidelines. By then, I had been experiencing mysterious and frightening musculoskeletal, cardiac, and neurologic symptoms for more than nine months after multiple rashes compatible with EM and had just been diagnosed with Lyme, complete with a positive antibody test. I was scared, but this doctor just seemed bored. And he didn't think I had Lyme. What about the positive blood test? This doctor thought it was likely a false positive. What about my prior response to antibiotics? He chalked that up to the placebo effect. But I couldn't possibly agree that the day after starting an antibiotic, the placebo effect would wake me up with chills, sweats, and my fingers locked in a bent position. These effects were signs of a Herxheimer reaction — toxins from the dying and stressed bacteria triggering a response — confirming the presence of the pathogen, and narrowing it down to the several that produce this reaction.

The ID doctor repeated the tests at his own lab, and wouldn't you know it, they were positive again. He wrote me a letter saying that since I was already taking tetracycline, he would just add two weeks of amoxicillin. I still have that letter. He didn't write "You have Lyme" or "I'm diagnosing you with Lyme" or "I'm sorry to tell you that you have Lyme." It just had my blood test results, the grudging agreement to prescribe two more weeks of amoxicillin, and the following admonishment: "I do not feel you have any evidence of advanced Lyme disease at present and therefore I would *not* recommend intravenous antibiotics." What was curiously lacking from the letter was a follow-up plan. What if I didn't get better? Shouldn't I see the doctor again to review my status after treatment? Would the same lack of follow-up have been doled out if I had a kidney infection, skin infection, or pneumonia? It's shocking that "Lyme" engenders so much bias that appropriate standards of medical care for infectious disease are abandoned. Our informal survey of over seven hundred Lyme patients concluded that two-thirds saw more than ten doctors to determine their diagnosis and begin treatment, and many saw upwards of forty over the course of decades.

ON THE ROAD TO BETTERLAND

Dr. Enid Haller, LCSW, PhD, is a clinical psychologist and Executive Director of Lyme Center of Martha's Vineyard. She describes the scenario well: "There is a complete sense of relief when you discover the mystery of your illness because then you experience a release from passive helplessness to a positive, proactive self-determination. The systematic denial of chronic Lyme is a black shame on our medical system, on our country, and on the individuals still engaged in denial."

We'll delve into a way of approaching treatment in the next chapter, but it's important to understand that healing from Lyme+ can feel like two steps forward, one step back. You may ask, "Will I ever get better? When? Why can recovery seem so slow?" Unless you're among the lucky few who respond nearly immediately to treatment, for my (Dr. Phillips) patients, the average duration of antibiotic therapy is usually about six to nine months total, spaced out across a year to eighteen months; most of my patients rate themselves at better than 90 percent back to normal after treatment.

Tracking symptoms is helpful for both patient and doctor. Everyone will have their preferred way of doing that. For example, you can grade the most troublesome symptoms on a scale from 1–5 or 1–10 once a week and compare them to the week before, and bring this list to your next appointment with your doctor. Keeping track of the worst ones helps doctors stay focused and makes things easier on patients who already feel overwhelmed. Another option is to color code your symptoms as red (really bad), yellow (manageable but still troubling), or green (better). With this method, you can see how you're doing in a glance (i.e., if symptoms are turning from red to yellow to green, you're improving).

We know this sounds basic, but you'd be shocked at how many people balk at keeping track of symptoms. When your doctor appointments are weeks or even months apart, you tend to forget symptoms and the memory of pain fades with time. It's likely a self-protection mechanism, insulating our psyches from bad memories. As it's said in medicine, if mothers accurately remembered the pain of childbirth, a lot of women would hesitate to have a second baby. These symptom notes can help inform ongoing treatment. We each found it hugely helpful to understand the ebb and flow of our illness this way and could celebrate as we saw evidence that symptoms were improving. After finally finding an effective regimen of antimicrobial therapy, I (Dr. Phillips) had a simple goal of driving to the supermarket alone, walking without crutches to the produce aisle at the back of the store, and buying a bag of lettuce. I drove there every day for weeks on end, and soon weeks turned into months. And every day I couldn't make it past the entrance to the store where the wagons were nested one inside the other like spoons. Until one day I could. With tears in my eyes, I called my mother: "I bought a bag of lettuce!" We should celebrate our personal victories, even if they seem small to others.

CHAPTER 7

The Road to Recovery

Healing is a matter of time,
but it is sometimes also a matter of opportunity.

—*Hippocrates*

NICOLE MALACHOWSKI SERVED more than twenty-one years as an officer and a career fighter pilot in the U.S. Air Force. She was among the first group of women to fly modern fighters and was the first female pilot selected to fly as part of the elite USAF Thunderbirds Aerial Demonstration Squadron. She's worked in the White House, first as a fellow for the U.S. General Services Administration and then as the executive director of the White House "Joining Forces" initiative. In 2019, she was inducted into the National Women's Hall of Fame. At the height of what would have been a long and promising career, her dream job came to an abrupt end when she was devastated by vector-borne disease, left struggling to speak fluently and walk safely for nine months. She was declared "100 percent unfit for duty," and forced to retire prematurely, and permanently, at forty-three years old.

Nicole's illness began in 2012 when, as the commander of an F-15E fighter squadron, she developed rapid onset of a multi-system illness, including intractable pain, insurmountable fatigue, cognitive dysfunction, and noticeable problems with speech, reading, writing, and short-term memory. Her symptoms would mysteriously wax and wane, baffling doctors. Repeated doctor visits yielded no answers, no diagnosis, no treatment—nothing. Nicole endured spatial disorientation, confusion, anxiety, and even moments of temporary paralysis. Unsafe to be left alone, she could not play with her children, care for herself, or interact with her husband, who had to take on the roles of both caregiver and single parent. Nicole had moments when she would have welcomed death. Despite her privileged status allowing access to any doctor she wanted—military and civilian physicians alike—diagnosing the root cause of her symptoms was difficult and destructively prolonged. "I thought I was tough, as a combat-proven fighter pilot. But tick-borne illness destroyed me, brought me to my knees, and ruthlessly broke me," Nicole says.

You'd think that someone like Nicole would have no trouble finding the source of her illness with the medical care available to her. But it took an unthinkable 1,525 days, to be exact, between her first doctor's visit and her accurate diagnosis. In those four-plus years, she saw over twenty-four doctors, both military and civilian, across eight specialties, and received three misdiagnoses. Often told she was just suffering from stress, Nicole felt patronized, discounted, and dismissed. She calls it "sheer luck" that she found herself at Harvard's Dean Center for Tick Borne Illness in Boston, Massachusetts, where she got her diagnosis and began treatment in coordination with a multi-disciplinary team at Massachusetts General Hospital. Only after that was she able to regain her abilities to stand safely, read and write, and speak fluently.

Today she works as an advocate for patients suffering from vector-borne disease and for the Congressionally Directed Medical Research Programs' Tick-Borne Disease Research Program to encourage the Departments of Defense and Veterans Affairs to take a leadership role in addressing the significant inadequacies in diagnostic testing and treatment options. She tells it like it is: "As a member of the military, every day, I was measured and held accountable to the highest, strictest standards of professionalism. That's as it should be." But that's not what's happening in the medical community. And even if a patient is lucky enough to encounter a doctor who thinks twice about Lyme and other tick-borne diseases, that may still be insufficient. That doctor may have heard of babesiosis and might even check for it, but that doctor would likely never have heard that there is more than one *Babesia* species and that the tests for one fail to diagnose the other. What's more, even though *Bartonella* likely wears the combined crown as the most common and destructive of the vector-borne illnesses to cause chronic illness, most physicians know almost nothing about it, can't evaluate for it properly, and in fact, miss it entirely. In addition to *Borrelia hermsii*, Nicole was infected with Lyme, *Anaplasma*, *Babesia microti*, and *Bartonella*, the latter of which was the major cause of her disease. She believes that *Bartonella* impacted her worse than anything else. So maybe we should restate it: in addition to *Bartonella*, she was also infected with *Borrelia hermsii*, Lyme, *Babesia*, and *Anaplasma*.

Nicole's harrowing story should sound familiar by now. We have to wonder if her military status hindered her diagnosis; the military is excellent at acute care and battlefield medicine, but patients with complex and chronic illnesses are often left behind due to the tempo of military operations. As we mentioned earlier, Lyme+ is overlooked and minimized on a wholesale basis by most government agencies. It also can be a career-killing diagnosis if you're in the military or even seeking a high-level government job. We spoke with someone off the record whose attempts to join the FBI were thwarted by her Lyme diagnosis. No one wants to talk about it in those halls. We hope that the Nicole Malachowskis of the world continue to fight the good fight, prompting real change in how vector-borne infections are handled in both military and civilian circles. Only then can we begin to treat these ailments with the right protocols and have patients receive the respect they deserve.

Now that you've gained a sense of testing techniques and the inherent challenges to making an accurate diagnosis, we're going to give you a toolkit by sharing how I (Dr. Phillips) approach these illnesses, individualizing treatment algorithms to each patient. This chapter will come from my perspective, based on the years I've spent creating a general framework for treating patients. I can't include my entire repertoire of methods and reasoning, as that would be a book unto itself, but I can share this overview of how I engage these infections and fine-tune treatments according to individual patient response, along with the tenets of pulse, or intermittent, antibiotic therapy.

This information is not offered as medical advice, simply a description of my approach, how my methods overlap and converge to quell these infections. And this is by no means the only way to treat the family of Lyme, *Bartonella*, and other microbes. Remember, there are no universally accepted treatment guidelines. IDSA's recommendations differ from those of ILADS, the latter of which I am more aligned with because they acknowledge persistent (chronic) infection for which long-term and repeated antimicrobial therapy needs to be considered.

Every patient must be treated in a highly individualized way based on their history, symptoms, and clinical and laboratory workup, as well as their personal preferences regarding how treatment fits into their lifestyle. Just as no two patients with a complex set of infections are alike, no two treatment protocols are identical. Patients who appear to have the identical clinical presentation can respond differently to the same drugs. I attribute this largely to differences in the mix of infections each person harbors, but there are also important differences among the patients themselves. It turns out that even though the ways that medications affect each of us are highly variable, this is due more to our many tiny and interrelated genetic differences than to any one major determinant. Although some of us have stronger reactions to certain pharmaceuticals, partly due to differences in rates of absorption of individual drugs, it's the genetically programmed biochemical differences that account for most of the variations among people, including toxic and allergic reactions.

It would be beyond the scope of this book to detail every possible treatment plan, but I want to give you a sense of how the beginnings of a regimen can shape up and play out. It's a combination of finding the right drugs by continuously fine-tuning as you go along, following symptoms, reactions, and side effects, while scrupulously checking blood work to make sure the patient isn't having serious side effects from the drugs to the liver or other organs. It's a mix of science and art attuned to an individual's unique biology and history. All drugs the patient has taken in the past, how they worked or failed, and whether they caused side effects, must also be considered. Such risk-benefit analyses must be taken into consideration every step of the way, and the treatment plan recalculated accordingly.

The information below is chiefly for adults (I don't see kids under the age of sixteen).

Failure rates are high when treating Lyme with one-month-long courses of antibiotics. Many of these patients will go on to develop a chronic form of Lyme that will be increasingly difficult to treat, possibly causing other conditions. Take it from the Harvard-trained infectious disease specialist Dr. Charlotte Mao: "Given the science that supports persistent Lyme, you would wonder why anyone thinks two to four weeks of antibiotics would do it for everyone. It's so individualized and complicated—it can't be a cookbook approach." Which is to say: If you're not getting the help you need and you continue to suffer after initial treatment, seek other opinions and find a doctor who will listen to you.

THE POWER OF PULSING

Pulsing means going off and on antibiotics in a predetermined manner, rather than taking them continuously day after day for months on end. For example, a patient would go on an antibiotic protocol for two weeks, then pause for two weeks before repeating it. Although it may sound counterintuitive and go against what many doctors have been taught about the treatment of bacterial infections—due to the concern of antibiotic resistance emerging in rapidly dividing and mutating bacteria — there's robust data published in the journal *Nature* in 2018 that a well-designed pulsed antibiotic regimen can actually reduce the emergence of antibiotic resistance compared to continuous antibiotic therapy.[1] That's the thing in medicine: we keep learning. Studies have shown that pulsing can work for Lyme when continuous antibiotics have failed.[2]

Pulsed antibiotics are not a panacea and they don't necessarily work for every infection in Lyme+. Moreover, we have no doubt the debate will continue about whether or not it worsens or mitigates the emergence of microbial resistance. Until there's definitive consensus, for now it's enough to know that pulsed antimicrobial therapy usually trumps long-term continuous antibiotics for many patients in my experience. Not all antibiotics can be pulsed, some because of long half-life issues (how long they stay in the body) and others because of increased risks of serious allergies and abnormal reactions. But for Lyme, pulsed antimicrobial therapy can often kill those stubborn persisters more effectively. Laboratory studies in test tubes with *B. burgdorferi* demonstrate that one application of the antibiotic ceftriaxone, for instance, does not eliminate persisters — the intransigent forms of the organism that put the "chronic" in chronic Lyme — but that pulsed therapy with ceftriaxone can.[3]

Spirochetes, the class of spiral-shaped bacteria that includes the Lyme-causing *B. burgdorferi*, are less likely to develop antibiotic resistance by spontaneous DNA mutation under the pressure of antibiotics. But antibiotic-resistant strains do exist, so if they're naturally present among a bacterial population in small numbers, they can emerge in the face of evolutionary pressure during large-scale antibiotic treatment, as we've seen in syphilis. *T. pallidum*, the spirochete that causes syphilis, remains sensitive to penicillin and hasn't mutated to develop resistance to this old, basic drug despite its extensive use as the treatment of choice since at least 1947. However, antibiotics derived from a class of drugs called *macrolides* (e.g., erythromycin, azithromycin, and clarithromycin) are increasingly ineffective against the syphilis-causing bacterium. This is largely due to evolution selecting out of the minority of strains that are inherently macrolide-resistant during mass antibiotic treatment programs for syphilis.[4] New genetic mutations causing resistance contribute in only a minor way.

Resistance and persistence don't mean the same thing: *Resistance* is the ability to mutate and actively grow in the presence of antibiotics, whereas *persistence* is the ability to enter into an altered metabolic state so as to "persist" despite antibiotics, but not actively grow in the same way. It's thought that *Bartonella*, like its cousin *Brucella* and probably other members of Lyme+, can develop resistance to antibiotics, but they tend not to develop it as quickly or as readily as the evolutionarily younger, more rapidly dividing organisms like staph or strep. I haven't seen the development of resistance in *Bartonella* patients, or other Lyme+ patients, as a significant problem in my practice but I believe that it can occur.

I've also used pulse therapy successfully in *Bartonella* patients in cases where long-term continuous antibiotics have failed. For example, I have a patient who had been on nearly continuous antibiotics for over twenty years by her prior doctors, including many rounds of IV formulas, before coming to see me. She could only work part-time, couldn't travel, was always on the brink of going on disability, and when she would try to stop the antibiotics she would become violently ill. Within eight months of pulsing under my guidance she was able to reduce her antibiotics down to a single two-week pulse every few months, and her functionality improved remarkably. Today she exercises, spends more time with friends and family, travels, drives, and lives a fairly normal, happy life. Having seen almost all of the major Lyme+ treating doctors in the U.S. before coming to see me, she asked one day, gobsmacked, "Why don't they all try pulsing?!" Old dogs, new tricks, and dogma don't mix well.

WHAT TREATMENT MAY LOOK LIKE

The following does not contain medical advice. Please consult your physician before embarking on any treatment regimen.

Before talking about antibiotics, I should talk about gut flora — the microbial communities that normally live in the stomach and intestines and play important roles in our physiology, especially with regard to our metabolism. Although I have designed my regimens to focus on fewer antibiotics and more non-antibiotic antimicrobials, antibiotics are usually a necessary component — and all of them can disrupt gut flora, which can lead to side effects like diarrhea. Tetracycline-class antibiotics, including tetracycline itself, are the backbone of many of my pulse regimens due to their safety and relatively mild impact on the microbiome compared with many other antibiotics. The pulses are usually two weeks on, two weeks off, or three weeks on, three weeks off. The timing depends on the other antimicrobials prescribed in the pulse, as some are slower to work so they require three weeks. Antibiotics that have longer half-lives also demand more time off in between pulses.

A severe example of antibiotic-associated diarrhea is *Clostridium difficile* colitis, or *C. diff* for short, an inflammation of the colon due to the proliferation of a certain bacterium (*C. difficile*). Probiotics, the friendly bacteria found in lots of fermented foods and yogurt, can help prevent this from happening. I recommend that my patients take an oral probiotic supplement that contains at least 10 billion colony-forming units (CFU) with any antibiotic regimen, taken at least two hours apart from the antibiotics but with food. In the rare instance that I must prescribe an antibiotic that comes with a higher risk for developing *C. diff*, I order a prescription-strength probiotic with a CFU of over 100 billion for the patient. Since 2013 (when I resumed my practice after my disability) I've seen two cases of *C. diff* among many thousands of patients. That said, I take *C. diff* colitis extremely seriously, and so should you. This condition is more dangerous in the very young, very old, and immune-compromised. My elderly grandmother died of it while I was in med school after she'd received antibiotics for pneumonia from her doctors. If only I'd known how to prevent and treat it then like I do now.

Doxycycline is usually the go-to antibiotic of choice among most physicians for treating Lyme, so if a Lyme patient hasn't had any prior doxycycline treatment, I start with that for one month. I also order certain blood tests ("safety labs") ten days in to check the patient's blood counts, levels of inflammation, and status of organs like the liver, kidneys, and pancreas, which can be compared to baseline safety labs that were drawn prior to treatment.

After the month of doxycycline, I typically prescribe pulsing with tetracycline, two weeks on/off for two rounds (one month total of antibiotics over two months of time). Safety labs are usually checked at ten days in if the baseline pancreatic enzyme (lipase) was normal. If the baseline lipase was even minimally elevated, safety labs are checked seven days into treatment. Such monitoring can also show signs of an underlying *Bartonella* infection and the need for other medications. It's not uncommon for bartonellosis to cause a low white blood cell count, elevated markers of inflammation like C-reactive protein, and an elevated pancreatic lipase, which is evidence of inflammation of the pancreas (more on that shortly).

Two weeks after stopping treatment with the second pulse of tetracycline, my patients follow up with me. Upon the second follow-up visit, the first thing to ascertain is which drug, in this case doxy versus tetra, was more effective with fewer side effects. And sometimes that's easier said than done: Herxheimers are frequently confused with side effects. As briefly mentioned in Part 1, a Herxheimer is a flare of prior and/or new symptoms in association with beginning an antibiotic therapy for certain types of infections, such as Lyme, *Bartonella*, *Brucella*, or *Coxiella*. Symptoms of a Herxheimer vary widely and can include flu-like symptoms, headaches, eye pain, muscle and joint pains, fatigue, sleep disturbance, tingling and numbness, psychiatric symptoms, and many others. They can also include worsening of the underlying lab abnormalities. For more specifics on distinguishing between Herxheimer reactions and side effects, see our website — we have downloadable guides. But let's take a closer look at The Dreaded Herx before describing more treatment.

THE DREADED HERXHEIMER

Anyone who has been treated for Lyme should know this term (and it's often used as a verb: "herxing"). Karl Herxheimer was a German dermatologist who completed his doctorate with a thesis on cerebral syphilis. He and fellow dermatologist Adolf Jarisch from Austria are credited with the discovery of the Jarisch–Herxheimer reaction, which often gets shortened to just "Herxheimer." Both Jarisch and Herxheimer observed reactions in patients with syphilis treated with mercury early in the twentieth century. The reaction was first seen following treatment with Salvarsan (an early anti-syphilis drug), mercury, or antibiotics. Jarisch thought that the reaction was caused by a toxin released from the dying spirochetes, and although he was right, this may be an oversimplification.

Herxheimers don't just occur with syphilis. They occur with other spirochetal infections like Lyme, leptospirosis, and relapsing fever, as well as some non-spirochetal infections, including but not limited to brucellosis, bartonellosis, tularemia, and Q fever. Herxheimer-like reactions even occur with treatment of some parasitic infections. Herxheimers for some infections, such as syphilis, leptospirosis, relapsing fever, and brucellosis, can be severe and some have even been published to be fatal. And they occur at different time points depending on the drug used and the infection(s) present, ranging from mild to very severe. A Herxheimer is often described as a die-off reaction when the bacteria are being destroyed, but this is an oversimplification which is not entirely accurate. If this were the case, then how could a chronic Lyme or *Bartonella* patient have Herxheimer after Herxheimer over many treatment cycles? How many bacteria could there be in such a patient to cause so many repeated Herxheimers? How many times can they be killed and how could a Herxheimer last many months? Wouldn't they be destroyed already if that description were accurate? How many times can they be killed? Chronic Lyme and *Bartonella* patients' experience with repeat or long-lasting Herxheimers could be due to the combination of a relatively small amount of bacterial destruction and a relatively larger amount of blebbing.

Blebs are like microbial dandruff, or more aptly put, can be thought of as decoys. They're small particles that are shed from the surface of a range of microbes, including Lyme, *Bartonella*, and *Brucella*. To the immune system, they appear the same as the intact organism. The ones involved in Lyme have been the most researched. But it's likely that the mechanisms demonstrated in Lyme blebs are similar to those in *Bartonella* and *Brucella*, as they're all ancient bacteria that have evolved their defense mechanisms over the same time frame, measured in eons. In Lyme, blebs occur as part of a microbial stress response and induce immune dysfunction by causing excess and abnormal stimulation that eventually results in what we have already defined as *anergy*: failure of the immune system to properly recognize the infection. This means that blebbing can occur upon initiation of antibiotics, as part of the observed transient flare in underlying symptoms, lumped in with the Herxheimer reaction.

More blebbing, causing a transient flare of symptoms, can then occur again upon discontinuation of the antibiotics. If blebbing does occur when the antibiotics are stopped, it's not another Herxheimer, as that only occurs upon starting antimicrobials and has to include some bacterial destruction. Rather, the blebbing reaction provides clinical evidence that the infection is still present, even if symptoms subsequently settle down, which they usually do in about a week or so after blebbing begins. The diagnosis of blebbing is made on clinical grounds, taking into account what we know of the behavior of these organisms. For example, the rapidity of onset of the flared symptoms that can occur when stopping antibiotics is not consistent with the division times of these organisms (that is, they don't grow fast enough to cause such a rapid increase in symptoms). These stealthy bacteria divide very slowly, but they can bleb very quickly. For these reasons, I prefer to space the pulsed antibiotics two to three weeks apart, depending on the regimen and the half-lives of the antibiotics involved. In my experience, it's best to wait until the blebbing has settled down before starting the next pulse of antibiotics.

Herxheimers can be scary and painful. I remember the case of a twenty-year-old woman who had been dealing with undiagnosed *Bartonella* since the age of ten, when she had severe body pains but her pediatrician was unable to find a cause. Her pain was so unbearable that by age sixteen she made the conscious decision to self-medicate with illicit oral narcotics, which she did for a few years. When her parents discovered this, they sent her to a rehab facility, and during her experience there it became very clear that something was very wrong with this girl — and that her drug addiction was an effect of a larger problem, rather than the sole cause.

They brought her to see me. I diagnosed her with a *Bartonella* infection, and she began antibiotic treatment. Although her Herxheimer on doxycycline was tolerable, the Herxheimer brought about by the first low-dose tetracycline pulse was anything but. Her father paged me because she was reduced to a fetal position on the floor, rocking herself back and forth in an effort to endure the pain. I advised that he call 911 and take her to the ER. He held the phone up to her ear so I could speak to her, and through gritted teeth and tears she said she realized she was going through a Herxheimer and that she planned to continue the tetracycline to see it through. I said, "I hear you, and I think you're very brave, but it's not necessary. I think that continuing would actually be counterproductive. Please stop the tetracycline now. We can try again in a couple of weeks, and it will probably be horrible for one or two more attempts, but after that, chances are good that it will be easier."

And that's exactly what happened. The general rule is that by the fourth pulse, even severe Herxheimers tend to get much easier. If it's not settling down by then, it's a clue that a different treatment may be indicated.

PRIMARY CARE MANAGEMENT
OF VECTOR-BORNE INFECTIONS

How do patients communicate effectively with the doctors who take their insurance to evaluate them thoroughly and provide treatment if necessary? We understand that most Lyme+ specialists don't take insurance and that paying out of pocket isn't always an option. An intellectually curious and motivated primary care doctor may be willing to consider treating complex vector-borne diseases with protocols from the ILADS guidelines (on ILADS.org website), which have been published in a peer-reviewed medical journal. The recommended treatments of antibiotics and antimicrobials are often covered by insurance.

WHEN TO GET IMMEDIATE HELP

I recommend a trip to the ER if any of the following happen, whether on or off medications: fever over 100.5°F; chest pain or shortness of breath; feeling faint; significant rash; bruising; bloody or black stools (although Pepto-Bismol causes very dark stools that are not serious and beets cause red stools that can be confused with blood); significant nausea, vomiting, or abdominal pain; watery, mucousy, or bloody diarrhea; hearing or vision loss; the worst headache of your life; and any other symptoms that the patient feels are severe. It's always better to be safe than sorry. Better to waste a few hours in the ER than miss a potentially life-threatening situation.

In the next chapter I'll offer some tips for dealing with the side effects of treatment as well as severe Herxheimers. There are lots of options to get through this difficult period.

BUILDING A REGIMEN

Pulsing with tetracycline is usually done for a couple of two-week pulses to make sure it works better than doxycycline. If doxycycline works better, however, that can be used as the backbone of treatment, and then a regimen can be built from there, adding other antimicrobial agents to doxycycline or tetracycline, pulse by pulse, changing one variable at a time to figure out what's working.

Note of caution: tetracycline can cause pancreatitis, an inflammation of the pancreas that can be life-threatening. People who have taken long-term corticosteroids (i.e., prednisone), are at higher risk for this happening. Interestingly, I've observed that if someone comes in on long-term corticosteroids that are discontinued when tetracycline is begun, this is a very risky situation for pancreatitis. In such situations, it's best to start with doxycycline, and if discontinuation of the steroids is warranted, to do so only at a glacial pace, weaning off them over a period of many weeks as dictated by an endocrinologist, while frequently checking safety labs (i.e., once weekly for the for first two pulses). To further muddy the waters, Lyme, *Bartonella*, and *Brucella* can all cause pancreatitis, and I think it's likely that many cases of pancreatitis related to tetracycline have a component of Herxheimer and blebbing in the pancreas as part of the disease process.

ORAL VERSUS IV ANTIBIOTICS: WHICH IS BETTER?

I do not prescribe IV antibiotics for Lyme because the comparative studies thus far do not show — on average — that IV antibiotics perform better than oral, and they come with higher risks for complications like blood clots, allergies, and infections that originate in the IV line. In the case of IV ceftriaxone, gallstones are known to develop. However, there will be the occasional patient who will respond better to IV antibiotics.

ADDING THE SECOND DRUG AND BEYOND

If we are to assume that this sample treatment plan is for the average chronic Lyme patient, upon starting the second round of pulsing, I usually consider the addition of a second agent. Studies have shown that combinations of antimicrobials against *B. burgdorferi* persisters can be helpful, and it's well known that combinations of effective antibiotics work better than single agents against *Brucella* and *Bartonella*.[5] The options for a second drug are usually liposomal oil of oregano (Lip OOO), monolaurin (Mono), fluconazole (FCZ), or azithromycin (Zmax), but sometimes clarithromycin (Biaxin) instead of Zmax. Briefly:

- **Oil of oregano** is an herbal antimicrobial that is known to have powerful activity against *B. burgdorferi*, as well as its biofilm, which is a viscous substance formed by colonies of bacteria.[6] The biofilm helps bacteria to survive antibiotics and the assault from the immune system. Oil of oregano has activity against *Bartonella* in the test tube as well,[7] and I've seen it work many times in *Bartonella* patients. *Oliveria decumbens*, a plant from the Middle East that contains many of the same components as oregano oil, is highly active against *Brucella*, *Bartonella*'s close cousin.[8]
- **Monolaurin** is a naturally occurring substance in breast milk with broad-range antimicrobial activity against a spectrum of bacteria, including Lyme bacteria, as well as viruses and even parasites.[9] Although no studies of its activity against *Bartonella* have yet been published, I've seen it work in *Bartonella* patients many times. Not an antibiotic per se, its broad range of activity is due to its detergent action, and its effectiveness at dissolving Lyme and other microbial biofilms has been published.[10] In my office, we use

a preparation that comes in granules; the maximum dose is 3,000 mg three times daily.

- **Fluconazole** is an antifungal that has been shown to be effective in treating patients with central nervous system Lyme who have failed IV antibiotics.[11] Researchers at Johns Hopkins have shown that it, along with numerous other antifungals, is active against both *B. burgdorferi* and *Bartonella* in the lab.[12] For this drug, I check safety labs at four days in, as it can cause rapid and potentially dangerous liver injury in a small minority of patients.
- **Biaxin and Zithromax** are related antibiotics derived from a class of antibiotics called macrolides. Some patients will respond better to one over the other, but Biaxin has far more drug interactions than Zithromax and both have risks for potentially serious heart arrhythmias. Biaxin also causes a metallic taste in the mouth that patients don't love. For this reason, it's not used as commonly as Zithromax.

In subsequent pulses going forward, some of these drugs can be combined and some cannot. For example, fluconazole cannot be combined with Zithromax or Biaxin due to potentially serious cardiac effects. Even on their own, fluconazole, Zithromax, or Biaxin can cause potentially life-threatening heart arrhythmias in patients with an abnormal EKG finding called a prolonged QT interval. I always make sure that patients have a normal EKG before starting any of these medications.

It's also important to take precautions when using any of these with other drugs in combination. Some common drug interactions can happen with medications like Xanax, Valium, statins, antidepressants, antipsychotics, and some cardiac drugs, but there are many more. Again, this is where an individual's risk factors and overall drug regimen must be carefully considered and discussed between doctor and patient, which is yet another reason to work with a doctor who is well versed in all the nuances to treatment and the adjustments that must be made on an ongoing basis.

MEPRON (ATOVAQUONE)

Mepron (generic name atovaquone) is an anti-parasitic drug that was FDA-approved in 1992 for the treatment of pneumocystis pneumonia, which was a common and life-threatening infection among AIDS patients before the advent of the more effective modern-day HIV medications. At first Mepron wasn't very popular due to its high cost, but then it was shown to be effective in treating babesiosis when used in combination with azithromycin, so today it is part of the go-to standard treatment for babesiosis.

Interestingly, in addition to babesiosis patients, I have also witnessed innumerable Lyme and *Bartonella* patients get better with Mepron. What's more, they frequently improve after experiencing major Herxheimers from the drug, which could mean that the drug is probably directly killing the bacteria. Although not yet published, Mepron has been demonstrated to kill *B. burgdorferi* in the test tube by researchers at Johns Hopkins.[13]

Patients have a variety of reactions to Mepron, but it's rarely boring. When Herxheimers occur, they often strike in the first three weeks. Some people develop a skin rash that looks like the measles and requires at least temporary discontinuation of the drug. Anyone who develops a rash should see an allergist familiar with Lyme+ and consult their ILADS doctor to help distinguish cutaneous Herxheimer from true allergy. Mepron can have neuropsychiatric effects as well, including anxiety and depression, which can be worse in those already vulnerable to these conditions. It can be difficult to distinguish neuropsychiatric Herxheimers from side effects, so I have a psychiatrist familiar with Lyme+ on board when needed. Caution: Mepron can cause serious liver damage and requires safety labs 10 and 20 days into a three-week treatment. I seldom use Mepron as part of a long-term continuous treatment, but when I do, I check safety labs monthly once it's been documented that blood tests were normal on day 20.

Some Lyme+ patients may also benefit from over-the-counter

herbal protocols and often combine them with antibiotics, but it's best to work closely with a doctor when doing so. Some of the more popular regimens are Zhang, Buhner, Byron White, and Cowden. Herbs can have powerful antimicrobial effects and can be considered "real medicine," with real Herxheimers and real side effects of their own. A doctor's supervision is therefore required, with routine blood monitoring.

If you remember nothing else from this book about how to treat these illnesses, remember that every treatment has to be given its fair shake and its expiration date, meaning that each treatment deserves to be given its minimum time to have an effect, to give it a chance at working, but not more than that, after which it's just a waste of precious time.

Even when there's laboratory and clinical evidence of Lyme+ infections, that knowledge alone doesn't provide a precise roadmap to treatment. For example, I have seen many *Bartonella* patients who did not respond to stereotypical treatments. I remember speaking to a new patient who was despondent. He had been told by his prior doctor that the single best treatment for *Bartonella* was doxycycline plus rifampin. She also told him to stay on those drugs for another few months, even though he'd already been taking them diligently for many months and was feeling worse than before he started. I advised him to stop taking the drugs for two weeks, after which I'd reassess him and consider a different course of treatment. This approach makes sense when you look at it through the lens of "the fair shake and the expiration date." But his previous doctor had rejected this approach because his illness was viewed dogmatically, which just made the patient feel hopeless. There isn't just a lack of flexibility among doctors who ignore vector-borne diseases, there can also be a rigidity among doctors who treat them too. Dogma is the enemy. Reason is key. Simple to say. Hard to follow.

So, generally speaking, when patients don't start improving following four to six weeks of antibiotic treatment (some medications like Bicillin shots take three to four months), it's time to consider changing the protocol. It's also time to think about other infections that have not been identified yet and which may call for a different plan of action. Two steps forward, one step back—it's to be expected. Don't deprive yourself of the hope that you deserve. Many people have recurrent symptoms between the first several pulses, which is typical. With continued pulses, most patients can go off antibiotics and remain stable without them.

How long do I treat? There's no single rule, but for those who have developed complex chronic illnesses, the average is about nine months of antibiotics, spaced over about one and a half years, because often much of it is pulsed therapy. And when does the protocol end? When patients feel better and symptoms come under management, the protocols can wind down, but stopping cold turkey is rarely a good idea. It's often best to gradually increase the time between pulses. I frequently have patients who are off antibiotics for four or more months in between pulses before they go off entirely.

A significant minority of people chronically relapse and require repeated treatment. Some people relapse within weeks to months to even years later, so if symptoms ever feel like they're coming back once treatment has ended, re-evaluation by your doctor is a good idea. Time is of the essence. Sometimes, patients will elect to give it some period of time before re-treating (say, one to two weeks), to see if it spontaneously resolves, but it's unwise to sit on the sidelines for too long. If it worsens for more than two weeks, it's best to seek care immediately.

A NOTE ABOUT
IMMUNOSUPPRESSIVE DRUGS

Immunosuppressant medications are often given to patients labeled with an autoimmune disorder. These are a class of drugs that suppress, or reduce, the strength of the body's immune system. As mentioned earlier, with an autoimmune disease, the immune system is purported to attack the body's own tissue, but why? It turns out that the body's own tissues are damaged like innocent bystanders in the war raged against the infections included in Lyme+. *Bartonella* tends to be a common bad apple among the bunch of infections that can cause autoimmune illness. Because immunosuppressant drugs weaken the immune system, they can suppress some components of this damage. Keep in mind that the majority of symptoms of Lyme+ are caused by the immune system going after the organisms. If you induce immune suppression, you can reduce symptoms in most patients, but at the huge cost of allowing the bugs to go deeper into tissues and become more evasive, entrenched, and ultimately hidden from the immune system. So it's no surprise that steroids given before, and even with, antibiotics increase the risk of a worsened prognosis in Lyme. Plus, the side effects of immunosuppression on its own can be very serious, including opportunistic infections and cancers, with well-documented fatalities. Further, immunosuppression can paradoxically cause additional chronic illness, such as inflammatory bowel disease and heart failure, which I believe may be due to worsening undiagnosed Lyme+ in patients labeled with autoimmune disease.

If you've been diagnosed with an autoimmune disorder and are taking immunosuppressants, you're not alone. These include a wide array of drugs, examples of which include prednisone (Orasone), adalimumab (Humira), etanercept (Enbrel), rituximab (Rituxan), and many others. It's a big business, an unending annuity for Big Pharma. Rather than providing a cure, these costly and dangerous treatments suppress symptoms over the life of the patient, only to allow them to quickly recur when the drugs are discontinued. It's striking to us that chronic autoimmune diseases are considered to be of unknown origin, yet so many have been linked in medical literature to infections, specifically Lyme and *Bartonella*, as we've seen. When people receive a diagnosis of fibromyalgia, MS, lupus, rheumatoid arthritis, Sjogren's, psoriatic arthritis, or another rheumatologic/inflammatory diagnosis, they are not getting an actual diagnosis, but rather a description of signs and symptoms that brings them no closer to an answer. Many doctors are not properly (and sometimes not at all!) evaluating these patients for the possibility of infections of the Lyme+ group, and it's disgraceful. To receive a negative Lyme ELISA as the sole test, instead of what should be an extensive workup for a complex set of vector-borne infections, and then sentence a patient to a lifetime of immunosuppressive drugs, is simply wrong.

Early on in my practice, a patient came in to see me with a common set of symptoms: fatigue, muscle pain, sleep disturbance, and cognitive problems. He had been diagnosed with fibromyalgia by his primary care doctor, despite his prior diagnosis of Lyme from that same doctor, who treated the Lyme with doxycycline. But when his Lyme symptoms returned after a few weeks of doxycycline, his primary care doctor defaulted to a diagnosis of fibromyalgia, which just happened to have the same symptoms as his recent Lyme. The doctor refused to prescribe further antibiotics. I re-treated him with a few months of antibiotics and he began feeling better and was able to discontinue treatment.

A couple of years later, this same patient was on the steroid prednisone to treat poison ivy. Within a few weeks of stopping the prednisone, his Lyme symptoms returned. He came back to see me to be re-treated, but this time, he didn't experience relief after a few months of antibiotics. Now it took over a year of treatment to get his symptoms under control. It's been more than fifteen years since I last saw the patient, but I've heard from him and he is still doing well.

HOW TO TREAT BARTONELLA

To refresh your memory, *Bartonella* is an infection caused by bacteria in the Lyme+ family that has multiple species and can be transmitted through ticks, fleas, lice, sand flies, spiders, and even ants. It belongs to the *Bartonella* genus and often travels with the *Borrelia* bacteria that causes classic Lyme. When doctors use the term "cat scratch disease," they are referring to just one of the many types of disease manifestations caused by *Bartonella* infection. It's noteworthy that cat scratch disease has been stereotypically associated with a mild course, but not only is this stereotype frequently wrong, it's caused some doctors to view other typically far more severe disease manifestations of *Bartonella* infection through the same "cat-scratch disease lens." Because of this mild stereotype, most cases of severe *Bartonella* infection get diagnosed as anything but *Bartonella*.

There is no standard best treatment for *Bartonella*. Many doctors still wrongly assume that it will resolve on its own and won't prescribe antibiotics at all. These doctors are not keeping abreast of the latest science demonstrating that *Bartonella* can cause a severe and debilitating range of illnesses, spanning from neurologic to psychiatric to rheumatologic to blood disease. The drugs that have been documented to be clinically beneficial in bartonellosis, the infection caused by *Bartonella*, include rifampin, Bactrim, quinolones, and aminoglycosides, all of which can have serious side effects. A portion of them are usually given in combination with doxycycline and sometimes Zithromax. (The many other drugs and herbals that I've seen to be beneficial are only now beginning to be officially studied.)

Dr. Ed Breitschwerdt is one of the world's leading experts on *Bartonella*, after having lost his father to this infection. Dr. Breitschwerdt is a veterinarian at North Carolina State University, where he is a professor of medicine and infectious diseases at the veterinary college and conducts cutting-edge research on vector-borne diseases in search of better diagnostics and treatments. "Vets are the best canaries in the coal mine," he likes to say, but dogs are apparently the best proxy for humans with *Bartonella*. "Eighteen different strains of *Bartonella* have caused disease in both dogs and humans. The tests for *Bartonella* are totally inadequate." He believes that *Bartonella* will be the next *Helicobacter pylori*—the stomach-infecting, stomach ulcer- and cancer-causing bacterium that changed the paradigm of how ulcers are treated and stomach cancers prevented—and that there will likewise be a paradigm shift in terms of how we diagnose and treat the many autoimmune conditions caused by *Bartonella*. He also states that *"Bartonella* can enter lots of cells and travel through tissues," which accounts for its wide range of symptoms, including neuropsychiatric, similar to the wide breadth of Lyme symptoms. He receives emails daily from dog owners reporting odd, suddenly aggressive behavior in their pets, for which *Bartonella* is ultimately found to be the cause. These scary psychiatric symptoms are also common in humans.

To get a sense of how this nasty infection can manifest in a human, consider the following case report published in the *Journal of Central Nervous System Disease*, authored by Dr. Breitschwerdt and his colleagues.[14] A fourteen-year-old boy from Ohio had been a gifted student, and an athlete on the fencing team. He was also the lead in his school play. That was, until his behavior suddenly changed. He declined rapidly, to the point where he was diagnosed with bipolar disorder and schizophrenia. His mother quit her job to help focus on her son, but his condition continued to worsen. Hallucinations set in and the boy went to Texas for institutionalization. The doctors there performed an extensive workup and diagnosed him with autoimmune encephalitis, cause unknown. Psychiatric medications for depression and schizophrenia didn't help but he continued to take them because nothing else was offered.

He then saw an integrative medicine doctor whose nurse noticed stretch marks, known as striae, on the boy's back. These can be the most obvious sign of a *Bartonella* infection. (In my experience, although they're common in younger *Bartonella* patients, they rarely happen in those more than twenty-five to thirty years old.) After a month of doxycycline prescribed by that doctor, which made a difference, his father contacted Dr. Breitschwerdt because of his renowned expertise. After multiple antimicrobials over the ensuing course of eighteen months, which included doxycycline, minocycline, clarithromycin, azithromycin, hydroxychloroquine, rifampin, and rifabutin, the boy was back to normal and able to discontinue all of his psychiatric drugs over six months.

And his schizophrenia? Gone.

CHAPTER 8

Mending Your Mind

Health is a crown that the healthy wear,
but only the sick can see it.

—*Egyptian proverb*

DEALING WITH MAJOR illness is traumatic under the best of circumstances. Worse is when it's discredited by doctors and loved ones. For people with Lyme+, trauma can be associated with any number of experiences along the complex journey from broken to better. You can encounter everything from stigma, mistreatment, and marginalization, to the often tortuously long road to proper diagnosis, to enduring treatments that usually make you feel worse before you feel better.

Managing a chronic and complex infectious disease can leave you perpetually fearful, waiting for the next shoe to drop. You may feel desperate and isolated, afraid to wake up to the horror of the next new symptom. How do you put faith in a new way of handling chronic illness—finding and treating the underlying cause rather than suppressing symptoms—when doctors herd you strongly down the rutted, dead-end roads they travel? Will you get better or will your disease worsen? If you get well, will you remain so? Living with Lyme+

can make you lose confidence in your body, too. You may look in the mirror asking, "Who am I? What happened to my life?" I (Dr. Phillips) recall one patient describing it as "It's like the disease was taking my body for a ride and I couldn't stop it and I couldn't get off."

We understand the mental merry-go-round you're on because we've been there, and we know the scars that can accrue by following that circular path. Our goal is to shine light on these dark mental wounds, healing the psyche as well as the body, and in so doing, helping to set you free.

Dr. Bessel van der Kolk, a trauma specialist and author of the best-selling book *The Body Keeps the Score*, believes that minds can't be healed if they're in bodies that have let them down unless they address the connection between the two. According to him, the single most important issue for traumatized people is finding a sense of safety in their own bodies. "Unfortunately, most psychiatrists pay no attention whatsoever to sensate experiences," he says. "They simply do not agree that it matters . . . Mindfulness, learning to become a careful observer of the ebb and flow of internal experience, and noticing whatever thoughts, feelings, body sensations and impulses emerge are important components in healing PTSD [Post-Traumatic Stress Disorder]."

We must become aware of our inner experience and "befriend" what's going on inside of us if we are to change how we feel. Dr. Van der Kolk spent his career studying how children and adults adapt to traumatic experiences and enlisted findings from neuroscience to develop effective treatments — ultimately helping people to feel safe again.

Everyone experiences and manifests trauma differently. We realize that there are many disparate forms of trauma, and that they don't always take stereotypical forms, such as war or child abuse. In this chapter, we're going to speak specifically to the healing of trauma that's arisen from dealing with chronic infections. We'll also speak to some general supportive measures. For example, it's important to know that attention to self-care and finding ways to keep stress at bay can help prevent the next symptoms from emerging. What works for us might not work for you, but the good news is there are lots of options today —

from simple relaxation techniques to dietary recommendations and exercises that stimulate our innate abilities to heal.

The sense of loss, doom, and shame often experienced by Lyme+ patients can cause severe Post-Traumatic Stress Disorder (PTSD), which is often exacerbated by the unacceptable care they've received from their prior physicians. Again, it's common for doctors to outright dismiss and demean symptoms that they don't understand, insinuate that patients are hypochondriacs, and send them to psychiatrists instead of getting them evaluated for common neurologic infections. One of my (Dr. Phillips') patients described her prior neurologist screaming and banging her fists down on her desk when my patient innocently reported that her illness recurred after antibiotics were stopped. "There's no such thing as chronic Lyme!" the neurologist screamed. My patient was so taken aback — it was as if she had been punched in the face. She held it together until she got into her car in the parking lot, and then broke down crying.

Recovering from any trauma you may have experienced is important to healing. In this chapter we'll cover the top three methods for treating trauma with licensed professionals, then we'll offer some basic strategies.

TREATING TRAUMA WITH PROFESSIONAL HELP

The area of trauma medicine dates back decades. One of the best-established techniques, well documented to help healing from trauma, is eye movement desensitization and reprocessing, known as EMDR. The therapy has been recognized as effective by numerous organizations, including the American Psychiatric Association, the World Health Organization, the Department of Defense, and the Department of Veterans Affairs. It was a life-changing tool for me (Parish), markedly reducing my anxiety and other symptoms, like nausea and even certain food sensitivities. In fact, more than thirty randomized controlled studies have evaluated EMDR therapy in the treatment of trauma, and an additional twenty-five studies have demonstrated its positive effects.[1] Some of the studies show that 84 to 90 percent of single-trauma victims no longer have PTSD after only three ninety-minute sessions. Another study found that 100 percent of the single-trauma victims and 77 percent of multiple-trauma victims were no longer diagnosed with PTSD after only six fifty-minute sessions.[2] Studies looking into its effects on combat veterans have been particularly illuminating, showing that it can eradicate PTSD in 77 percent of patients in as few as twelve sessions.[3] Given its positive effects on military personnel returning from combat — who experience some of the most extreme forms of trauma — one can easily see how it can treat other forms of trauma that similarly lead to deeply psychological and physical challenges.

The technique was developed in 1990 by Francine Shapiro, Ph.D., who is a Senior Research Fellow Emerita at the Mental Research Institute in Palo Alto, California, and Executive Director of the EMDR Institute in Watsonville, California. The goal of EMDR is to reformulate negative memories and reduce the physiological arousal in the nervous system that can trigger physical symptoms — in other words, to bring the charge down. Sessions are conducted by a certified clinician. During EMDR, the individual relives emotionally disturbing memories while focusing on an external stimulus, such as an object moving back and forth.

At the heart of this therapy is an eight-phase treatment. Eye movements (or other bilateral stimulation, as patients with vertigo frequently cannot tolerate the eye movements) are used during one part of the session. After the practitioner has determined which memory to target first, she asks the patient to hold different aspects of that event or thought in mind and to use her eyes to track either the therapist's hand or a visual "EyeScan" board as it moves back and forth across the patient's field of vision. The patient also can choose to keep their eyes closed, to follow audio with headphones that beep ear to ear, or to hold small sensors in both hands that vibrate alternately. As this happens, internal associations arise and the patient begins to process the memory and disturbing feelings.

I (Parish) saw immediate benefits with EMDR. My most oppressive symptoms at the time were constant nausea accompanied by strange food reactions, and crippling anxiety. After the first session, I felt half of my nausea fall away, after eight months of relentless queasiness that was not relieved by any medication. By session three, my panic attacks had stopped and my anxiety level, rated on a scale of 1 to 10, had gone from an 8 to a 3. Within ten sessions, my symptoms of nausea, anxiety, and food sensitivities were at a 0 or a 1. EMDR felt like a miracle, but there's hard data to support its beneficial effects.

In successful EMDR therapy, the meaning of painful events is transformed on an emotional level. For example, a Lyme+ patient shifts from feeling powerless and victimized by the system to holding the firm belief that "I am strong and healthy." Unlike traditional talk therapy, the insights people gain in EMDR result more from their own intellectual and emotional processing — not so much from the therapist's interpretation. The net effect is that people end up feeling empowered by the very experiences that once devastated them. While there is debate about how exactly this method works and what the underlying mechanism is, some of the explanations stem from accessing the biological mechanisms involved in rapid eye movement (REM) sleep. Dr. Shapiro hypothesizes that EMDR therapy helps access the neural network associated with the traumatic memory, so that information processing is enhanced, with new associations forged between the traumatic memory and more adaptive memories or information. For more information about EMDR, go to www.EDMR.com (there are lots of YouTube videos on it, although we recommend doing this with therapist supervision), or visit emdria.org to find a practitioner near you. We are firm believers in this method because it's helped so many heal from the stresses of combatting Lyme+ when other methods have failed.

SOMATIC EXPERIENCING

Dr. Peter A. Levine developed an approach called Somatic Experiencing (SE) more than forty years ago. He is the founder of the Somatic

Experiencing Trauma Institute in Boulder, Colorado. He received his PhD in medical biophysics from the University of California in Berkeley. His bestselling book, *Waking the Tiger: Healing Trauma*, has been published in twenty-four languages since its initial publication in 1997. SE is a form of alternative therapy aimed at relieving the symptoms of trauma-related health problems by focusing on the person's perceived body sensations. (He and Dr. Van der Kolk have collaborated a lot through the years and headline workshops and speaking engagements together.)

The word "somatic" is derived from the word "soma," which is of ancient Greek origin and means "body." Somatic therapy studies the relationship between the mind and the body in regard to one's psychological past. The theory behind somatic therapy is that trauma symptoms are the effects of instability of the autonomic nervous system (ANS). Your ANS is a control system that acts unconsciously to regulate bodily functions such as heart rate, digestion, respiratory rate, urination, and sexual arousal. It is also the main mechanism in control of your famous fight-or-flight response. It's one of the body's oldest, most primitive "technologies." We are hard-wired to respond swiftly and powerfully to any signs of threat, be it a predator nearby or the fear that accompanies a serious medical diagnosis. The fight-or-flight system evolved about 300 million years ago. When it's overreacting or not in balance with the body's other systems (and not communicating properly to your higher-order executive functions of the brain that are logical and calming), trouble can develop, in the form of physical symptoms like pain, digestive issues, hormonal imbalances, immune system dysfunction, and medical issues including depression, anxiety, and even addiction.

According to Dr. Levine, "Trauma is when we are overwhelmed, terrified, and unable to respond effectively to a given situation. What one person experiences as trauma may not happen to another. So it has to do with *perceptions*. These are deeply unconscious. If we are tuned to perceive something as a severe threat, then we will potentially become traumatized. Everybody has a breaking point. If there were a drug to cure trauma, it'd be a bestseller. Because threat has been with us for millions of years, the nervous system is not easily fooled," he told us.

Somatic Experiencing is not something we can teach you through this book; it's best done with a certified practitioner. A therapy session typically involves the patient tracking his or her experience of sensations throughout the body. There are many forms that this can take. It may include awareness of bodily sensations, dance, breathing techniques, voice work, physical exercise, movement, and healing touch. The goal is to reframe the trauma so it has less of an impact on the body. You're not actually exposing the person to more trauma — you're restoring the responses that were overwhelmed, which is what led to the trauma in the first place. Like EMDR, it builds resilience and hope — and confidence in the body.

Dr. Levine initially developed his ideas about trauma locked in the body when he was studying stress on the animal nervous system in the 1970s. He noted that animals in the wild are constantly under threat of death, yet show no symptoms of trauma. He then realized that trauma has to do with the "third survival response to perceived life threat, which is 'freeze'. When fight and flight are not options, animals can freeze and immobilize, like 'playing dead.'" This makes the animal less of a target, but the reaction should not be ongoing. It's time-limited — it should run its course, after which the animal unfreezes and discharges the pent-up energy for fighting or fleeing by shaking and trembling. "If the immobility phase doesn't complete, then that charge stays trapped, and, from the body's perspective, it is still under threat. Somatic Experiencing works to release this stored energy and turn off this threat alarm that causes severe dysregulation and dissociation."

Many studies have shown that Somatic Experiencing is effective, including a 2017 randomized controlled study of the effectiveness of the therapy for PTSD.[4] The sample in this study consisted of men and women who experienced a variety of traumas an average of four years before entering treatment; most trauma was civilian in nature, such as car accidents, assault, medical trauma, or the death of a family member. A small percentage of people had experienced combat in war (the study was conducted in Israel during a time when several highly stress-ful national events also occurred, including terrorist attacks that everyone was exposed to, either directly or indirectly). The people were split into two groups, one that received fifteen weekly one-hour sessions of SE immediately and another that were treated later, thereby allowing the researchers to compare the two groups after the first fifteen weeks. After those first fifteen weeks, the untreated group underwent treatment for the same amount of time (fifteen weekly one-hour sessions), after which a final evaluation was conducted. These evaluations involved questionnaires and interviews by trained clinical examiners. The therapists used in the study were all SE practitioners with extensive previous experience treating PTSD. The results at the end of the study—from both the earlier-treated and the later-treated groups—showed that the level of post-traumatic symptoms had declined, and the diagnosis of PTSD was actually reversed for a little more than 44 percent of participants.

In 2018, a study of SE therapists themselves revealed how significant the technique can be in their own lives. They experience "a significant improvement in self-reported measures associated with resiliency including: quality of life (well-being) and psychological symptoms (anxiety and somatization)."[5] SE therapists can be found throughout the world. You can go to www.somaticexperiencing.com or www.healingtrauma.org to learn more.

DYNAMIC NEURAL RETRAINING SYSTEM (DNRS)

The Dynamic Neural Retraining System is another method based on retraining the brain's stress response system to help people recover from many chronic illnesses, Lyme+ among them. It's based on the concept of neuroplasticity—the brain's ability to rewire itself and thereby change its function and structure. The goal is to reshape the part of the brain that's largely responsible for our emotions (e.g., fear reactions), the memories we make in response to experiences, and our anxiety "switch." This ancient part of our brains is called the limbic system, and it's often referred to as the seat of our social and emotional intelligence. This system is closely tied to the immune, hormonal, and autonomic systems, the latter of which controls things like blood pressure, digestion, and breathing (the actions we don't have to think about). When the limbic system is disrupted or impaired (by, say, the trauma of Lyme+), it can become hypersensitive and react to stimuli that it wouldn't otherwise interpret as dangerous. The limbic system essentially misfires, producing effects on the body's immune, hormonal, and nervous systems, which leads to more chronic illness.

Annie Hopper developed DNRS in 2008 after her own experience of suffering from a mysterious illness. The science of neuroplasticity was well documented by then, and she used it to create a healing program whose goal is to reorganize the brain's neural connections for healthy functioning rather than being stuck in a trauma cycle. It involves visual, spatial, movement, language, and emotional restructuring exercises that are led by certified instructors trained in this type of therapy. Three formats are available: five-day interactive training seminar "boot camps" at various locations throughout the year in the U.S. and Canada; a fourteen-hour instructional video series; and a fourteen-hour online course. It may seem unusual at first, but we've heard lots of success stories from people who've benefited from this technique. Many doctors endorse this program and we invite you to check out more about it at www.retrainingthebrain.com. It's not meant to be completed once for a quick fix. It teaches a practice that requires a daily commitment. The program is highly experiential in nature and incorporates components from other types of therapy, from mindfulness-based cognitive restructuring to cognitive behavior therapy — which is where we go next.

COGNITIVE BEHAVIORAL THERAPY

Cognitive behavioral therapy (CBT) is recommended for a range of problems, including depression, anxiety disorders, and PTSD. Dr.

Aaron T. Beck pioneered the approach in the 1960s while he was a psychiatrist at the University of Pennsylvania. CBT has the goal of changing beliefs and thought patterns that result in uncomfortable reactions in the body. Some studies show that it can be at least as effective as other forms of psychological therapy or psychiatric medications for conditions like depression and anxiety. But we should add that there's controversy today over CBT's effectiveness for trauma in particular. Dr. van der Kolk discourages this method based on his opinion that trauma has nothing to do with cognition. And he may be right, but we still think it's important to include it, since it may help certain individuals. There are different levels of severity when it comes to trauma, and for mild trauma, CBT could be helpful to some people, or used in combination with other forms of therapy.

Cognitive behavioral therapy, which is endorsed by the American Psychological Association, focuses on how certain thought patterns are related to emotions and behaviors. It aims to change those patterns that can trigger challenges in how a person functions and feels. If you have a thought process, for example, that makes you feel bad about yourself and engage in unhealthy behavior, such as binge eating, CBT tries to stop the mental chatter that causes those thoughts and triggers the resulting behavior. CBT is less about leveraging physical movements, as in SE and EDMR, and more about reframing thoughts through simple mental exercises that challenge one's beliefs. By altering a person's self-sabotaging thinking, what are sometimes called cognitive distortions ("I'll never survive this; I am ruined; I must be a bad person to have to suffer through this; I am so ashamed by this diagnosis and my condition"), the door is more open to healthier behaviors in general and improved emotion regulation. You can begin to think differently, to re-evaluate your thinking patterns and assumptions, so you can reframe your understanding of traumatic experiences, as well as your understanding of yourself and your ability to cope.

Therapists trained in CBT use a variety of techniques to help patients in reducing symptoms and improving functioning. A therapist will provide mental exercises to practice so that thought patterns can be reframed and given a different context. It can take time to become proficient in using CBT on oneself, which is why ongoing therapy is often needed. But some people can pick up the habit of reframing thoughts with practice. CBT is not for everyone—in some individuals, the trauma of illness is not helped by CBT. Part of the protocol also entails managing stress and planning for potential crises in the future. In other words, with a foundation of CBT education, it may be possible to more easily navigate those moments of vulnerability to flare-ups and recurrences of symptoms, and possibly resolve them sooner. The American Psychological Association maintains an abundance of information and resources for patients on CBT; we recommend that you go to their website (www.apa.org). Still, in our experience, and from talking to others who are managing the trauma of their Lyme+ illness, EMDR, SE, and DNRS can be far superior tools to CBT.

SUPPLEMENTAL AND ALTERNATIVE TREATMENTS

We are often asked about the need to "detox," which is not a traditional medical term unless you're referring to medical detox from substance abuse. But the word "detox" has gained an alternative connotation in the lay public and often refers, generally, to cleansing the body of toxicants that can be harmful—which are thought by some to contribute to things like weight gain, fatigue, and pain. Everyone has a different idea of what "detox" means. But the basic tenet is that we're all trying to feel better and ease the suffering produced by these infections and the side effects of treatment. In addition to the prescription protocol, there are many other complementary therapies to consider. Some patients report that herbals like parsley, pinella, and burbur extract help them, as do liposomal glutathione or lemon water. Others swear by Epsom salt baths, infrared saunas, and CBD oil.

Here is a list of popular supplemental strategies to consider. It's best to work with a doctor in finding the ideal way to incorporate these into a traditional drug regimen. It's prudent to give the body time to adjust to a prescription protocol before adding anything else to the mix.

Some ideas, however, like eating an anti-inflammatory, grain-free diet (such as paleo), or a vegan diet, could be commenced today.

While we're all for exploring, please understand that some of the following methods could make us feel worse and most are not proven to be effective from a scientific standpoint. For some the risks are not well studied or not studied at all. Most should be considered an unknown entity, viewed as an alternative medical treatment, and all should be discussed with one's doctor before starting. Blood tests should be considered to ensure that they are not producing any obvious toxic side effects. Everyone responds to these strategies differently, as no two bodies are exactly alike.

Herbals that have been shown to be effective in the test tube against *B. burgdorferi* include grapefruit seed extract, banderol, samento, and artemisinin, along with the following essential oils: oil of oregano, cinnamon bark oil, clove bud oil, citronella oil, and wintergreen oil.[6] Again, discuss these options with your practitioner before taking them. There is no one-size-fits-all and these need to be considered within the context of other medications being taken.

A 2017 study conducted by researchers from major universities, including Harvard and Johns Hopkins, demonstrated that the essential oils listed above killed Lyme bacteria more effectively than pharmaceutical antibiotics.[7] In particular, oils from oregano, garlic cloves, myrrh trees, thyme leaves, cinnamon bark, allspice berries, and cumin seeds were shown to have strong killing activity against "persister" forms of the Lyme bacterium. Bear in mind that since some of these may be stronger than antibiotics, it would not be advisable to add any in to your MD-prescribed protocol on your own. Don't be fooled into thinking something isn't potent because it can be bought over the counter. Please, always ask your doctor first.

For *Bartonella*, the effects of some herbals are largely anecdotal. Houttuynia is thought by many to work, and artemisinin may be quite likely effective due to its mechanism of action involving iron and *Bartonella*'s affinity for iron and heme, the iron-containing molecule of red blood cells. Both of us have used these at different times during treatment and found liposomal artemisinin to be highly effective. Dana's stubborn foot numbness resolved with houttuynia. Again, please discuss safety issues with your treating physician before trying any of these formulations. An Iranian herb, *Oliveria decumbens*, components of which are contained in oil of oregano, have also been shown to be effective against *Brucella* in laboratory studies.[8] Since *Brucella* is so closely related to *Bartonella*, it's always been our assumption that oil of oregano would be effective against *Bartonella* as well, and now, at the time of this writing, this has just been demonstrated by researchers at Johns Hopkins, along with cinnamon bark oil and mountain savory oil.[9] Also, in general, it's unknown whether activity observed in a lab setting for any of the herbals adequately translates to activity in the body.

I (Dr. Phillips) have seen many cases where liposomal oil of oregano made a huge difference in my patients. I've seen similar responses to liposomal artemisinin, although it can have greater toxicity (i.e., the rare instance of possible neurotoxicity and the infrequent case of liver damage, both of which could have been serious if we didn't have scrupulous monitoring). Remember, just because it's herbal, don't assume that it's safer.

That all said, we think the following strategies can be considered by most people suffering from Lyme+ if they obtain prior approval from their physician:

A better diet. The best choice is a whole-foods, low-glycemic vegan diet, though it can be hard to part with a good steak. For the carnivorous among us, an anti-inflammatory Mediterranean-style diet is better than our traditional Western diet that's high in processed foods made with refined sugars and flours. The Mediterranean style, on the other hand, emphasizes fresh fruits and vegetables high in antioxidants (e.g., dark leafy greens, berries, avocados); lean proteins (mostly wild), oily fish (e.g., salmon, herring, sardines) and less meat; nuts and seeds; fiber-rich whole grains (e.g., brown rice); legumes; and healthy fats like extra virgin olive oil, eggs, and flaxseed. This diet minimizes foods that can promote inflammation: processed products high in refined grains, sugars, and vegetable oils. Sugary drinks, desserts, margarine, and processed snack foods are avoided. Recently published data shows that a whole-foods, low-glycemic vegan diet is even less inflammatory than the American Heart Association's recommended diet, which is similar to the Mediterranean diet.[10] In view of this data, it's a generally good idea to reduce our intake of animal products when possible, as there's evidence that we consume way too much meat. We also think it's important to eat warm foods, as this induces relaxation.[11] There are lots of online resources for help in following an anti-inflammatory diet, such as www.chewfo.com, www.drweil.com, www.vegan.com, and www.drperlmutter.com/the-best-diet/.

Activities that induce the relaxation response. According to Dr. Herbert Benson, of the Benson-Henry Institute for Mind-Body Medicine at Boston's Massachusetts General Hospital, the relaxation response is "a physical state of deep rest that changes the physical and emotional responses to stress." The response can be achieved through various forms of meditation, yoga, tai chi, breathing exercises, and progressive muscle relaxation. Deep breathing and meditation in particular seem to trigger the relaxation response in ways that prevent the body from translating psychological worry into physical inflammation. The experience of the relaxation response also appears to change cellular connections in areas of the brain associated with the stress response.

We should mention the lymphatic system here, too, which circulates lymph, a clear fluid filled with immune cells, throughout the body through a system of vessels. Pivotal to your immune system, it delivers nutrients and collects cellular waste while helping to destroy pathogens. Unlike your circulatory system, which has a heart to pump blood, the lymphatic system has no built-in pump, so it relies on your breathing, and the muscle contractions as you move, to get around the body. It has long been known that exercise stimulates this movement of lymphatic fluid, and when scientists finally managed to photograph lymphatic flow, we learned that breathing plays an important role in its motion as well. Deep breathing in particular causes lymph to rush through the lymphatic vessels.

Restful, routine sleep and adequate exercise throughout the week. The benefits of restorative sleep and exercise are numerous (and explaining them could take up a whole book). The quality and quantity of sleep you get has an astonishing impact on every system in your body. Sleep is not a state of inactivity or a zone in which your body momentarily presses the pause button. A lot goes on during sleep at the cellular — and even genetic, molecular — level to ensure that you can live another day. Nocturnal shifts in the stress hormone cortisol result in increased immune cell activity at night. Sleep, particularly deep sleep, supports adaptive immunity — the memory defense that works in concert with the front-line innate immune system. By activating two response systems, the fight-or-flight "adrenergic" system and the stress response hormonal system or HPA axis, lost sleep can skew immune system function. If you've ever noticed that you get sick more often, such as catching the common cold, when you're sleep-deprived, now you know why: Sleep disruption can leave you more vulnerable to infection.

Sleep disturbance is a common symptom of Lyme+. Dr. Bransfield told us that 100 percent of his Lyme+ patients have sleep disorders that can include non-restorative sleep, insomnia, hypersomnia, and a number of other sleep disorders. There are many prescription medications for sleep but some are addictive. Supplements that have helped some of my (Dr. Phillips) patients include the amino acids glycine and L-theanine, and a combination of an immediate and time-release melatonin, which is the hormone released at night naturally in our bodies to prepare us for sleep. The latter has to be taken with care because melatonin can augment the immune response and increase symptoms of Lyme+ if it's not well enough under control. Since many of the symptoms of Lyme+ are caused by the immune system going after the microbes, making the immune system stronger, although ultimately a good thing, can also make the symptoms worse if too many microbes are still present early on during treatment. Some people can only tolerate time-release melatonin at first and have to work their way up to tolerating immediate-release melatonin because of this.

Another popular over-the-counter supplement that can induce sleep and relaxation is GABA (gamma-aminobutyric acid), an amino acid that occurs naturally in the brain and reduces neuronal activity.

GABA is generally well tolerated at recommended dosages and is said to help alleviate pain, balance mood, reduce stress, and induce sleep. Please check with your doctor before taking it, especially if you are on blood pressure medications, antidepressants, or neurally active medications, as GABA can interfere with them.

Exercise is also a natural anti-inflammatory, pro-immunity activity (among its many other benefits, including being a natural antidepressant!). After obtaining approval from your doctor that it's safe to begin or change an exercise regimen, it's a good general rule to do what you comfortably can and be gentle with your body. Multiple biological events take place in the body when we charge up a hill, take a group fitness class, or go for a brisk walk. We know that exercise can be the last thing on your mind when you're not feeling well. We also realize that some may not be able to exercise at all. For those who are able to walk but have been sedentary, it's prudent to start with just five to ten minutes of mild exercise and work up to twenty minutes at least three times per week. This can be done any number of ways: walking outside, varying speed and levels of intensity with hills, using classic gym equipment, or following online videos to perform a routine in the comfort of home. For those who already maintain a fitness regimen and are in reasonably good shape, a goal would be to exercise for a minimum of thirty minutes a day, at least five days a week. And again, listen to your body and back off when you feel it's getting too intense. People can experience significant flares of symptoms after intense exercise, so be careful. Once your exercise tolerance is improving, a goal would be to limit the minutes spent sitting down, which slows everything down biologically.

Acupuncture. This centuries-old practice uses hair-thin needles inserted into the body at specific points, which in Eastern medicine is thought to change the body's flow of energy, or "qi." According to the WHO, there are more than thirty diseases or conditions for which this ancient method is recommended. Followers of Eastern medicine believe that illness is often couched in terms of energy imbalances in the body, and that acupuncture needles stimulate the body's fourteen major meridians, or energy-carrying channels, to rebalance and return the body to health. From a scientific perspective, it's believed that acupuncture works by targeting points that are close to nerves, and can decrease pain by stimulating the release of endorphins—those natural morphine-like chemicals that block pain. Acupuncture has gone mainstream in many places today, so finding an acupuncturist is pretty easy. Very often, physicians have referrals from their own experience or that of their patients. I (Parish) went weekly during the most intense part of my treatment and got great relief from it, physically and mentally. Earlier in my life, acupuncture significantly reduced my interstitial cystitis pain.

Epsom salt baths. These can be a powerful tool in reducing the symptoms associated with Lyme+. Epsom salt consists of magnesium sulfate, which is absorbed through the hair follicles.[12] While the magnesium can improve inflammatory arthritis,[13] reduce depression[14] and anxiety,[15] lower blood pressure,[16] and protect nerves from damage,[17] the sulfate is also helpful in a number of cellular biochemical systems.

As surprising as this may sound, the following should be approved by one's treating doctor prior to use as well. This is because Lyme+ patients with dysautonomia/POTS can be become faint from taking a bath, and some patients have very sensitive skin and can't tolerate a dry skin brush.

To take an Epsom salt bath, a bathtub is filled with warm water (not too hot, as this can worsen symptoms) deep enough that the whole body can be submerged. If a bathtub is small, alternating between submerging the legs and then bending the legs to submerge the upper body can do the trick. Once the bathtub is filled, two cups of Epsom salt are added, stirred, and allowed to dissolve; the bath is then ready for a twenty-minute soak. Some patients begin to feel better immediately, but the effects of an Epsom salt bath are frequently felt in the hours after the bath.

To help make an Epsom salt bath more effective, some patients use a dry skin brush before getting in. A dry skin brush helps to stimulate the lymphatic system, which, again, is where a lot of biological waste from the body's metabolism ends up before the body removes it.

Monolaurin. We mentioned this supplement in the previous chapter but want to reiterate it here, since it worked wonders for me (Dr. Phillips), outperforming the antibiotics in many ways. This is a substance that's naturally occurring in breast milk, but in supplement form it's derived from lauric acid in coconut oil, a saturated fatty acid. It acts like soap and kills a wide array of pathogens, including harmful bacteria, viruses, and parasites. Also like soap, bacteria can't become resistant to it because its mechanism of action is so overwhelming: utter destruction by washing away the lipid membranes of the bugs, rather than an antibiotic working on a small target that can become resistant by a gene mutation. And monolaurin does something that antibiotics can't: It dissolves the viscous biofilms that make chronic Lyme+ infections so difficult to eradicate. We should note: Monolaurin's antimicrobial action means it can cause serious Herxheimer reactions. We should also note that monolaurin tends to be easier on the microbiome compared to antibiotics, so it's not apt to destroy as much of the good bacteria. The benefits of its powers on disease-causing bacteria, coupled with the relatively mild effect on the friendly microbiome and its excellent safety profile, make it a triple win.

Gentle sauna and gentle massage. Both of these can be helpful as long as they are not too intense. For patients who are not accustomed to sauna therapy, it pays to go slowly. I (Dr. Phillips) feel strongly that, as a general rule, patients should visit a cardiologist for medical clearance before beginning sauna therapy. Some of you will be in good cardiovascular shape, but we know that others will be barely able to sit up. If you're in that group, sauna is not for you — yet. When I was at my sickest, I had heart rates that were spontaneously going up to 160 at rest and I felt like I was going to pass out every day just trying to stand up. There was no way that I would have attempted sauna in that state! I only began after months of antibiotics, after which I was much better and able to tolerate its stress. Even then, when I started, I couldn't go over 90°F for more than ten minutes. I slowly worked my way up to a maximum of 115°F for twenty minutes. The temperature and duration of therapy have to be tailored to what the individual patient can tolerate, and it's vitally important to bring plenty of water to drink into the sauna.

Some patients who have problems regulating their blood pressure and pulse rate due to Lyme+ are at risk of being too aggressive with sauna, so please take these warnings to heart. I believe that the sauna should be no hotter than 130° if it's a traditional sauna, or 115° for infrared, and the duration over 100°F should be no longer than twenty minutes. Just like I don't believe in lifting heavy weights in the gym to get good benefits, I also don't believe that sauna has to be excessive to derive benefits. I'm all about minimizing risks in the pursuit of getting well.

For massage, my patients initially avoid deep tissue and "sports" massages and go instead for gentler versions, such as Swedish massage. If this type of massage is easily tolerated, more vigorous techniques can be cautiously investigated. Some patients have reported flares of their symptoms with both sauna and massage, which is another reason to go slowly with both.

METHODS WITH MORE CAUTIONARY NOTES

Electromagnetic field machines. An example of such devices is a Rife machine, which imparts radio frequencies to patients. It's named after the microbiologist and microscopist Royal Raymond Rife, who invented it in the early 1930s and studied it for the treatment of a variety of chronic illnesses, including cancer. Rife machines have been the subject of fierce controversy[18] for many decades since the death of its inventor — for example, in 1994 the American Cancer Society was strongly urging cancer patients not to seek treatment with such devices.[19] At present, there are many iterations of these machines that fall under the general umbrella of electromagnetic therapy devices, some of which use radio waves and some of which use pulsed electromagnetic fields. Some pulsed electromagnetic field machines are currently FDA-approved for the treatment of a range of diseases, including non-healing wounds, depression, and ironically, given the American Cancer Society's prior strong protestation against such devices, certain cancers. Cancers that can be treated with FDA-approved electromagnetic field machines include the brain tumor known as glioblastoma[20] and the lung cancer known as mesothelioma.[21] The original Rife machines were well studied in infections and cancer, and many of the non–FDA approved electromagnetic field machines are currently marketed to treat these same conditions. There is considerable scientific evidence that the application of electromagnetic frequencies can reduce tumor growth in the test tube,[22] as well as in both animal and human studies. Some scientists suggest that specific frequencies may modulate the immune system and boost its natural ability to fight off cancerous cells, but studies on this have been mixed.[23] In terms of treating other ailments, the science shows that a variety of even low-power electromagnetic energies, including radiofrequency, magnetic fields, and both direct and alternating low-voltage electric currents, can effectively kill microbes in the test tube, which is why they may have a place in treating Lyme+ and other infections.[24] Serious side effects or adverse outcomes are not frequently reported in the short term, but long-term safety data does not exist. Since long-term cell phone use has been demonstrated to be a risk for brain tumor,[25] we are concerned about whether electromagnetic field devices, including Rife, could pose similar risks.

Unfortunately, it's not likely that these questions of safety will be answered any time soon, given the lack of research funding for such topics. The non–FDA approved machines are not regulated, so they can vary in design and quality. If electromagnetic field machines are to be considered as a treatment option, it should be understood that there is no published data specifically proving efficacy for the treatment of Lyme+, and that their long-term safety is unknown, with a potential concern being the development of cancer. As with any alternative treatment, it's generally a reasonable policy to view them as an addition to traditional treatments and not as replacements. It's imperative to get approval from one's doctor before considering such a treatment.

Disulfiram (brand name Antabuse). This decades-old FDA-approved compound has many potential uses, including antimicrobial, but is most commonly prescribed to help alcoholics resist alcohol consumption. It works by changing how alcohol is metabolized; it causes extremely unpleasant reactions if you drink alcohol while taking it.

With a grant funded by Bay Area Lyme Foundation, scientists from Stanford, led by Dr. Jayakumar Rajadas, have discovered that disulfiram is also effective in the test tube at killing *Borrelia burgdorferi* — both the actively replicating bacteria and the relatively quiescent persister forms.[26] It's being investigated as a potential treatment for Lyme. There is a promising case series published by Dr. Kenneth Liegner, which posits that it also kills *Babesia*. Clinical trials are now underway.[27] There are serious potential side effects from this drug. It cannot be used in combination with certain other drugs, and obviously alcohol must be avoided. It also can result in severe liver and brain damage. There have been rare published reports of fatal liver injury on this drug, and the rare development of brain lesions causing parkinsonism, a Parkinson's-disease-like movement disorder, which would be permanent.

Dapsone. This drug has been used since the 1940s to treat leprosy and a few other conditions. Leprosy is a bacterial infection that has long been known to evade treatments by antibiotics. Sound familiar? Dr. Richard Horowitz has conducted his own preliminary trials on patients and found that their symptoms can improve dramatically on the drug in combination with other antibiotics or agents.[28] Potential side effects include anemia, abnormal blood counts, and other bone marrow damage, all of which can be life-threatening. Of note: Chinese patients are at an increased genetic risk of Dapsone Hypersensitivity Syndrome, which can be fatal in approximately 10 percent of cases.[29] There is a genetic test to see if patients may be at risk.[30]

Methylene blue. Methylene blue is a medication that has historically been used for methemoglobinemia, which can be a side effect from medications such as dapsone or lidocaine. It has activity in the test tube against Lyme and *Bartonella* persisters,[31] but there have been no human studies on these infections. Side effects may be numerous and include nausea, chest pain, lightheadedness, and confusion. A serious potential side effect is serotonin syndrome, when levels of serotonin are increased, which can be dangerous. The likelihood of this occurring is increased when taking medications that raise serotonin levels, such as some antidepressants.

Although methylene blue has antioxidant activity,[32] it also induces DNA mutations in the test tube and caused pancreatic cancer in a two-year rat study.[33] Humans haven't typically taken it long-term, so there is insufficient data for long-term use.

Immune-modulating therapies

Drugs that affect the immune system, and that have been traditionally used to treat autoimmune conditions and neurodegenerative diseases, are increasingly finding their way into treatments for Lyme+. Among them:

- **Low-dose immunotherapy, or LDI:** Classically used to treat chronic allergies, LDI is an alternative therapy now used for a spectrum of chronic illnesses, mostly those that trigger an inappropriate, overreactive immune response and its associated symptoms. LDI is thought to turn the volume down on the abnormal aspects of immune system's response, which may help it fight pathogens more effectively. LDI is a relatively safe therapy and may be useful against a variety of microbes in the Lyme+ family.

- **Low-dose naltrexone, or LDN:** This drug was FDA-approved in 1984 to treat drug addiction; it blocks opioid receptors in the brain, preventing patients from experiencing a high when they take opioid drugs. Soon it became known that the drug—at much lower doses than what's typically prescribed—could help AIDS and cancer patients thanks to the drug's effect on the immune system. Today it's being used to treat a wide array of ailments, Lyme+ included.

Medical cannabis (marijuana) and CBD oil. Some people may not have access to medical cannabis depending on where they live, but more and more states are changing laws to make it legal and more available (i.e., in some states, cannabis can be purchased without a prescription). In particular, cannabidiol (CBD) oil formulations, which are legal everywhere now, in various ingestible and topical forms, have benefited lots of patients—helping to lessen their physical pain, improve their sleep, and even reduce anxiety. CBD is not the compound of the marijuana plant that causes a "high"; the psychoactive part of cannabis is THC (tetrahydrocannabinol). A lot of formulas, however, have these two ingredients in combination. More research is needed to understand cannabis's therapeutic effects (and potential downsides) in treating Lyme+, but many doctors are already encouraging patients to experiment with CBD-rich products if they wish. The challenge, however, is knowing which formulas will work for which patients and avoiding any adverse reactions. Responses to cannabis can vary greatly. There are countless different types of cannabis oils on the market; it's important to buy only from a reputable retailer who can report how and where the cannabis was grown. This is a rapidly changing industry, and we trust that these products will only continue to advance and become more readily available throughout the country.

Psychedelic plants. The medical benefits of psychedelic plants that contain mind-altering, psychoactive compounds (e.g., psilocybin, ayahuasca) are being studied for treating things like depression, drug addiction, anxiety, chronic pain, PTSD, and much more.[34] Michael Pollan wrote about his own exploration of the subject in his 2018 bestseller *How to Change Your Mind: What the New Science of Psychedelics Teaches Us about Consciousness, Dying, Addiction, Depression, and Transcendence.* Pollan takes the skepticism out of the subject and calls for more research, which is needed to move this conversation forward in serious medical circles. The use of these drugs has its place in modern medicine; they can be safe and effective when used in the right setting and under the guidance of a professional. Some of them, however, are currently in legal gray zones; the tropical plant ayahuasca, for example, is not illegal, but its active, hallucinogenic ingredient— dimethyltryptamine (DMT)—is. If use of these medicinal plants is contemplated, it should only be done within the context of a study, as there can be risks involved. Pilot studies are underway at some of our finest medical institutions.

STRATEGIES TO PREVENT COGNITIVE DECLINE

As we explained earlier, some forms of dementia, including Alzheimer's disease, have been shown to possibly be the result of long-term infection. There is new science emerging that certain supplements might help prevent the occurrence of memory loss and cognitive impairment:

- *Curcumin*: Rural India has among the lowest rates of Alzheimer's and other dementias in the world, despite high rates of chronic infections that can cross into the brain. These infections should increase the rate of dementias, according to our newest science, and yet the global scourges of Alzheimer's and Parkinson's are a relative rarity there. Tons of in vitro and animal data show that curcumin, the compound found in the turmeric plant that gives curry its quintessential flavor and yellow color, can be helpful (this is the same compound shown to have anti-HSV-1 effects, as we described in Chapter 5). But it's poorly absorbed from the GI tract in its native form. The reason that it's well absorbed from curry is that it's cooked over time with ghee, clarified butter — the fat making it easier to absorb. The key is to choose a curcumin product that's easily absorbed by the body. Although many claim to be bioavailable and better absorbed, at the time of this writing, one trademarked formula, called Theracurmin, had been the subject of a well-designed study demonstrating that it helped improve cognition in patients with both normal cognitive decline of aging and mild cognitive impairment, or pre-dementia.[35] You can find this online just by Googling "theracumin."
- *Nicotinamide riboside*, or NR, goes by the trademarked name

Niagen (not regular nicotinamide, which is flush-free niacin): NR is a form of vitamin B_3 and a precursor compound to nicotinamide adenine dinucleotide (NAD+), which our cells need to regulate DNA repair and other key signaling pathways. Because NAD+ declines with age, scientists have wondered whether boosting the level of NAD+ through its precursor NR could help aging brain cells (neurons) to function better. In animal studies, NR can improve cognitive performance, extend lifespan and healthspan (the length of time lived in good health), and reverse other age-related findings, such as fatty liver.[36] This supplement can also be found online. Dr. David Sinclair of Harvard Medical School is studying NAD+ extensively for its role in improving physiology in many parts of the body, including how it fixes epigenetic DNA damage, thereby preventing cancers and other ailments.

▪ *Lithium orotate*: In low doses, lithium has been shown to be neuroprotective in many studies.[37] Over-the-counter lithium orotate is not the same as the prescription lithium carbonate that's used to treat bipolar disorder. Although it contains the same active element, with standard low doses of lithium orotate, i.e., 5 mg, total elemental lithium is much less than in prescription lithium. Prescription lithium can cause serious side effects to the kidneys and thyroid. Lithium orotate is generally safer, but it should still only be taken under a doctor's supervision.

STAYING ENGAGED WITH FRIENDS

It's important to note that scheduling social interactions with others is key to recovery. Managing a chronic illness can be incredibly isolating. Some days you can't imagine leaving home. You don't want to accept invitations to parties and other events. But it's not always a good idea to stay holed up in your bed or on the couch. Until you're strong enough to put yourself together for an outing, ask a friend to come over when you feel terrible. Watch uplifting stories of recovery online and read inspirational books. The goal is to find ways to feel like you're in control and to believe that you WILL get better in time.

In Our Own Words: Here's how we each relax and enjoy the health we're so grateful to have.

Dr. Phillips: "I relax by exercising at the gym, and going for long walks. I see as many sci-fi movies as possible, even the embarrassingly bad ones. In the summer, I paint pictures outside with the sun on my face and go out on the deck at night and feel small beneath the stars. And when I can get away, I like to go far away, forgetting my worries for a bit. And most importantly, I feel a sense of connectedness when I'm with interesting, good people, especially the ones I love."

Dana: "I live in New York City and love wandering with no destination, day or night. Sometimes I bring my angel, Lucy, who's a Tibetan Terrier rescue from Puerto Rico. She lights people up (including me) and gets treats everywhere she goes. One day a guy snuck her his bagel and cream cheese. I find it therapeutic to travel, but I always return to my 'happy place,' Santa Ynez Valley in California, with its Tuscan-like landscape, relaxed vibe, zillions of beautiful, grazing animals, and close friends. You'll also catch me singing a lot, which has always given me a peace I can't describe."

PREVENT FUTURE BITES

It goes without saying that preventing more tick and other bug bites is essential. We are huge proponents of using permethrin insecticide on clothes (especially shoes and socks, since ticks tend to travel upward), which is so effective at killing ticks and other bugs that the military purchases uniforms that are pretreated with it. Permethrin comes from the pyrethroid family, a class of synthetic chemicals that act like natural extracts from the chrysanthemum flower. Permethrin is used to treat head lice and scabies, and topical forms require a prescription. You can buy permethrin as a spray, however, that you can use on clothing. This form should not be used directly on skin, so if you're applying it to clothing yourself, please wear gloves, do it in a well-ventilated area that's not windy (it's not good to get a face full of permethrin from a gust of wind!), and give it twenty-four hours to dry. After that, it's considered generally safe to wear and will stay potent for several washes. It not only repels ticks, mosquitos, and a whole host of other insects, but it kills them, too. Instructions on the bottle are easy to follow and will tell you how long the treatment will last. Other classic bug repellants can also be considered, such as the chemical sprays DEET (diethyltoluamide) and picaridin, and natural essential oils such as lemon and eucalyptus oil. Permethrin is most effective.

It's also important to realize that it's not just ticks that can spread serious infections. Remember, I (Dr. Phillips) got infected by spider bites while I was sleeping in my own bed. Some steps I took after that were to move the head of the bed six inches away from the wall and spray the legs of the beds with insecticide during the warmer months. There are also tips that may help reduce entrance of bugs into the house, about which a contractor can further advise. For example, I had the sill plate area in my basement sprayed with a foam insulation to seal the basement from the outside more effectively. There are various types of foam insulation and some have toxic odors, so it's best to get the opinion of an expert if you're considering this.

Dr. Richard (Rick) Ostfeld is a disease ecologist who focuses on the interactions among organisms that influence the risk of human exposure to vector-borne diseases. One of his projects, The Tick Project, is testing whether environmental interventions, such as treating areas around people's homes with a fungus that kills ticks, can prevent tick-borne diseases in our communities.[38] Unfortunately, "cleaning up woodpiles won't help," he says. According to him, some of the best ways of prevention today are the old-fashioned methods of avoiding brushy areas, checking yourself for ticks when coming in from the outside, and taking a shower right away. Put exposed clothes in the dryer on high heat to kill leftover ticks. And he, too, lists permethrin-treated clothing as among the best strategies for avoiding bites.

CHAPTER 9

COVID

W ITH SO MUCH division in the world today, I think we can all agree: 2020 was a terrible year. A new virus called SARS-CoV-2 tore across our planet within a few short months, causing the disease COVsID-19, and reaping a heavy toll in human suffering and loss of life.

As we each became aware of the pandemic's unfolding, country by country, creeping ever closer and eventually landing in our own communities, there was a sense of unreality. It was hard to believe what we were witnessing—a chaotic scramble to understand this new infection and rally the best of science to find treatments and cures. At the same time, we watched in horror as healthcare systems buckled and patients died in droves. Some perished at home, unable to receive treatment in time. Worse yet, many died in isolation in hospital beds, separated from their loved ones, due to fear of spreading the disease. The climbing numbers of infections, hospitalizations, and deaths became mind-numbing. By the end of 2020, the U.S. had more COVID-related deaths than any other nation.

We completed this manuscript before the pandemic hit, hence the omission of the word "COVID" until now. But in this final chapter, we want to bring this new scourge into the fold and reveal the painful similarities that COVID has with the gallery of infections covered in the book. They share many of the same issues — unreliable testing, questionable treatments, and a large number of patients developing chronic illness after the acute infection. Not unlike individuals saddled with Lyme+, many of these patients have also been marginalized by mainstream medicine, and their numbers are so large, and growing every day, that they constitute their own pandemic within this pandemic. Many of the challenges we've faced combatting COVID have been the same ones we've been tackling for decades with Lyme+. All those lessons learned from years spent in the war rooms, unraveling the complexities of vexing infections, have led us to this point. Here. Now. Through not only our own experiences, but with the help of countless others, we hope that the skill set we've cultivated can help shine a light into the many shadows of this pandemic — and help us be better prepared for the next one.

As we say with Lyme+, you don't get it till you get it. It was the same with COVID. In New York City and its suburbs, where COVID first hit the hardest in the U.S., many experienced an existential crisis. Life for the most part went on as usual in the rest of the country, where the "it can't happen to me" mentality was pervasive until the virus finally hit their own backyards and living rooms. I (Dana) moved out of New York City early in the pandemic and many thought I was a fearmonger. I (Dr. Phillips), changed my practice to telemedicine about a month sooner than my colleagues, many of whom thought I was an alarmist. Unfortunately, many doctors, nurses, and other frontline caregivers didn't have that same degree of professional flexibility. Some were terrified to go to work each day, out of concern both for themselves and for what they might bring home to their families, but they couldn't stop working out of financial necessity. I also know some who closed their practices not knowing when they'd open again, if ever.

Because we want to focus on exploring the complexities of COVID and proposing solutions, we will purposely not spend much time bemoaning the failures of our government and healthcare authorities in handling the pandemic. That is another book. Still, we'd be remiss not to highlight a few of the epic errors in the U.S. that helped the virus infect far too many people. We, meaning the U.S., were the architects and authors of the best-laid pandemic plans in the world, yet ignored our own playbook. Ironically, we exported that playbook to many countries with far fewer resources, and many of them successfully gained control of the virus. It was hard to watch certain countries ring in the new year of 2021 with a semblance of normalcy, while we experienced rising cases, with one American dying every minute.[1]

On multiple fronts, the grave mismanagement of this pandemic presents déjà vu moments for Lyme+ patients. We often felt helpless shouting from the sidelines, trying to share our hard-won knowledge with the public. Take, for example, the initial mixed messaging around masks that quickly grew into a political statement and remained a sticking point throughout the pandemic. The confusion sowed doubt that could never be fully expunged, with resulting damage that can't be overstated. Doubt also fell upon patients who complained of symptoms months after the acute phase of the infection had passed and were dismissed by many doctors who didn't think it was possible for infections to rage on, despite an ever-growing body of evidence to the contrary. Another problem was the CDC's insistence on developing its own testing, rather than using verified tests from other countries. This delayed the establishment of a U.S. test-and-trace program, which could have stemmed the spread of the disease. After the CDC finally distributed its homegrown tests, it was discovered that they were contaminated[2] and unreliable. A subsequent investigation showed that officials knew[3] they were bad, yet they sent them out anyway. For those outside of the Lyme+ community, the rapidly evolving scenario seemed unbelievable. To the Lyme+ community, it was, wearily, more of the same.

The CDC's lack of transparency and consistency further sowed distrust. When its hospital and ICU bed data suddenly vanished[4] on July 14, 2020, the move thwarted communities from effectively managing their scarce resources. There wasn't even a clear consensus about the most basic and imperative information — how COVID spread — droplet vs. airborne transmission. Droplets are small drops of saliva and mucus we expel when we cough, sneeze, or talk, but they're too heavy to stay suspended in the air. They fall to the ground pretty quickly, so they can only infect people within a short distance. This is why you've heard so much about staying six feet apart. Airborne transmission is when even smaller particles, referred to as aerosols, are expelled, also by coughing, sneezing, and talking, but these stay suspended in the air for long periods, floating around a room, and potentially farther, like smoke. Both droplets and aerosols can infect people through the eyes, nose, or mouth, but aerosols can do so at a much greater distance and are far more insidious. For example, aerosols can get around gaps in a poorly fitting mask. Even though Chinese health officials[5] and WHO's director general, Dr. Tedros Adhanom,[6] characterized COVID as airborne by early February, the U.S. public was still being told to wear gloves but not masks, so they went about their business doing the exact opposite of what they could and should have been doing to protect themselves. The CDC and many others acknowledged far too late that the virus spreads primarily through airborne transmission. The CDC's continual revisions and back-pedaling on guidance made for pervasive division, skepticism, and distrust. The standard answer is that as they learned more, their guidance was updated, but there was sound evidence of airborne transmission early on and using masks for airborne infections is a well-established and effective policy.

Molecular biologist and assistant secretary at the U.S. Department of Energy, Dr. Ali Nouri,[7] expressed similar frustrations when he spoke to us: "We have seen over and over how, as a country, we have failed to follow science and evidence when it comes to things like how severe is the pandemic? Is it airborne? Are masks going to be helpful? Those are basic issues where we have failed. Going forward, we really need to think about how we communicate public health to the public."

And we can't forget to mention the race for a vaccine that, while admirable and necessary, left behind what should have been an equally ferocious race for early treatments. At this writing—a year into the pandemic—in the U.S. alone we have approximately 4,000 people dying per day and no early, at-home treatments sanctioned by our health officials, other than the usual advice to stay in bed, stay away from others, keep hydrated, and use over-the-counter pain relievers like Tylenol. And even as vaccines have been rolled out in the U.S. and other privileged countries,[8] millions around the globe still don't have access to them.

Clearly, even those with the highest honors, credentials, and responsibilities are fallible and make mistakes. If there is anything to be gained from this enormous tragedy, it's that the same failures and gaslighting the Lyme+ community has suffered at their hands have now played out on the world's stage for all to see. If not for the horror of COVID, it would have been a hard sell.

Next, we'll put those fallibilities behind us and turn to what you need to know going forward. We assume you've already learned about prevention — wear a mask, watch your distance around others outside your household, and wash your hands routinely — but we'd like to add a few more tips. There is varying data on different types of masks, but we prefer N95 respirators, when available. Since they filter out tiny viral particles so well, they're associated with a lower infection rate. They were in short supply early on but are now more widely available to the public. Proper fit with a good seal is imperative, so please seek out one of the "how-to" videos from OSHA[9] or other trusted sources for at-home instructions on how to use them. Eye protection (glasses or goggles) also lowers risk. And finally, we feel that it's also crucial to highlight the importance of ventilation. Dr. Shelly Miller, environmental engineer at the University of Colorado Boulder, told us, "COVID primarily spreads indoors, and it's the long-range exposure that's concerning since infectious aerosols can float for hours in a poorly ventilated room. Ventilation is key. We like to use the cigarette smoke analogy so people can visualize this and understand how to keep themselves safe indoors. Simply opening windows and using air cleaners with HEPA filters can help prevent transmission." Though she warns against fogging unsafe chemicals into the air, Miller says that as long as a space is unoccupied, using an ozone machine to clean the air is okay. Still, even if we do everything right, not everyone will escape this beast.

THE NEW CORONAVIRUSES

Seasonal coronaviruses have been infecting us for eons, with studies concluding that "coronaviruses appear to be an ancient viral lineage."[10] While the early strains have remained relatively innocuous human pathogens, causing mild upper respiratory symptoms comparable to the common cold, in the last few years, things have changed.

The word "changed" doesn't seem to quite do it justice. "Quantum leap" might be a more accurate term. SARS was first discovered in Asia in 2003.[11] With a 15 percent case fatality rate,[12] terror gripped most of the continent, and almost overnight, inhabitants of Asian countries started wearing surgical masks for protection. WHO's official consensus statement[13] straddled the fence on how the virus was spread, saying that airborne transmission was "plausible" and "could not be excluded." Unlike COVID, patients with SARS were not infectious before the development of symptoms, and by 2004, the pandemic was largely contained. SARS was demonstrated to be spread by airborne transmission in the analysis that followed the pandemic.[14]

In 2012, another coronavirus, Middle East Respiratory Syndrome (MERS), sprang up in Saudi Arabia. The case fatality rate of this coronavirus was a staggering 35 percent.[15] Fortunately, it proved to be less contagious than SARS[16] and the worst of it was contained quickly, but it continues to smolder to this day, with small numbers of cases still occurring. Despite its reduced transmissibility, evidence of airborne transmission has also been demonstrated in MERS.[17]

And then in 2020, when the now infamous third iteration from this same coronavirus lineage began ravaging us, theories as to its provenance began circulating in scientific circles. At first, COVID-19 was viewed as simply a severe upper respiratory virus with an average incubation period of 5 to 6 days (with a range of 2 to 14 days), but it quickly became clear that its clinical features were multi-systemic and alarmingly severe. Doctors were told to be on the lookout for fever, cough, and shortness of breath. They didn't know about the nausea and diarrhea, as well as a set of more ominous features: heart failure with fatal arrhythmias, kidney failure, hepatitis, loss of taste and smell, heart attacks, strokes, and pulmonary embolisms. The medical community was left reeling.

One of the puzzling features of COVID-19 was that patients who had incredibly low blood oxygen saturations didn't feel short of breath. In ordinary pneumonias, patients with similarly low oxygen levels would be gasping for air. Doctors have called this "happy hypoxia," and it's mainly due to numerous small blood clots developing in the lungs.

We now know that vascular injury resulting in abnormal clotting is arguably the most significant part of COVID's ability to cause disease. When Dr. William Li, president and medical director of the Angiogenesis Foundation, looked at tissue from autopsies of people who died from COVID, what he found astounded him: "It wasn't just lung destruction, inflammation, and pneumonia. The virus was invading and infecting blood vessel cells in the lungs and every other organ in the body. We saw it in the brain, heart, the kidneys, testicles, lymph nodes. Seeing microscopic blood clots everywhere was really a Eureka moment to understanding how some of the damage that this disease causes is beyond simple pneumonia or respiratory distress."[18]

THE LONG HAUL

Today, there are a staggering number of reports on "recovered" COVID patients who are saddled with months of debilitating, chronic symptoms, many of which can be serious, even resulting in organ damage.[19] There is also an ever-growing number of patients with "mild" cases that initially resolve, but who become extremely ill weeks or months later. The presence of such a latency period is eerily reminiscent of what happens in many Lyme+ infections, and it begs the question of whether acute COVID can turn into a chronic, insidious infection. A study of protracted illness after initial COVID documented a whopping 205 symptoms across ten body organs.[20]

These patients have been referred to by a growing group of monikers: "long-haulers," "long-COVID," and "long-term COVID." Some doctors refer to their condition as "post-COVID syndrome," a name that implies, perhaps erroneously, that the virus is gone. The list of those affected, and their symptoms, is terrifying in both its breadth and its randomness. Even young, otherwise healthy patients are being struck down.[21]

Diana Berrent, founder of Survivor Corps, the largest long-term COVID movement in the world, tells us, "We have seen an untold number of heart-wrenching pediatric COVID cases that are experiencing the same devastating manifestations as their adult counterparts."

Berrent's 12-year-old son is a perfect example. She described his February case of COVID as extremely mild. Yet nine months later, one of his adult front teeth fell out spontaneously while he was watching TV.[22] The oral surgeon was stunned and said it should have looked like "a bloodbath," yet there was no blood at all. Berrent said, "There had evidently been vascular damage, but we still don't know whether it was to the tooth, the gum, or the jaw," and there were no warning signs. He felt just fine. "The data varies between 10 to 80 percent, but we're seeing that about a third of those who contract COVID become long-haulers — and those are the people who *have* symptoms. We don't know how many have invisible damage, like my son. We don't know how many may have an internal time bomb about to go off, or if we'll even hear it if it does. For example, my case of COVID-onset glaucoma was found accidentally when I went in for complaints of blurry vision."

Twelve-year-old Maggie Flannery, a Manhattan sixth-grader, and her family, had a three-week bout with COVID in early March. They all recovered, but Maggie soon suffered a horrific relapse that left her with trouble breathing, extreme fatigue, nausea, joint pain, and light-headedness. She can no longer walk to school or participate in her beloved virtual ballet classes. Yet, since she had no positive COVID-19 test to prove she had the disease, doctors initially suggested this once-healthy girl's debilitating symptoms may be psychological.[23] (Sound familiar?)

Dr. Natalie Lambert, an associate professor at Indiana University School of Medicine, has analyzed thousands of COVID patients' health narratives. She's a leading expert in how COVID impacts health and works closely with Survivor Corps. She tells us it's not unusual for those with serious symptoms to be written off as psychosomatic. "One of the most common complaints that COVID patients have is that they go to their doctor to get help with ongoing symptoms and go home in tears. Many quickly realize that they'll have to prove that they're ill; that their joint pain, their racing hearts, their blurry vision, their inability to remember words is not some form of mass-pandemic anxiety. These patients are reluctant to seek care as they don't want to be re-exposed to COVID, yet the fact that they know their own bodies and know that something's really wrong is still often dismissed."

Lambert said the most shocking part in all of this is that COVID is still talked about in certain circles as "the flu." "This is nothing like the flu, with its vast neurologic, psychiatric, and vascular complications. It can even cause autoimmune disorders. It's an incredibly serious disease and people need to understand that there *are* long-term, terrible health impacts that can affect anyone — even young, healthy marathon runners."

So, how do we understand those who experience such an array of prolonged symptoms? From our perspective, the terms "post-viral syndrome," "post-infectious syndrome," and "post-COVID" are misleading. They leave patients floating in a sea of uncertainty, with no clear path back to health. Damage to the body from the acute infection is perhaps the easiest potential cause of long-term COVID for most of us to grasp, but it's not the only one, and it wouldn't explain people developing long-term symptoms after a latency period of feeling fine, or after mild cases.

We don't claim to have all the answers, but as is often the case, missing links tend to hide in plain sight. As described in the book, there is precedent for chronic infections as the cause of ongoing symptoms in a multitude of chronic disease states. Aside from the vector-borne infections that have been the focus of this book, persistent infection has been documented as a potential root cause in illnesses ranging from ulcers[24] to back pain.[25] We're concerned by the echo chamber in the medical community that defaults patients who develop chronic illness after an acute infection to a "post-viral" or "post-infectious" syndrome, without deep exploration into the likelihood of ongoing infection. We fear that long-term COVID patients will be relegated to the same fate.

Many viruses, including coronaviruses,[26] set up persistent infection in various cell lines, organs,[27] and body fluids,[28] in some cases long after presumed recovery from the acute phase. For coronaviruses, this has been known since at least 1979.[29] So, it's not surprising that SARS-CoV-2 has been found not only within the brain,[30] spleen,[31] and many other sites[32] distant from the lungs, but also that it's been shown to persist[33] for many months[34] after apparent recovery from acute COVID infection. An immune-suppressed man experienced a series of multiple confirmed COVID relapses[35] after thinking he was free of the virus, and he ultimately died from COVID after a grueling 154 days. All of this is deeply troubling, especially when we realize that the pharmaceutical industry has succeeded in putting more of us on lifelong immunosuppressants than at any time in history. And to add salt to this wound, the virus itself also induces a degree of immunosuppression.[36]

And then there are those like Chris Long,[37] who was not immunosuppressed but was still admitted to the hospital seven times after contracting COVID in March of 2020. Hospital readmissions after acute COVID are shockingly common.[38] Unlike the aforementioned cases that have had documented SARS-CoV-2 persistence, in Long's case we don't have proof that the virus is persistent—but we also don't have proof that it's not. Nature isn't fickle. If the virus can persist in some and cause chronic illness, why assume that it's gone in others who have had similar chronic illness after acute COVID? Documenting persistent SARS-CoV-2 infection isn't as simple as a repeat throat swab PCR or simple blood test. It has taken invasive and painstaking measures to confirm its presence, which aren't available to patients outside of a research setting.

Harvard neuroscientist Dr. Michael VanElzakker points out, "Blood tests produce both false negatives and false positives. There was a tragic case of a woman with COVID-19 losing her pregnancy in the third trimester. Her blood and urine tested negative, but the placenta tested positive. Chronically ill people often have a blood test come back negative, and doctors assume this must mean infection isn't involved and the issues must be psychological. It's absurd to think that everything happening in the human body is represented in 1 milliliter of blood."

We expect that drug trials for long COVID will be a burgeoning field over the next few years.[39] One drug being studied, leronlimab,[40] is an immunomodulator — meaning it can help support immune function. Accumulating data shows that SARS-CoV-2 can persist long after the acute phase of illness has resolved. So, in addition to drugs that work on the immune system, it would be logical to also study medications with direct anti-SARS-CoV-2 activity. Given the institutional denial of the overwhelming evidence of active infection in chronic Lyme+, if persistent viral infection is a major cause of long-term COVID, we fear that history may repeat itself.

In addition to persistent infection with SARS-CoV-2, another potential explanation for COVID long-haulers is that the insult from the initial infection upsets the immunologic apple cart, allowing other asymptomatic chronic infections to manifest as disease, which has already been documented with COVID.[41] It's a hard notion to get your head around, that we're all walking around with a bunch of hidden infections. Lyme is a perfect example — random blood testing of healthy individuals in the northeastern U.S. routinely reveals that almost 10 percent[42] of the population has been infected with this organism, often unbeknownst to the infected healthy person. Studies from Italy demonstrate that 11 percent of healthy adults have been infected with *Bartonella*,[43] another common but widely overlooked bacterium whose spectrum of illness, including Lyme,[44] ranges from asymptomatic infection to debilitating and even deadly. Could a tip of the scales turn asymptomatic infection into symptomatic infection? Could this be the cause of chronic symptoms in a subset of COVID long-haulers?

It's going to take a lot of objective research to solve the riddle of what's causing chronic suffering in long-haulers. We believe that both of the above theories warrant exploration. What should be stricken from the medical lexicon is the term "post-infectious syndrome," as no good ever comes from this characterization. It only serves to stifle further research into the cause of ongoing symptoms. Uncovering the root cause of disease is the clearest path to a lasting remedy. Simply describing a set of symptoms and providing symptom relief is an unacceptable substitute.

EARLY TREATMENT SAVES LIVES

Let's say you slice your finger with a knife while cooking in the kitchen. The next day it gets infected and you call your doctor. By that point, your finger is red and throbbing and you have a low-grade fever. Would your doctor tell you to stay home and take no action until your entire arm gets infected? To do nothing until you're in septic shock and need ICU treatment? Of course not. And if you ever get advice like that from a doctor, please find a new doctor. That's not the way infections are managed. From bacterial infections like typical community-acquired pneumonia and syphilis, to viral infections like herpes or HIV, treating early leads to better outcomes.

This is especially true in COVID-19. The disease has two main phases. The first part is the viral replication phase. But after about five days or so, the later stages of the illness can be characterized by a hyper-inflammatory phase, more commonly referred to as a cytokine storm, causing vascular damage leading to dangerous blood clots resulting in heart attacks, pulmonary embolisms, strokes, and multi-organ failure. Vascular injury and clotting are the main mechanisms of disease and death in COVID-19.

An ounce of prevention during the viral replication phase, with the goal of heading off the hyper-inflammatory phase, is worth a thousand pounds of cure. But the corollary is also true: A thousand pounds of cure won't work as well as an ounce of prevention once the disease has gotten to the latter phase. Like so many infectious diseases, there is a window of opportunity during which anti-pathogen treatment can be most helpful.

But in this dystopian era, decades of accumulated medical wisdom dissipated like a puff of smoke. In its place, reason has been tainted by harmful mixed messaging, which has spread through the U.S. and Western Europe as insidiously as an aerosol. Doctors are not being widely informed that there are early, outpatient treatment options, so patients are being advised to only take action when they're sick enough to go to the hospital. By this time, the disease is advanced, and the odds of dying are markedly increased. Politicians and celebrities have had access to early treatment; everyday patients have the right to these options as well.

It's beyond the scope of this book to offer treatment protocols for every type of COVID patient in this rapidly changing landscape. The take-home message is that at-home treatments and those administered in hospital settings exist and that they may help reduce loss of life when used properly for COVID-19. The treatments listed here are for informational purposes only and do not constitute medical advice. Please consult with your physician before considering any treatments for COVID-19.

Information on COVID-19 treatment options is an evolving area, so we invite you to visit our website (https://www.thechronic book.com/) for more specifics.

COVID-19 treatments can be grouped into several categories: antiviral, immunologic, and anti-clotting. Antiviral treatments generally work best early on, before the hyper-inflammatory phase begins. Many agents that are not typically thought of as "antivirals" have antiviral activity against COVID. Immunologic treatments serve to calm the inflammatory pathways leading to cytokine storm, and anti-clotting strategies are used in order to mitigate what's now accepted to be a major cause of COVID-related pathology. And some treatments have activity that falls within more than one category — they can have both antiviral and immunologic effects. Different drugs are used at different phases of the disease, with some requiring a hospital setting, and others recommended off-label by doctors who take an individual's symptoms and personal risk factors into account when prescribing and creating a treatment protocol. Others are over-the-counter medications and supplements. Vitamin D is a great example of this. Vitamin D deficiency has been associated with worse outcomes in many infections, and in COVID-19 it's associated with an almost quadrupling of mortality.[45] A letter from over 4,000 experts was sent to world leaders, imploring them to increase vitamin D intake recommendations in order to mitigate COVID-19.[46] A randomized controlled trial of vitamin D in early COVID-19 demonstrated improved viral clearance. More is not always better, however, as too much vitamin D can be toxic.[47] Ideally, supplementation should be taken under the supervision of a doctor.

In October 2020, the FDA approved the first treatment for COVID-19—the antiviral drug remdesivir. This drug has a dubious track record. One randomized controlled trial failed to demonstrate improved survival rates in COVID-19 patients.[48] In another study, surviving patients treated with remdesivir recovered more quickly, but the study failed to demonstrate a statistically significant survival benefit.[49] In a subsequent clinical trial of 11,000 people from 30 countries, remdesivir also failed to prevent death.[50] The WHO recommends against using remdesivir for COVID-19.[51] Notably, Gilead Sciences, the maker of remdesivir, spent more money lobbying in the first quarter of 2020 than it ever had before,[52] and remdesivir is still the only antiviral drug approved for the treatment of COVID-19 in the United States.[53]

If there is any silver lining to the pandemic, it's the breakdown of long-standing silos in medicine and the forced collaboration among the sciences. Many drugs that have long been on our shelves for use in other areas of medicine are currently being explored for COVID-19.

I (Dr. Phillips) have treated more than sixty COVID-19 patients, most at high risk due to underlying medical conditions, with early, outpatient combination therapies that have demonstrated benefits in clinical studies throughout the world. All did exceptionally well, and none required hospitalization or developed long-term COVID. My only long-term COVID patient is one who came to me several months into her illness. Her primary care doctor's treatment was, "Stay home and rest." Weighing the pros and cons of treating early with drugs I deem safe for my patients, in my opinion, has ultimately kept them out of the hospital and alive.

More people should have access to early treatments to potentially change the course of their disease. Even monoclonal antibodies meant for the early stages of infection in those at high risk for severe illness are too rarely being used. Convalescent plasma, a blood component from recovered COVID-19 patients that contains antibodies against the virus, has demonstrated some benefits[54] but is still being evaluated. Other drugs that warrant more attention and study within the context of COVID-19 include ivermectin, which, in a WHO-sponsored meta-analysis of eleven randomized controlled trials, reduced COVID-19 mortality by an average of 83 percent among 1,452 patients.[55] More studies are underway to cover a greater number of patients. The controversial drug hydroxychloroquine is also still being studied, as a meta-analysis of chloroquine and HCQ demonstrated about a two-thirds reduction in mortality,[56] although some of these studies also included other antiviral therapies. Then there are over-the-counter medicines such as bromhexine, zinc, quercetin, vitamin C, bromelain, NAC, glutathione, melatonin, and aspirin, which all show promise in research studies. We expect many more will come into the spotlight as more data accumulates.

Our point being: Early treatment is key to surviving COVID-19 and may be able to reduce the risk of becoming a long-hauler. But, as with Lyme+, we need to advocate for ourselves (or a loved one). There are scores of possible treatment protocols out there being used by physicians in both academic settings and private practice. When it comes to COVID, subscribing to the notion that we should "ride it out" and hope to avoid dire consequences just doesn't cut it. We've heard horror stories from people — young and old — who were sent home from their doctor with no treatments whatsoever other than a "prescription" for isolation, a bed, and chicken soup. And they go on to suffer mightily or, worse, end up in the ICU.

By the time you read this, vaccines will have been deployed globally and on a massive scale. You may have received one already. We are likely going to have to learn how to live with this virus in our environment for the rest of our lives, and it remains to be seen how effective the vaccines will be as the virus mutates and changes. But even with a vaccine, there will be "breakthrough" infections in those who are not vaccine candidates or whose immune systems may not respond well enough to protect them. Effective early treatments are absolutely essential.

We believe that there are crucial lessons from the Lyme+ world scattered throughout this book that could prove invaluable to COVID-19 patients. First, prevention is key. Second, early treatment is associated with better outcomes. Third, advocate for yourself if you're not being heard by your doctor. And, most importantly, don't give up. Never in the history of the world has science moved at such lightning speed with the goal of unraveling complex, chronic illness caused by infection. We are hopeful that COVID-19 will inspire the global scientific community and clinicians to view chronic illness in a new and treatable light.

CONCLUSION:

Hope Around the Globe

There is a crack in everything. That's how the light gets in.

—*Leonard Cohen*

The things you do for yourself are gone when you are gone,
but the things you do for others remain as your legacy.

—*Kalu Ndukwe Kalu*

I T'S DIFFICULT TO bring this book to a close because every day
we field calls, texts, and emails from people around the world desperate for help for themselves or for a loved one. Immense suffering
that began with a painless, minuscule bite. And we increasingly receive
correspondence from people in parts of the world without any awareness of Lyme+, yet these infections lurk and dismantle innocent lives
everywhere.

Joe Adjei is one such special soul. He came across Dana's story in
the Huffington Post and was amazed that his symptoms matched hers.[1]
It was the first time he felt he had a name for his years-long illness.
He reached out to us online and we started corresponding a few years
ago. Joe hails from Ghana, Africa, where he's a nurse and a science stu-

dent. Although there is evidence of Lyme in Africa, we had no idea if Joe had Lyme per se, or perhaps a different Lyme+ infection, but what we cannot stress enough is that there are innumerable similar infections worldwide. For example, in Brazil, there is a borrelial Lyme-like illness called Baggio-Yoshinari Syndrome that is now gaining a lot of attention.[2]

We equipped Joe with knowledge, data, and an evaluation protocol from the ILADS website for Lyme+, which he'd never heard about in his country. Sadly, many Ghanaians who suffer from chronic illness, including those who have serious psychiatric conditions such as psychosis or severe depression — and which could very well be rooted in an infection — are confined to enormous prayer camps, where they are warehoused by the thousands. Ghana is one of the most religious societies in the world. Mental illness can be seen as a problem of supernatural evil, driving the families of those with mental problems to seek spiritual solutions. The stage is thus set for these camps to attract thousands of desperate patients seeking salvation and respite from their pain. They are established by self-proclaimed prophets, usually without any medical training; human rights abuses are rife in these camps. It's not uncommon for visitors to spend months there and experience physical abuse, forced starvation, chaining, and other human rights violations.

Joe passed through a few of these camps during the height of his illness in order to show respect toward senior members of his family so they'd keep supporting him, but he knew there must be something better. And he found it in two physician friends who evaluated him and diagnosed him with Lyme. Joe kept us in the loop and, over the course of six months with antibiotic treatment, he returned to health. Today he is thriving. But we're haunted by all the Joes who are still wandering through prayer camps. The realization of the global impact these infections have on human suffering is almost too much to bear.

The teen with whom we opened this book is also thriving today. Although it took two years and fifty doctors to arrive at the correct diagnosis of *Bartonella*, and seven more years of treatment, Marna's son recovered. After a harrowing decade, he's enjoying a beautiful life and is on his way to becoming a kindergarten teacher. He recently got married and can't wait to be a dad.

As for Lisa, who contracted Lyme+ in France soon after graduating from Wellesley College, the disease stole ten years of her life, included a trip to the psych ward, and cost her the dream of becoming an FBI agent. She's now in remission and revisiting the possibility of that dream job.

It's never a good time to develop strange neurologic symptoms, let alone in the prime of your life. Imagine going to your doctor, who appropriately suspects Lyme and orders a Lyme antibody test, which comes back positive. And think how you'd feel when, instead of being offered antimicrobial treatment for Lyme, you're told by your neurologist that the positive Lyme test is "really negative." And when brain lesions are found on an MRI, which Lyme can do in many published studies, your neurologist suggests a lifetime of treatments for MS at age forty-three. This happened to Kim of Connecticut, who ultimately responded well to antibiotic therapy, with resolution of most neurologic symptoms for more than five years.

Adrienne from New Jersey had already suffered through three back surgeries for scoliosis and a shoulder surgery for a labral tear by the time she was twenty-one years old. The pain then deepened to other joints, stomach, and head, with sensitivity to light, cognitive problems, and sleep disturbances. A slim person without weight gain, stretch marks spontaneously appeared on her hips. Nothing made sense—a healthy young woman's body shouldn't just start breaking down. She saw a great many doctors—an endocrinologist, pain management specialist, primary care physician, cardiologist, gastroenterologist—all of them to no avail. Then she found me (Dr. Phillips), and thankfully, she responded very well to treatment. She's now back to a full life with great health.

Even the most well-connected among us can experience a merciless road to recovery. David Leite is a memoirist, cookbook author, food writer, and publisher of the two-time James Beard Award–winning website Leite's Culinaria.[3] He's also a long-time sufferer from bipolar disorder. When two tick bites led to worse manifestations of the disorder, coupled with a long list of symptoms such as pain and burning in his feet, headaches, diarrhea, profuse sweating, and distractibility, he sought help from numerous doctors. But those doctors attributed his symptoms to being overweight and to the side effects of the medication he took for his bipolar disorder. It took him six years to find Dr. Phillips and relief. During this period, he saw a parade of doctors — cardiologists, dermatologists, gastroenterologists, neurologists, headache specialists, acupuncturists, massage therapists, and chiropractors — and not one uttered the words "Lyme disease." Among the more insulting diagnoses he received: "an overexcited nervous system," hypochondria, overactive imagination, and psychological releasing of trauma after having written his memoir. He was told more than once that he was "too smart for his own good." Now he advises people who find themselves where he was years ago to keep searching for answers, trust yourself, and push onward. And when you can, pay it forward. Help others to consider Lyme disease and its associated Lyme+ infections as a possible cause of mysterious illnesses.

In David's words: "These days, I find my mood to be greatly improved. I remember one morning looking out the kitchen window and thinking, 'I haven't felt this good in years and years.' And it wasn't just the relief of physical symptoms but also the lift in my mood. The passion for my work returned, I had energy to tackle my to-do lists, I could focus better, and, the biggest sign of mental health for me: I wanted to socialize. My partner and I returned to the days of entertaining and cooking for friends several times a month, having weekend guests, and going places with friends. Also, a resiliency returned. I've been better able to cope with the ups and downs of life. Most important, I've been able to get so much more out of therapy than I had in years."

Nick is a corporate executive and former investment banker with an economics degree from Harvard and a law degree from a great Southern university. When he was suddenly struck by psoriasis in 2001, he was given steroids and biologic immunosuppressants. His wife, a close friend of Dana's, became suspicious after hearing about all the skin conditions Lyme+ can cause. She encouraged him to see a Lyme doctor, especially once he couldn't bend his index finger and sharp pains were migrating throughout his body. Nick had been a varsity runner

in high school and college, but now had trouble walking. His dermatologist, who'd pushed for more immunosuppressants, scoffed: "Lyme
doctors are quacks. We just need to get you back on Humira and all
this stuff will go away." A week or two after that exchange, tests came
back from another doctor: Nick was infected with more than one vector-borne illness, including *Bartonella*, which was thought to be causing his psoriasis. He has no idea when he became infected but recalls
many tick bites as a kid growing up down South. Notably, Nick's psoriasis largely cleared with several rounds of antibiotics and he's been off
of Humira for many months. He tells it like it is: "The medical community is a name-and-prescribe profession. Rheumatologists and dermatologists are glorified drug-pushers."

That doctors tend to dole out palliative medicine without looking
at the bigger picture, as well as discredit or belittle patients who beg for
their symptoms to be taken seriously, is not an American phenomenon. The challenges of Lyme+ are a global problem.

According to a 2016 survey by NorVect, the Nordic Network for
Vector-borne Diseases, 88 percent of Norwegian patients feel that
they're not taken seriously in their health care system; 76 percent said
their general practitioner was unwilling or unable to prescribe antibiotics due to strict guidelines; and a whopping 92 percent were sick
for longer than twelve months.[4] Sissel Davidsson, who is now in remission in Norway and is involved with Lyme+ disease awareness, got
to the point where she was bedridden, paralyzed, and in a wheelchair
when tests showed she had multiple vector-borne infections — from
Lyme and *Bartonella* to tularemia, *Rickettsia*, *Anaplasma*, *Ehrlichia*,
and *Babesia*. Prior to these tests, doctors rejected her suggestion that
she could have Lyme and told her to "think positive thoughts." She
eventually received proper treatment from a combination of specialists from her home country, as well as Germany and New York. One of
her most salient points: "What puzzles me is that when I had rosacea
when I was young, I was offered years of treatment with doxycycline,
but when I was paralyzed and in a wheelchair, I was denied the same
antibiotic treatment."

Jack Lambert is a Scottish infectious disease doctor who is currently working as an infectious disease consultant in a public hospital in Dublin, Ireland. He started treating Lyme+ patients more than twenty years ago in the U.S. He sees many similarities between HIV, hepatitis C, transplant medicine, and the many complications that patients with Lyme and co-infections live with. He told us: "We need to better train primary care doctors, those who would see such patients early in their infection, so they have a high degree of suspicion, and to consider these infections where the history and examination are suggestive. The testing can sometimes be helpful, but the art of medicine continues to require a good, inquiring doctor who asks the right questions. As we currently only have imperfect, indirect measures to test patients in most clinical settings worldwide, we must continue to use our clinical skills and clinical suspicion to initiate treatment and to evaluate response to treatment . . . The even greater challenge is for those who have 'long-standing infection' or 'partially treated infection' with Lyme borreliosis, and possibly other 'co-infections.' In this situation it is much more complex, and there is a well-recognized cascade of immunological and inflammatory responses that are part of these persistent infections. Such complex interactions have been described for other infections including HIV and billions of research monies have been invested to better understand them. The debate of whether these clinical conditions are truly 'post-infectious' and just immunological and inflammatory in nature without persistent infection is not a helpful debate in our quest for 'better science.' Nor is it helpful to the sick patients with suspected but not proven tick-borne infections.

"There are volumes of published studies to support a better understanding of these complex interactions between vector-borne infections and the host response to invasion by the multiple pathogens inoculated by these vectors. However, reading the medical literature on Lyme disease over the last thirty years shows very little progress, as we continue to be caught in the debate, rather than investing our energy and resources into better understanding of these 'cryptic' infections. Without such changes in approach, new science will never be invested in, and sick patients will accumulate. Clearly this is an unacceptable position to take."

Dr. Christian Perronne is one of the most prominent medical scientists in Europe. He takes the Lyme+ epidemic seriously and has helped many French Lyme+ patients in his hospital near Paris. He is Professor of Infectious and Tropical Diseases at Versailles Saint-Quentin-en-Yvelines University. Before 2015, discussion of chronic Lyme disease and other "crypto-infections" in the French media was constrained. But when a brave journalist wrote about it in July 2016, the Lyme cause reached a fever pitch, landing on the cover page of a weekly magazine with an eye-popping headline: "Lyme Disease, This Epidemic That Is Hidden From You! 100 Physicians Raise the Alarm." In September that year, the minister of health, director general of health, and High Authority for Health (Haute Autorité de Santé, HAS) acknowledged that Lyme is a great public health problem and that diagnostic methods and treatment strategies should be revised. The minister of health acknowledged publicly that many chronic Lyme patients are abandoned and rejected by the health system. She announced a national plan against Lyme disease and other vector-borne diseases. For the first time, public funds were made available for research. A research project of a national cohort of patients was planned. In 2017, the European Centre for Disease Prevention and Control published a handbook and manual for the prioritization of infectious disease threats, which includes Lyme among the thirty most threatening diseases in public health.

According to Perronne, "The medical condition of many Lyme patients improves with prolonged anti-infectious treatments following the short-term antibiotic treatment officially recommended. Journalists were convinced by their medical history, especially when they were cured after years or decades of medical errancy. In 2014, the French High Council for Public Health (Haut Conseil de la Santé Publique) has acknowledged the lack of sensitivity of Lyme serologies and has recommended that, in the absence of reliable diagnostic tests, an empiric antibiotic treatment is to be given to patients with a probable Lyme borreliosis or another crypto-infection. However, the situation is blocked, despite the fact that the persistence of *Borrelia* after antibiotic treatment is now evident in the literature. Not a single study has evaluated a really prolonged antibiotic or anti-infectious treatment versus placebo. In four published randomized studies, the duration of treatment evaluated versus placebo was short, from four weeks to three months maximum . . . The time has come to stop discussing any more and to act to save lives."[5]

In Africa, Professor Oladapo Adenrele Ashiru is sounding the alarm on Lyme+. He is the CEO of the Institute of Reproductive Medicine in Lagos, Nigeria. He is one of the world's most eminent specialists in the field of fertility treatment and recognizes the link between infertility in both men and women and undiagnosed Lyme. As we mentioned, Lyme is rarely discussed in Africa, where concerns about malaria continue to take center stage. Dr. Ashiru writes, "What if we tell you that there are other insects [in Africa] biting us and giving us even more deadly diseases than malaria? There are many different insects biting us and giving us illnesses, which have been classified as Lyme disease . . . The difficulty is that, unlike malaria that shows signs and symptoms like fever and headache within a few days of the bite, Lyme is a more intelligent pathogen that shows no signs until later stages when fully developed inside the body, in places like the joints or the spinal cord or the reproductive system."[6] He adds: "The same is true of infertility due to Lyme infections that affects both male and female infertility. In most cases, it is not diagnosed. If pregnant women are infected, they sometimes pass Lyme to their unborn children. Some doctors believe other types of human to human transmission are possible." "Intelligent pathogen," indeed — more like "evil genius."

But still, when we think about the future of Lyme+, we feel hopeful. Every day there seems to be a piece in the news about it. The world is finally waking up to the pandemic and the denialism cannot be sustained. The data speaks and will inform how we deal with this pandemic and search for better treatment options and preventative strategies.

Our friend and colleague Dr. Neil Spector at Duke University is on the cutting edge of the research and is exploring how revolutions in cancer medicine could apply to Lyme+. As he told us: "Having been involved in cancer research for nearly thirty years, I have been fortunate to have led the translational research programs for two molecular targeted cancer therapies, which are both FDA approved, one for the treatment of women with advanced stage HER2+ breast cancer and the other for pediatric acute lymphoblastic leukemia. I decided that the successful lessons in translating cancer research into targeted and immunotherapies that have transformed clinical outcomes in children and adults with previously rapidly lethal cancers could be applied to changing the paradigm of therapeutics for the treatment of tick and other vector-borne diseases." Dr. Spector is using genomic and proteomic information on different species and strains of *Borrelia* and *Bartonella* to develop non-antibiotic, molecular targeted therapies that are directed at the Achilles heel of these microbes, sparing normal tissue and the microbiome. His team is also interested in the development of immunotherapies that will re-educate an individual's immune response to recognize and eliminate *Borrelia* and *Bartonella* (for starters), in a manner similar to the immunotherapies that have transformed the treatment of a wide variety of cancers.

In the process of developing these targeted therapies, he has identified a compound that appears to specifically target a *Borrelia* protein, which has enabled him to use the compound in combination with an imaging substance to image *Borrelia* in infected animals. He is extremely hopeful that this approach can lead to a *Borrelia* "scan" to diagnose individuals with suspected Lyme and also to monitor the efficacy of treatment—something that is currently lacking. Dr. Spector says, "My personal experience, and hearing from folks around the globe on a near daily basis about their horror stories, has only strengthened my resolve and commitment to develop more reliable diagnostics, and safer and more effective therapeutics using scientific rationale rather than empiricism to transform the lives of those suffering the debilitating consequences of *Borrelia*, *Bartonella* and other infections related to vector-borne pathogens."

In May 2018, I (Dr. Phillips) was lucky enough to be awarded the Emerging Leader Scientific Grant from The Bay Area Lyme Foundation, an eminent non-profit that has funded some of the most innovative and translational research in the area of Lyme+. The grant was awarded to study and develop an innovative therapy I devised for the treatment of *Bartonella* and Lyme. To this end, I've organized a study protocol whereby we're evaluating white blood cells that harbor infection with *B. burgdorferi* and *B. henselae* to see if the study medication clears the infections. If so, we plan to move on to animal studies. Dana and I are working to move this project forward together, along with researchers from Duke and Stanford, and many others.

We take for granted today the lower rates or total eradication of many of the infectious diseases that once decimated populations and frightened people: cholera, plague, smallpox, and polio, to name a few. But we can no longer ignore the expanding pandemic of zoonotic infections. The truth of this should not be politicized. The lunacy of Lyme+ reminds us of a story about a nineteenth-century doctor who discovered something that should have revolutionized medicine at the time but would take several decades to be adopted.

Ignaz Semmelweis is not a household name, but the habit he championed more than 150 years ago should be. Semmelweis was a prickly Hungarian obstetrician who had long abandoned the idea that illness was caused by an imbalance of bad air or evil spirits — an idea that was embraced for centuries until medicine caught up to knowledge about the real origins of disease, such as pathogens. He started to collect data in the maternity ward of the clinic where he worked at the General Hospital of Vienna. He wanted to know why so many women in one of the maternity wards were dying from puerperal fever, also known as childbed fever. In the ward where doctors and medical students tended to patients, the patients died at a rate nearly five times higher than women in the maternity ward staffed by midwives. Semmelweis realized that the big difference between the two wards was that the doctors were doing autopsies and the midwives weren't. That was a clue. Semmelweis hypothesized that the students were picking up particles from cadavers they were dissecting and that these particles would end up in the women whose babies they were delivering. He ordered his medical staff to start cleaning their hands and instruments, not just with soap, but with a chlorine solution. We all know that chlorine is a great disinfectant, but Semmelweis didn't know anything about germs. He merely chose chlorine because he thought it would be the best way to get rid of any smell left behind by the corpse particles. Soon after he imposed this new rule, the rate of childbed fever plummeted dramatically.

On May 15, 1850, Semmelweis stepped up to the podium of the Vienna Medical Society's lecture hall, where some of medicine's greatest discoveries were first announced, and told his colleagues to start washing their hands. But on that day, his "discovery" would not be heard. Nobody wanted to listen to Semmelweis; many were outraged at the suggestion that they were the cause of their patients' miserable deaths. And they never did listen to him — Semmelweis died in 1865, at only forty-seven years old, never having lived to see the acceptance of his ideas. Just a couple of years later, in 1867, the Scottish surgeon Joseph Lister, whom we mentioned earlier, presented the theory and practice of antiseptic surgery, which included washing the hands with carbolic acid to prevent infection. He apparently had never heard of Semmelweis. The germ theory of disease had just been born through the work of Louis Pasteur between 1860 and 1865. By 1876, the German physician Robert Koch had successfully linked a germ, *Bacillus anthracis*, to a specific infectious disease, anthrax. How many people could have been saved if doctors had listened to Semmelweis? He was right. Mainstream medicine, steeped in bias toward doing things the old ways based on entrenched dogma, was wrong.

Today millions of people around the world are paying a heavy price for the failure of our medical community to recognize the pandemic in plain sight, and to address and treat Lyme+ properly. Those who subscribe to the wrong narrative may as well be subscribing to the "bad air and evil spirits" theory of disease. We need more Semmelweises. We need to wash our hands clean of the dirty politics of medicine and forge ahead with resolve to end the scourge of chronic and autoimmune diseases with science. After all, science is truth found out.[7] May that truth prevail for the sake of us all.

Bibliography

Abbott, Alison. 2005. "Medical Nobel Awarded for Ulcers." *Nature* (October 3). https://www.nature.com.

Abelson, Reed. 2020. "Covid Overload: U.S. Hospitals Are Running Out of Beds for Patients." *New York Times,* November 27. https://www.nytimes.com/2020/11/27/health/covid-hospitals-overload.html.

Aberer, E., M. Kehldorfer, B. Binder, and H. Schauperi. 1999. "The Outcome of Lyme Borreliosis in Children." *Wiener Klinische Wochenschrift* 111: 941–944.

Adams, Anthony J. 1948. "The Rural Life Crusade." *American Journal of Economics and Sociology,* vol. 8, no 1, 37.

Ahmadi, M. H., A. Mirsalehian, M. A. Sadighi Gilani, et al. 2017. "Asymptomatic Infection with *Mycoplasma hominis* Negatively Affects Semen Parameters and Leads to Male Infertility as Confirmed by Improved Semen Parameters after Antibiotic Treatment." *Urology* 100: 97–102.

Alabiad, C. R., T. A. Albini, C. I. Santos, and J. L. Davis. 2010. "Ocular Toxocariasis in a Sero-negative Adult." *Ophthalmic Surgery, Lasers, and Imaging Retina* (April): 1–3.

Alsolamy, Sami, and Yaseen M. Arabi. 2015. "Infection with Middle East Respiratory Syndrome Coronavirus." *Canadian Journal of Respiratory Therapy* 51, no. 4: 102. https://www.ncbi.nlm.nih.gov/pmc/articles/PMC4631129/.

American Cancer Society. 1994. "Questionable Methods of Cancer Management: Electronic Devices." *CA: Cancer Journal for Clinicians* 44, no. 2 (March–April): 115–127.

American Psychological Association. 2018. "Can Psychedelic Drugs Heal?" Public release, August 9. https://www.eurekalert.org

Anderson, Pauline. 2013. "Low Back Pain Linked to Bacterial Infection." Medscape, May 8. https://www.medscape.com/viewarticle/803858#:~:text=New%20research%20suggests%20that%20some,relief%20by%20taking%20an%20antibiotic.

The Angiogenesis Foundation. https://angio.org/who-we-are/.

Arbour, Nathalie, et al. 1999. "Acute and Persistent Infection of Human Neural Cell Lines by Human Coronavirus OC43." *Journal of Virology* 73, no. 4 (April): 3338–3350. https://www.ncbi.nlm.nih.gov/pmc/articles/PMC104098/.

Arbour, Nathalie, et al. 2000. "Neuroinvasion by Human Respiratory Coronaviruses." *Journal of Virology* 74, no. 19: 8913–8921. doi: 10.1128/JVI.74.19.8913-8921.2000.

Argyriou, A. A., P. Karanasios, A. Papapostolou, et al. 2018. "Neurobrucellosis Presenting as Clinically Definite Amyotrophic Lateral Sclerosis." *International Journal of Neuroscience* 128, no. 7.

ASCO Post. 2019. "FDA Approves the NovoTTF-100L System in Combination with Chemotherapy for Malignant Pleural Mesothelioma." Posted May 28. https://www.ascopost.com

Ashiru, Oladapo. 2019. "Managing Problems Caused by Lyme Disease." *The Punch Newspaper,* January 16.

Aung-Din, D., D. R. Sahni, J. L. Jorizzo, and S. R. Feldman. 2018. "Morgellons Disease: Insights into Treatment." *Dermatology Online Journal* 24, no. 11.

Azoulay, Pierre, Christian Fons-Rosen, and Joshua S. Graff Zivin. 2019. "Does Science Advance One Funeral at a Time?" *American Economic Review* 109, no. 8: 2889.

Azuma, K., I. Uchiyama, M. Tanigawa, et al. 2019. "Chemical Intolerance: Involvement of Brain Function and Networks after Exposure to Extrinsic Stimuli Perceived as Hazardous." *Environmental Health and Preventive Medicine* 24, no. 61.

Bachmaier, K., and J. M. Penninger. 2005. "Chlamydia and Antigenic Mimicry." *Current Topics in Microbiology and Immunology* 296: 153–163.

Baker, Christopher M., Matthew J. Ferrari, and Katriona Shea. 2018. "Beyond Dose: Pulsed Antibiotic Treatment Schedules Can Maintain Individual Benefit while Reducing Resistance." *Scientific Reports* 8: 5866.

Balandraud, N., J. Roudier, and C. Roudier. 2004. "Epstein-Barr Virus and Rheumatoid Arthritis." *Autoimmunity Reviews* 3, no. 5 (July): 362–367.

Banerjee, B., and L. Petersen. 2009. "Psychosis Following Mycoplasma Pneumonia." *Military Medicine* 174, no. 9 (September): 1001–1004.

Battafarano, D. F., J. A. Combs, R. J. Enzenauer, et al. 1993. "Chronic Septic Arthritis Caused by *Borrelia burgdorferi.*" *Clinical Orthopedics and Related Research* 297: 238–241.

Bauer, Lucy. 2015. "The Great Willy Burgdorfer." The NIH's Intramural Research Program, February 2. https://irp.nih.gov/

Beatman, E.L., A. Massey, K.D. Shives et al. 2015. "Alpha-Synuclein Expression Restricts RNA Viral Infections in the Brain." *J Virol* 90, no. 6: 2767–82.

Belluck, Pam. 2020. "He Was Hospitalized for COVID-19. Then Hospitalized Again. And Again." *New York Times,* December 30. https://www.nytimes.com/2020/12/30/health/covid-hospital-readmissions.html.

Bennet, L., and J. Berglund. 2002. "Reinfection with Lyme Borreliosis: A Retrospective Follow-up Study in Southern Sweden." *Scandinavian Journal of Infectious Diseases* 34: 183–186.

Berk, Michael, Lana J. Williams, Felice N. Jacka, et al. 2013. "So Depression Is an Inflammatory Disease, but Where Does the Inflammation Come From?" *BMC Medicine* 11: 200.

Bharathan, B., L. Backhouse, D. Rawat, et al. 2016. "An Unusual Case of Seronegative, 16S PCR Positive Brucella Infection." *JMM Case Reports* 3, no. 5 (October): e005050.

Billeter, S. A., M. G. Levy, B. B. Chomel, and E. B. Breitschwerdt. 2008. "Vector Transmission of *Bartonella* Species with Emphasis on the Potential for Tick Transmission." *Medical and Veterinary Entomology* 22: 1–15.

Blankenship, Kyle, 2019. "Enbrel." fiercepharma.com/special-report/3-enbrel.

Boggs, Dierdre. 2001. Interview with Dr. Willy Burgdorfer. National Institutes of Health. https://history.nih.gov

Boyle, N. B., C. Lawton, and L. Dye. 2017. "The Effects of Magnesium Supplementation on Subjective Anxiety and Stress: A Systematic Review." *Nutrients* 9, no. 5 (April): E429.

Bozbaş, G. T., A. İ. Ünübol, and G. Gürer. 2016. "Seronegative Brucellosis of the Spine: A Case of Psoas Abscess Secondary to Brucellar Spondylitis." *European Journal of Rheumatology* 3, no. 4 (December): 185–187.

Bozkurt, B., E. G. Dumlu, M. Tokac, et al. 2015. "Methylene Blue as an Antioxidant Agent in Experimentally-induced Injury in Rat Liver." *Bratislavske Lekarske Listy* 116, no. 3: 157–161.

Bradley, W. G., R. X. Miller, and T. D. Levine. 2018. "Studies of Environmental Risk Factors in Amyotrophic Lateral Sclerosis (ALS) and a Phase I Clinical Trial of L-Serine." *Neurotoxicity Research* 33, no. 1 (January): 192–198.

Brant, S. V., and E. S. Loker. 2009. "Schistosomes in the Southwest United States and Their Potential for Causing Cercarial Dermatitis or 'Swimmer's Itch.'" *Journal of Helminthology* 83, no. 2 (June): 191–198.

Breitschwerdt, Edward B., Rosalie Greenberg, Ricardo G. Maggi, et al. 2019. "*Bartonella henselae* Bloodstream Infection in a Boy with Pediatric Acute-onset Neuropsychiatric Syndrome." *Journal of Central Nervous System Disease* 11 (March): 1179573519832014.

Breitschwerdt, Edward B., Ricardo G. Maggi, Peter Farmer, and Patricia E. Mascarelli. 2010. "Molecular Evidence of Perinatal Transmission of *Bartonella vinsonii* subsp. *berkhoffii* and *Bartonella henselae* to a Child." *Journal of Clinical Microbiology* 48, no. 6 (June): 2289–2293.

Briones-Vozmediano, E., and E. Espinar-Ruiz. 2019. "How Do Women Suffering from Multiple Chemical Sensibility Experience the Medical Encounter? A Qualitative Study in Spain." *Disability and Rehabilitation* (Aug. 13): 1–11.

Brom, D., Y. Stokar, C. Lawi, et al. 2017. "Somatic Experiencing for Posttraumatic Stress Disorder." *Journal of Traumatic Stress* 30, no. 3 (June): 304–312.

Brorson, O., S. H. Brorson, T. H. Henriksen, et al. 2001. "Association between Multiple Sclerosis and Cystic Structures in Cerebrospinal Fluid." *Infection* 29: 315–319.

Bullmore, Edward. 2018. *The Inflamed Mind: A Radical New Approach to Depression*. New York: Picador.

Burgdorfer, W., A. G. Barbour, S. F. Hayes, et al. 1982. "Lyme Disease — A Tick-borne Spirochetosis?" *Science* 216, no. 4552 (June): 1317–1319.

Cabello, F. C., H. P. Godfrey, J. V. Bugrysheva, and S. A. Newman. 2017. "Sleeper Cells: The Stringent Response and Persistence in the *Borreliella* (*Borrelia*) *burgdorferi* Enzootic Cycle." *Applied and Environmental Microbiology* 19, no. 10 (October): 3846–3862.

Callahan, Patricia, and Trine Tsouderos. 2010. "Chronic Lyme Disease: A Dubious Diagnosis." *Chicago Tribune*, December 8.

Cartter, M. L., and J. L. Hadler. 1989. "Reinfection with *Borrelia burgdorferi*." *Connecticut Medicine* 53: 376–377.

Caskey, J. R., N. R. Hasenkampf, D. S. Martin, et al. 2019. "The Functional and Molecular Effects of Doxycycline Treatment on *Borrelia burgdorferi* Phenotype." *Frontiers in Microbiology* 10, no. 690.

Center for Food Security and Public Health. No date. "Brucellosis: *Brucella melitensis*." Fact Sheet. http://www.cfsph.iastate.edu/Factsheets/pdfs/brucellosis_melitensis.pdf

Centers for Disease Control and Prevention. No date. "Heartland and Bourbon Virus Diseases." https://www.cdc.gov/ticks/tickbornediseases/heartland-virus.html

Centers for Disease Control and Prevention. 2011. "National Notifiable Diseases Surveillance System, Lyme Disease." https://wwwn.cdc.gov/

Centers for Disease Control. 2013. "CDC SARS Response Timeline." April 26. https://www.cdc.gov/about/history/sars/timeline.htm.

Centers for Disease Control. 2013a. "CDC Provides Estimate of Americans Diagnosed with Lyme Disease Each Year." Press release, August 19. https://www.cdc.gov/

Centers for Disease Control. 2013b. "Diagnosis and Management of Q Fever — United States, 2013." *Morbidity and Mortality Weekly Report* 62, no. 3 (March 29).

Centers for Disease Control. 2015. "U.S. Public Health Service Syphilis Study at Tuskegee." December 22. https://www.cdc.gov/tuskegee/timeline.htm

Centers for Disease Control. 2019a. "Lyme Disease: Data and Surveillance." February 5. https://www.cdc.gov/lyme/datasurveillance/index.html

Centers for Disease Control. 2019b. "Parasites — Toxocariasis." September 3. https://www.cdc.gov/parasites/toxocariasis/epi.html

Centers for Disease Control. 2019c. "Q Fever." January 15. https://www.cdc.gov/qfever/symptoms/index.html

Centers for Disease Control. 2019d. "What You Need to Know about Lyme Carditis." October 23. https://www.cdc.gov/lyme/signs_symptoms/lymecarditis.html

Chaignat, Valérie, Marina Djordjevic-Spasic, Anke Ruettger, et al. 2014. "Performance of Seven Serological Assays for Diagnosing Tularemia." *BMC Infectious Diseases* 14: 234.

Chamberlain, S. R., J. Cavanagh, P. de Boer, et al. 2019. "Treatment-resistant Depression and Peripheral C-reactive Protein." *British Journal of Psychiatry* 214, no. 1 (January): 11–19.

Chandrasekaran, N. C., W. Y. Sanchez, Y. H. Mohammed, et al. 2016. "Permeation of Topically Applied Magnesium Ions through Human Skin Is Facilitated by Hair Follicles." *Magnesium Research* 29, no. 2 (June): 35–42.

Chen, Min, Zhi-Yun Du, Xi Zheng, et al. 2018. "Use of Curcumin in Diagnosis, Prevention, and Treatment of Alzheimer's Disease." *Neural Regeneration Research* 13, no. 4 (April): 742–752.

Cheslock, M. A., and M. E. Embers. 2019. "Human Bartonellosis: An Underappreciated Public Health Problem?" *Tropical Medicine and Infectious Diseases* 4, no. 2 (April): E69.

Cheung, Chun Chau Lawrence, et al. 2020. "Residual SARS-CoV-2 Viral Antigens Detected in Gastrointestinal and Hepatic Tissues from Two Recovered COVID-19 Patients." *MedRxiv,* November 3 (preprint). doi: https://doi.org/10.1101/2020.10.28.20219014.

Choi, Bina, et al. 2020. "Persistence and Evolution of SARS-CoV-2 in an Immunocompromised Host." *New England Journal of Medicine,* November 11. doi: 10.1056/NEJMc2031364.

Chomel, B. B., H. J. Boulouis, E. B. Breitschwerdt, et al. 2009. "Ecological Fitness and Strategies of Adaptation of *Bartonella* Species to Their Hosts and Vectors." *Veterinary Research* 40: 29.

Chomel, B. B., R. W. Kasten, K. Floyd-Hawkins, et al. 1996. "Experimental Transmission of *Bartonella henselae* by the Cat Flea." *Journal of Clinical Microbiology* 34: 1952–1956.

Chopra, Vineet, et al. 2020. "Sixty-Day Outcomes among Patients Hospitalized with COVID-19." *Annals of Internal Medicine,* November 11. doi: https://doi.org/10.7326/M20-5661.

Chou, R., L. H. Huffman, R. Fu, et al. 2005. "Screening for HIV: A Review of the Evidence for the U.S. Preventive Services Task Force." *Annals of Internal Medicine* 143, no. 1 (July): 55–73.

Chu, K., W. Chen, C. Y. Hsu, et al. 2019. "Increased Risk of Rheumatoid Arthritis among Patients with Mycoplasma Pneumonia: A Nationwide Population-based Cohort Study in Taiwan." *PLoS One* 14, no. 1 (January): e0210750.

CNBC Television. 2020. "World Health Organization Holds News Conference on Coronavirus Outbreak." February 11. https://www.youtube.com/watch?v=edvsh6x_f4Q.

Condemi, J. J. 1992. "The Autoimmune Diseases." *JAMA* 268, no. 20 (November): 2882–2892.

Cong, W., X.X. Zhang, N. Zhou, et al. 2014. "*Toxocara* Seroprevalence among Clinically Healthy

Individuals, Pregnant Women and Psychiatric Patients and Associated Risk Factors in Shandong Province, Eastern China." *PLoS Neglected Tropical Diseases* 8, no. 8 (Aug): e3082.

Constantino, G., A. Rivera, D. Banuelos, et al. 2009. "Presence of *Mycoplasma fermentans* in the Bloodstream of Mexican Patients with Rheumatoid Arthritis and IgM and IgG Antibodies Against Whole Microorganism." *BMC Musculoskeletal Disorders* 10: 97.

Cook, Michael J. 2015. "Lyme Borreliosis: A Review of Data on Transmission Time after Tick Attachment." *International Journal of General Medicine* 8: 1–8.

Cox, F. E. 2001. "Concomitant Infections, Parasites and Immune Responses." *Parasitology* 122: Suppl. S23–38.

Cox, P. A., R. M. Kostrzewa, and G. J. Guillemin. 2018. "BMAA and Neurodegenerative Illness." *Neurotoxicity Research* 33, no. 1 (January): 178–183.

Craft, J. E., D. K. Fischer, G. T. Shimamoto, and A. C. Steere. 1986. "Antigens of *Borrelia burgdorferi* Recognized During Lyme Disease: Appearance of a New Immunoglobulin M Response and Expansion of the Immunoglobulin G Response Late in the Illness." *Journal of Clinical Investigation* 78, no. 4: 934–939.

Crocetti, S., C. Beyer, G. Schade, et al. 2013. "Low Intensity and Frequency Pulsed Electromagnetic Fields Selectively Impair Breast Cancer Cell Viability." *PLoS One* 8, no. 9: e72944.

Crossland, Nicholas A., Xavier Alvarez, and Monica E. Embers. 2018. "Late Disseminated Lyme Disease." *American Journal of Pathology* 188, no. 3 (March): 672–682.

Croxatto, A., N. Rieille, T. Kernif, et al. 2014. "Presence of Chlamydiales DNA in Ticks and Fleas Suggests that Ticks Are Carriers of *Chlamydiae*." *Ticks and Tick-Borne Diseases* 5, no. 4 (June): 359–365.

Dattwyler, Raymond J., David J. Volkman, Benjamin J. Luft, et al. 1988. "Seronegative Lyme Disease." *New England Journal of Medicine* 319: 1441–1446.

Davidsson, Marcus. 2018. "The Financial Implications of a Well-hidden and Ignored Chronic Lyme Disease Pandemic." *Healthcare* (Basel) 6, no. 1 (March): 16.

de Jager, C. A., A. Oulhaj, R. Jacoby, et al. 2012. "Cognitive and Clinical Outcomes of Homocysteine-lowering B-vitamin Treatment in Mild Cognitive Impairment: A Randomized Controlled Trial." *International Journal of Geriatric Psychiatry* 27, no. 6: 592–600.

Delong, A.K., B. Blossom, E.L. Maloney, et al. 2012. "Antibiotic Retreatment of Lyme Disease in Patients with Persistent Symptoms." *Contemp Clin Trials* 33, no. 6 (Nov):1132–42.

DeLong, A., M. Hsu, and H. Kotsoris. 2019. "Estimation of Cumulative Number of Post-treatment Lyme Disease Cases in the US, 2016 and 2020." *BMC Public Health* 19 (April): 352.

Dennis, D. T., and E. B. Hayes. 2002. "Epidemiology of Lyme Borreliosis." In *Lyme Borreliosis: Biology, Epidemiology and Control*, edited by O. Kahl, J. S. Gray, R. S. Lane, and G. Stanek, 251–280. Oxford: CABI Publishing, 2002.

Derrick, E. H. 1983. "'Q' Fever, a New Fever Entity: Clinical Features, Diagnosis and Laboratory Investigation." *Reviews of Infectious Diseases* 5, no. 4 (July–August): 790–800.

Dias De Melo, Guilherme, et al. 2020. "COVID-19-Associated Olfactory Dysfunction Reveals SARS-CoV-2 Neuroinvasion and Persistence in the Olfactory System." *BioRxiv*, November 18. doi: https://doi.org/10.1101/2020.11.18.388819.

El-Diasty, M., G. Wareth, F. Melzer, et al. 2018. "Isolation of *Brucella abortus* and *Brucella melitensis* from Seronegative Cows Is a Serious Impediment in Brucellosis Control." *Journal of Veterinary Sciences* 5, no. 1 (March): E28.

Diethelm, Pascal, and Martin McKee. 2009. "Denialism: What Is It and How Should Scientists Respond?" *European Journal of Public Health* 19, no. 1 (January): 2–4.

Diniz, Breno Satler, Rodrigo Machado-Vieira, and Orestes Vicente Forlenza. 2013. "Lithium and Neuroprotection: Translational Evidence and Implications for the Treatment of Neuropsychiatric Disorders." *Neuropsychiatric Disease and Treatment* 9: 493–500.

Donta, S.T. 1997. "Tetracycline Therapy for Chronic Lyme Disease," *Clin Infect Dis.* Suppl 1 (Jul): S52–6.

Douaud, G., H. Refsum, C. A. de Jager, et al. 2013. "Preventing Alzheimer's Disease-related Gray Matter Atrophy by B-vitamin Treatment." *Proceedings of the National Academy of Sciences of the United States of America* 110, no. 23: 9523–9528.

Drago, Francesco, et al. 2020. "Human Herpesvirus-6, -7, and Epstein-Barr Virus Reactivation in Pityriasis Rosea during COVID-19." *Journal of Medical Virology*, September 24. doi: https://doi.org/10.1002/jmv.26549.

Drummond, M. R., L. S. dos Santos, M. N. da Silva, et al. 2019. "False Negative Results in Bartonellosis Diagnosis." *Vector-Borne and Zoonotic Diseases* 19, no. 6: 453–454.

Dysautonomia International. No date. "Instructions for POTS Exercise Program—Children's Hospital of Philadelphia." https://www.dysautonomiainternational.org/pdf/CHOP_Modified_Dallas_POTS_Exercise_Program.pdf

Dysautonomia International. No date. "Lifestyle Adaptations for POTS." https://dysautonomiainternational.org/page.php?ID=44

Dysautonomia International. No date. "Postural Orthostatic Tachycardia Syndrome (POTS)." http://dysautonomiainternational.org/conditions.php?ID=1

Ebel, G., and L. Kramer. 2004. "Short Report: Duration of Tick Attachment Required for Transmission of Powassan Virus by Deer Ticks." *American Journal of Tropical Medicine and Hygiene* 71, no. 3 (September): 268–271.

Eddie, B., F. J. Radovsky, D. Stiller, and N. Kumada. 1969. "Psittacosis-lymphogranuloma Venereum (PL) Agents (Bedsonia, Chlamydia) in Ticks, Fleas, and Native Mammals in California." *American Journal of Epidemiology* 90, no. 5 (November): 449–460.

Embers, Monica E., Nicole R. Hasenkampf, Mary B. Jacobs, et al. 2017. "Variable Manifestations, Diverse Seroreactivity and Post-treatment Persistence in Non-human Primates Exposed to *Borrelia burgdorferi* by Tick Feeding." *PLoS One* 12, no. 12: e0189071.

EMDR Institute. No date. "Research Overview." www.EMDR.com.

Endo, Y., T. Shirai, M. Saigusa, and E. Mochizuki. 2017. "Severe Acute Asthma Caused by *Chlamydophila pneumoniae* Infection." *Respirology Case Reports* 5, no. 4 (July): e00239.

Endresen, G. K. 2003. "Mycoplasma Blood Infection in Chronic Fatigue and Fibromyalgia Syndromes." *Rheumatology International* 23, no. 5 (September): 211–215.

Facco, F., G. Grazi, S. Bonassi, et al. 1992. "Chlamydial and Rickettsial Transmission through Tick Bite in Children." *Lancet* 339, no. 8799 (April): 992–993.

Fainardi, E., M. Castellazzi, S. Seraceni, et al. 2008. "Under the Microscope: Focus on *Chlamydia pneumoniae* Infection and Multiple Sclerosis." *Current Neurovascular Research* 5, no. 1 (February): 60–70.

Fallon, B., and J. A. Nields. 1994. "Lyme Disease: A Neuropsychiatric Illness." *American Journal of Psychiatry* 151, no. 11 (November): 1571–1583.

Farmer, Aaron, Thomas Beltran, and Young Sammy Choi. 2017. "Prevalence of *Toxocara* Species Infection in the U.S.: Results from the National Health and Nutrition Examination Survey, 2011–2014." *PLoS Neglected Tropical Diseases* 11, no. 7: e000518.

Fatmi, S. S., R. Zehra, and D. O. Carpenter. 2017. "Powassan Virus—A New Reemerging Tick-borne Disease." *Frontiers in Public Health* 5: 342.

Feldman, K.A., D. Stiles-Enos, K. Julian, et al. 2003. "Tularemia on Martha's Vineyard: Seroprevalence and Occupational Risk." *Emerging Infectious Diseases* 9, no. 3 (Mar): 350–354.

Feng, Jie, Paul G. Auwaerter, and Ying Zhang. 2015. "Drug Combinations against *Borrelia burgdorferi* Persisters in Vitro: Eradication Achieved by Using Daptomycin, Cefoperazone and Doxycycline." *PLoS One* 10, no. 3: e0117207.

Feng, J., J. Leone, S. Schweig, et al. 2019. "Evaluation of Natural and Botanical Medicines for Activity Against Growing and Non-growing Forms of *B. burgdorferi*." *bioRxiv* 652057 (May).

Feng, Jie, Tingting Li, Rebecca Yee, et al. 2019. "Stationary Phase Persister/Biofilm Microcolony of *Borrelia burgdorferi* Causes More Severe Disease in a Mouse Model of Lyme Arthritis." *Discovery Medicine* (March 28).

Feng, J., M. Weitner, W. Shi, et al. 2015. "Identification of Additional Anti-persister Activity against *B. burgdorferi* from an FDA Drug Library." *Antibiotics (Basel)* 4, no. 3 (Sept): 397–410.

Feng, J., S. Zhang, W. Shi, et al. 2017. "Selective Essential Oils from Spice or Culinary Herbs Have High Activity against Stationary Phase and Biofilm *Borrelia burgdorferi*." *Frontiers in Medicine* (Lausanne) 4 (October): 169.

Feng, Jie, Shou Zhang, Wanliang Shi, and Ying Zhang. 2016. "Ceftriaxone Pulse Dosing Fails to Eradicate Biofilm-like Microcolony *B. burgdorferi* Persisters Which Are Sterilized by Daptomycin/Doxycycline/Cefuroxime without Pulse Dosing." *Frontiers in Microbiology* 7: 1744.

Feuer, Will. 2020. "Coronavirus Data Has Already Disappeared after Trump Administration Shifted Control from CDC." CNBC, last modified July 17. https://www.cnbc.com/2020/07/16/us-coronavirus-data-has-already-disappeared-after-trump-administration-shifted-control-from-cdc-to-hhs.html.

Filardo, S., M. Di Pietro, A. Farcomeni, et al. 2015. "*Chlamydia pneumoniae*–mediated Inflammation in Atherosclerosis: A Meta-analysis." *Mediators of Inflammation*: 378658.

Fillaux, J., and J.-F. Magnaval. 2013. "Laboratory Diagnosis of Human Toxocariasis." *Veterinary Parasitology* 193, no. 4 (April): 327–336.

Finkelstein, J. L., T. P. Brown, K. L. O'Reilly, et al. 2002. "Studies on the Growth of *Bartonella henselae* in the Cat Flea." *Journal of Medical Entomology* 39: 915–919.

Fox, D. A. 2005. "Etiology and Pathogenesis of Rheumatoid Arthritis." In *Arthritis and Allied Conditions: A Textbook of Rheumatology*, 15th ed., vol. 1, edited by W. J. Koopman, 1089–1107. Philadelphia: Lippincott Williams & Wilkins, 2005.

Fraser, D. D., L. I. Kong, and F. W. Miller. 1992. "Molecular Detection of Persistent *Borrelia burgdorferi* in a Man with Dermatomyositis." *Clinical and Experimental Rheumatology* 10, no. 4 (July–August): 387–390.

Freedberg, A. S., and L. E. Baron. 1940. "The Presence of Spirochetes in Human Gastric Mucosa." *American Journal of Digestive Disorders* 7: 443–445.

Garcia-Monco, J. C., J. Miro Jornet, B. Fernandez Villar, et al. 1990. "Multiple Sclerosis or Lyme Disease? A Diagnosis Problem of Exclusion." *Medicina Clinica* 94, no. 18 (May): 685–688.

Garfield, Eugene. 1989. "Lyme Disease Research Uncovers a Case of Delayed Recognition: Arvid Afzelius and His Successors." In *Essays of an Information Scientist: Creativity, Delayed Recognition, and Other Essays*, vol. 12, p. 345.

Garin, C., and A. Bujadoux. 1922. "Paralysie par les tiques." *Journal de Médecine de Lyon* 71: 765–767.

Garson, Jeremy A., Louise Usher, Ammar Al-Chalabi, et al. 2019. "Quantitative Analysis of Human Endogenous Retrovirus-K Transcripts in Postmortem Premotor Cortex Fails to

Confirm Elevated Expression of HERV-K RNA in Amyotrophic Lateral Sclerosis." *Acta Neuropathologica Communications* 7, no. 45 (March).

Gerber, M. A., E. D. Shapiro, G. S. Burke, et al. 1996. "Lyme Disease in Children in Southeastern Connecticut, Pediatric Lyme Disease Study Group." *New England Journal of Medicine* 335: 1270–1274.

Global Lyme Alliance. No date. "Lyme Disease Testing." https://globallymealliance.org/about-lyme/diagnosis/testing/

Global Lyme Alliance. No date. "What Is Lyme?" https://globallymealliance.org/about-lyme/

Goc, A., A. Niedzwiecki, and M. Rath. 2015. "In Vitro Evaluation of Antibacterial Activity of Phytochemicals and Micronutrients against *Borrelia burgdorferi* and *Borrelia garinii*." *Journal of Applied Microbiology* 119, no. 6 (December): 1561–1572.

Goc, A., A. Niedzwiecki, and M. Rath. 2017. "Reciprocal Cooperation of Phytochemicals and Micronutrients Against Typical and Atypical Forms of *Borrelia* spp." *Journal of Applied Microbiology* 123, no. 3 (September): 637–650.

Golde, W. T., B. Robinson-Dunn, M. G. Stobierski, et al. 1998. "Culture-confirmed Reinfection of a Person with Different Strains of *Borrelia burgdorferi sensu stricto*." *Journal of Clinical Microbiology* 36: 1015–1019.

Gompels, L.L., A. Smith, P.J. Charles, et al. 2006. "Single-blind Randomized Trial of Combination Antibiotic Therapy in Rheumatoid Arthritis." *J Rheumatol.* 33 no. 2 (Feb):224–7.

Gonzalez Gompf, Sandra, Lily Jones, and Charles Patrick Davis. No date. "Middle East Respiratory Syndrome Coronavirus Infection (MERS-CoV Infection)." Medicinenet. https://www.medicinenet.com/mers_middle_east_respiratory_syndrome/article.htm.

Gunnarsson, L. G., and L. Bodin. 2019. "Occupational Exposures and Neurodegenerative Diseases — A Systematic Literature Review and Meta-analyses." *International Journal of Environmental Research and Public Health* 16, no. 3 (January): E337.

Gupta, Aakriti, et al. 2020. "Extrapulmonary Manifestations of COVID-19." *Nature Medicine* 26: 1017–1032. doi: https://doi.org/10.1038/s41591-020-0968-3.

Gürtler, L., U. Bauerfeind, J. Blümel, et al. 2014. "*Coxiella burnetii* — Pathogenic Agent of Q (Query) Fever." *Transfusion Medicine and Hemotherapy* 41, no. 1 (Feb): 60–72.

Guru, P. K., A. Agarwal, and A. Fritz. 2018. "A Miraculous Recovery: *Bartonella henselae* Infection Following a Red Ant Bite." *BMJ Case Reports.* pii: bcr-2017-222326

Gustafson, R., B. Svenungsson, M. Forsgren, et al. 1992. "Two-year Survey of the Incidence of Lyme Borreliosis and Tick-borne Encephalitis in a High-risk Population in Sweden." *European Journal of Clinical Microbiology and Infectious Disease* 11: 894–900.

Gutierrez, R., B. Krasnov, D. Morick, et al. 2015. "*Bartonella* Infection in Rodents and Their Flea Ectoparasites: An Overview." *Vector-Borne and Zoonotic Diseases* 15, no. 1 (January): 27–39.

Hahn, D. L., and R. McDonald. 1998. "Can Acute *Chlamydia pneumoniae* Respiratory Tract Infection Initiate Chronic Asthma?" *Annals of Allergy, Asthma, and Immunology* 81, no. 4 (October): 339–344.

Hakim, Danny, and Matt Richtel. 2019. "Warning of 'Pig Zero': One Drugmaker's Push to Sell More Antibiotics." *New York Times,* June 7.

Halperin, J. J., G. P. Kaplan, S. Brazinsky, et al. 1990. "Immunologic Reactivity against *Borrelia burgdorferi* in Patients with Motor Neuron Disease." *Archives of Neurology* 47, no. 5: 586–594.

Halperin, J. J., B. J. Luft, A. K. Anand, et al. 1989. "Lyme Neuroborreliosis: Central Nervous System Manifestations." *Neurology* 39, no. 6 (June): 753–759.

Han, H., X. Fang, X. Wei, et al. 2017. "Dose-response Relationship between Dietary Magnesium Intake, Serum Magnesium Concentration and Risk of Hypertension." *Nutrition Journal* 16, no. 1 (May): 26.

Hancocks, Nikki. 2020. "Experts Send Vitamin D and Covid-19 Open Letter to World's Governments." Nutraingredients, last modified December 21. https://www.nutraingredients.com/ Article/2020/12/21/Experts-send-Vitamin-D-and-Covid-19-open-letter-to-world-s -governments#.

Hänsel, Y., M. Ackerl, and G. Stanek. 1995. "ALS-like Sequelae in Chronic Neuroborreliosis." *Wiener medizinische Wochenschrift* 145, no. 7: 186–188.

Harrill, Rob. 2000. "Magnetic Fields May Hold Key to Malaria Treatment, UW Researchers Find." *UW News*, March 30.

Hasanjani Roushan, M. R., M. Mohrez, S. M. Smailnejad Gangi, et al. 2004. "Epidemiological Features and Clinical Manifestations in 469 Adult Patients with Brucellosis in Babol, Northern Iran." *Epidemiology and Infection* 132, no. 6 (December): 1109–1114.

Hassler, D., K. Riedel, J. Zorn, and V. Preac-Mursic. 1991. "Pulsed High-dose Cefotaxime Therapy in Refractory Lyme Borreliosis." *Lancet* 338, no. 8760 (July): 193.

Haupl, T., H. Hahn, M. Rittig, et al. 1993. "Persistence of *Borrelia burgdorferi* in Ligamentous Tissue from a Patient with Chronic Lyme Borreliosis." *Arthritis and Rheumatology* 36, no. 11 (November): 1621–1626.

Healio. 2019. "Ebola RNA Persists for Months in Breast Milk, Semen of Survivors." November 19. https://www.healio.com/news/infectious-disease/20191118/ebola-rna-persists-for-months-in-breast-milk-semen-of-survivors.

Herman, Bob 2019. "Humira Sales Approach $20 Billion." axios.com/abbvie-humira-2018-sales-20-billion-e4039176-baeb-44ff-b4fe-1b63005283b9.html

Herwaldt, B., D. H. Persing, E. A. Précigout, et al. 1996. "A Fatal Case of Babesiosis in Missouri: Identification of Another Piroplasm that Infects Humans." *Annals of Internal Medicine* 124, no. 7 (April): 643–650.

Hill, Andrew. 2020. "Unitaid, Part of the World Health Organization Funding Ivermectin Research Targeting COVID-19 Led by British Expert." *TrialSite News* (blog), December 29. https://trialsitenews.com/unitaid-part-of-the-world-health-organization-funding-ivermectin-research-targeting-COVID-19-led-by-british-expert/.

Hokynar, K., J. J. Sormunen, E. J. Vesterinen, et al. 2016. "Chlamydia-like Organisms (CLOs) in Finnish *Ixodes ricinus* Ticks and Human Skin." *Microorganism* 4, no. 3 (Sept): 28.

Hollström, E. 1958. "Penicillin Treatment of Erythema Migrans Afzelius." *Acta Dermato-Venereologica* 38: 285–289.

Honegr, K., D. Hulinska, V. Dostal, et al. 2001. "Persistence of *B. burgdorferi sensu lato* in Patients with Lyme Borreliosis." *Epidemiologie Mikrobiologie Immunologie* 50, no. 1 (Feb): 10–16.

Hook, Sarah A., Christina A. Nelson, and Paul S. Mead. 2015. "U.S. Public's Experience with Ticks and Tick-borne Diseases: Results from National HealthStyles Surveys." *Ticks and Tickborne Diseases* 6, no. 4: 483–488.

Hornig, M., M. A. Bresnahan, X. Che, et al. 2017. "Prenatal Fever and Autism Risk." *Molecular Psychiatry* 23, no. 3 (Mar): 759–766.

Horowitz, Richard I., and Phyllis R. Freeman. 2019. "Precision Medicine: Retrospective Chart Review and Data Analysis of 200 Patients on Dapsone Combination Therapy for Chronic Lyme Disease/Post-treatment Lyme Disease Syndrome: Part 1." *International Journal of General Medicine* 12: 101–119.

Iacobucci, Gareth. 2020. "Long COVID: Damage to Multiple Organs Presents in Young, Low Risk Patients." *BMJ,* November 7: 371. doi: https://doi.org/10.1136/bmj.m4470.

Infectious Diseases Society of America. No date. "IDSA Practice Guidlines." https://www.idsociety.org/practiceguidelines#/date_na_dt/DESC/0/+/

Itzhaki, Ruth F., Richard Lathe, Brian J. Balin, et al. 2016. "Microbes and Alzheimer's Disease." *Journal of Alzheimer's Disease* 51, no. 4: 979–984.

Jacquet, L., and A. Sézary. 1907. "Des formes atypiques et dégénératives du tréponème pale." *Bulletins et mémoires de la Société Médicale des Hôpitaux de Paris* 24: 114.

Jensen, T. B., D. Dalsgaard, and J. B. Johansen. 2014. "Cardiac Arrest Due to Torsades de Pointes Ventricular Tachycardia in a Patient with Lyme Carditis." *Ugeskrift for Læger* 176, no. 35.

Johns Hopkins Newsroom. 2018. "Study Shows Evidence of Severe and Lingering Symptoms in Some after Treatment for Lyme Disease." HopkinsMedicine.org news release, February 1.

Johnson, Lorainne. 2016. "LymePolicyWonk: Misdiagnosis of Lyme Disease as MS." April 19. https://www.lymedisease.org/lymepolicywonk-lyme-neurologic-misdiagnosis/

Johnston, Sebastian L. 2001. "Is *Chlamydia pneumoniae* Important in Asthma? The First Controlled Trial of Therapy Leaves the Question Unanswered." *American Journal of Respiratory and Critical Care Medicine* 164, no. 4 (August).

Joyner, Michael J., et al. 2021. "Convalescent Plasma Antibody Levels and the Risk of Death from Covid-19." *New England Journal of Medicine,* January 13. doi: 10.1056/NEJ Moa2031893.

Kalish, R. A., G. McHugh, J. Granquist, et al. 2001. "Persistence of Immunoglobulin M or Immunoglobulin G Antibody Responses to *Borrelia burgdorferi* 10–20 Years after Active Lyme Disease." *Clinical Infectious Diseases* 33, no. 6 (September): 780–785.

Kanjwal, K., B. Karabin, Y. Kanjwal, and B. P. Grubb. 2011. "Postural Orthostatic Tachycardia Syndrome Following Lyme Disease." *Cardiology Journal* 18, no. 1: 63–66.

Kaplan, Sheila. 2020. "C.D.C. Labs Were Contaminated, Delaying Coronavirus Testing, Officials Say." *New York Times,* last modified May 7. https://www.nytimes.com/2020/04/18/health/cdc-coronavirus-lab-contamination-testing.html.

Katoh, T. 2018. "Multiple Chemical Sensitivity (MCS): History, Epidemiology and Mechanism." *Nihon Eiseigaku Zasshi* 73, no. 1: 1–8.

Keller, A., A. Graefen, M. Ball, et al. 2012. "New Insights into the Tyrolean Iceman's Origin and Phenotype as Inferred by Whole-genome Sequencing." *Nature Comm* 3, no. 698.

Khademvatan, Shahram, Niloufar Khajeddin, Sakineh Izadi, and Elham Yousefi. 2014. "Investigation of Anti-*Toxocara* and Anti-toxoplasma Antibodies in Patients with Schizophrenia Disorder," *Schizophrenia Research and Treatment* 2014: 230349.

Kim, Tae. 2018. "Goldman Sachs Asks in Biotech Research Report: 'Is Curing Patients a Sustainable Business Model?'" CNBC.com, April 11.

Klempner, M.S., R. Noring, and R.A. Rogers. 1993. "Invasion of Human Skin Fibroblasts by the Lyme Disease Spirochete, *Borrelia burgdorferi.*" *J Infect Dis* 167, no. 5 (May): 1074–81.

Klempner, M. S., L. T. Hu, J. Evans, et al. 2001. "Two Controlled Trials of Antibiotic Treatment in Patients with Persistent Symptoms and a History of Lyme Disease." *New England Journal of Medicine* 345, no. 2 (July): 85–92.

Kloppenburg, M., F.C. Breedveld, J.P. Terwiel, et al. 1994. "Monocycline in Active Rheumatoid Arthritis." *Arthritis & Rheumatism* 37, no. 5: 629–636.

Kohler, J., U. Kern, J. Kasper, et al. 1988. "Chronic Central Nervous System Involvement in Lyme Borreliosis." *Neurology* 38, no. 6 (June).

Kolata, Gina. 2016. "Could Alzheimer's Stem from Infections? It Makes Sense, Experts Say." *New York Times*, May 25.

Kraaijeveld, Huib. 2017. "My Fight for the Recognition of Chronic Lyme Borreliosis and Other Crypto-infections: Interview with Professor Perronne." Posted October 14. https://on-lyme.org/

Krause, P. J., D. T. Foley, G. S. Burke, et al. 2006. "Reinfection and Relapse in Early Lyme Disease." *American Journal of Tropical Medicine and Hygiene* 75: 1090–1094.

Krause, Peter J., et al. 2020. "*Borrelia miyamotoi* sensu lato Seroreactivity and Seroprevalence in the Northeastern United States." *PubMed* 7: 1183–1190. doi: 10.3201/eid2007.131587.

Kuchynka, P., T. Palecek, S. Havranek, et al. 2015. "Recent-onset Dilated Cardiomyopathy Associated with *Borrelia burgdorferi* Infection." *Herz* 40, no. 6: 892–897.

Kuhn, M., and R. Bransfield. 2014. "Divergent Opinions of Proper Lyme Disease Diagnosis and Implications for Children Co-morbid with Autism Spectrum Disorder." *Medical Hypotheses* 83, no. 3 (September): 321–325.

Kuhn, P., and G. Steiner. 1917. "Über die Ursache der M.S." *Medizinische Klinik* 13 (1017): 1001.

Kuhn, P., and G. Steiner. 1920. "Über die Ursache der multiplen Sklerose." *Zeitschrift für Hygiene und Infektionskrankheiten* 90, no. 3: 417–422.

Kumar, D. K., S. H. Choi, K. J. Washicosky, et al. 2016. "Amyloid-β Peptide Protects Against Microbial Infection in Mouse and Worm Models of Alzheimer's Disease." *Science Translational Medicine* 8, no. 340 (May): 340ra72.

Landford, Cameron. 2017. "Insurers Accused of Conspiring to Deny Lyme Disease Coverage." Courthouse News Service, November 14. www.courthousenews.com.

Lapenta, Jose. 2018. "Congenital Transmission of Erythema Migrans or Lyme Disease, Myth or Reality?" *Investigative Dermatology and Venereology Research* (September).

Latov, N., A. T. Wu, R. L. Chin, et al. 2004. "Neuropathy and Cognitive Impairment Following Vaccination with OspA Protein of *B. burgdorferi*." *Journal of the Peripheral Nervous System* 9, no. 3 (September): 165–167.

Lavelle, Marianne. 2014. "Mothers May Pass Lyme Disease to Children in the Womb." *Scientific American*, September 22.

Lawrence, C., R.B. Lipton, F.D. Lowy et al. 1995. "Seronegative Chronic Relapsing Neuroborreliosis." *Eur Neurol* 35:113–117.

Lawton, Samuel, and Abhilasha Sharma. 2017. "Psychiatric Manifestations of *Toxocara*." *Progress in Neurology and Psychiatry* 21 (January–March).

Lee, S. H., J. E. Healy, and J. S. Lambert. 2019. "Single Core Genome Sequencing for Detection of Both *Borrelia burgdorferi sensu lato* and Relapsing Fever *Borrelia* Species." *International Journal of Environmental Research and Public Health* 16, no. 10 (May): E1770.

Li, T., J. Feng, S. Xiao, et al. 2019. "Identification of FDA-approved Drugs with Activity against Stationary Phase *Bartonella henselae*." *Antibiotics* (Basel) 8, no. 2.

Liegner, Kenneth B. 2019. "Disulfiram (Tetraethylthiuram Disulfide) in the Treatment of Lyme Disease and Babesiosis." *Antibiotics* (Basel) 8, no. 2 (June): 72.

Liu, Hong, Zhenzhen Wang, Fangfang Bao, et al. 2019. "Evaluation of Prospective HLA-B*13:01 Screening to Prevent Dapsone Hypersensitivity Syndrome in Patients with Leprosy." *JAMA Dermatology* 155, no. 6: 666–672.

Liu, Jie, et al. 2020. "A Comparative Overview of COVID-19, MERS and SARS: Review Article." *National Center for Biotechnology Information* 81: 1–8. doi: 10.1016/j.ijsu.2020.07.032.

Lobraico, J., A. Butler, J. Petrini, and R. Ahmadi. 2014. "New Insights into Stages of Lyme Disease Symptoms from a Novel Hospital-based Registry." *Primary Care Community Health* 5, no. 4 (October): 284–287.

Lonn, E., S. Yusuf, M. J. Arnold, et al. 2006. "Homocysteine Lowering with Folic Acid and B Vitamins in Vascular Disease." *New England Journal of Medicine* 354, no. 15: 1567–1577.

Lorber, B. 1996. "Are All Disease Infectious?" *Annals of Internal Medicine* 125, no. 10 (November): 844–851.

Loria-Kohen, V., C. Gómez-Candela, S. Palma-Milla, et al. 2013. "A Pilot Study of Folic Acid Supplementation for Improving Homocysteine Levels, Cognitive and Depressive Status in Eating Disorders." *Nutrición Hospitalaria* 28, no. 3: 807–815.

Loria-Kohen, V., H. Marcos-Pasero, R. de la Iglesia, et al. 2017. "Multiple Chemical Sensitivity: Genotypic Characterization, Nutritional Status and Quality of Life in 52 Patients." *Medicina Clínica* 149, no. 4: 141–146.

Luft, B. J., C. R. Steinman, H. C. Neimark, et al. 1992. "Invasion of the Central Nervous System by *Borrelia burgdorferi* in Acute Disseminated Infection." *JAMA* 267, no. 10 (March): 1364–1367.

Luger, S. W., P. Paparone, G. P. Wormser, et al. 1995. "Comparison of Cefuroxime Axetil and Doxycycline in Treatment of Patients with Early Lyme Disease Associated with Erythema Migrans." *Antimicrobial Agents and Chemotherapy* 39: 661–667.

Lulu, A.R., G.F. Araj, M.I. Khateeb, et al. 1988. "Human Brucellosis in Kuwait: A Prospective Study of 400 Cases." *Q. J. Med.* 66 no. 249 (Jan): 39–54.

Lupkin, Sydney. 2020. "Gilead Lobbying Increased as Interest in COVID-19 Treatment Remdesivir Climbed." WGBH, May 2. https://www.wgbh.org/national-news/2020/05/02/gilead-lobbying-increased-as-interest-in-covid-19-treatment-climbed.

Lyme Disease Association. 2002. "Special Report: LDA Meets with FDA on Lymerix." January 22. https://lymediseaseassociation.org

LymeDisease.org. 2015. "Is Lyme Disease the New AIDS?" November 3.

Ma, X., W. Shi, and Y. Zhang. 2019. "Essential Oils with High Activity against Stationary Phase *Bartonella henselae*." Preprints.org, October 16.

Macdonald, A. B., and J. M. Miranda. 1987. "Concurrent Neocortical Borreliosis and Alzheimer's Disease." *Human Pathology* 18, no. 7 (July): 759–761.

Manouélian, Y. 1930. "Gommes syphilitiques et formes anormales du treponemes: Ultra-virus syphilitiques." *Comptes Rendus des Séances de la Société de Biologie et de ses Filiales* 104: 249–251.

Manouélian, Y. 1935. "Syphilis tardive: Formes minuscules du *Spirochaeta pallida*, spirochetogène syphilitique." *Annales de l'Institute Pasteur* 55: 698–708.

Mansueto, Pasquale, et al. 2012. "Prevalence of Antibodies anti-*Bartonella henselae* in Western Sicily: Children, Blood Donors, and Cats." *PubMed* 33, no. 1: 18–25. doi: 10.1080/15321819.2011.591476.

Marcin, Ashley. 2019. "What You Need to Know about the MTHFR Gene." *Healthline*, August 14.

Marcus, S., P. Marquis, and C. Sakai. 1997. "Controlled Study of Treatment of PTSD Using EMDR in an HMO Setting." *Psychotherapy* 34: 307–315.

Al-Mariri, A., and M. Safi. 2013. "The Antibacterial Activity of Selected Labiatae (Lamiaceae) Essential Oils against *Brucella melitensis*." *Iranian Journal of Medical Sciences* 38, no. 1 (March): 44–50.

Marks, D. H. 2011. "Neurological Complications of Vaccination with Outer Surface Protein A (OspA)." *International Journal of Risk Safety in Medicine* 23, no. 2: 89–96.

Martens, Christopher R., Blair A. Denman, Melissa R. Mazzo, et al. 2018. "Chronic Nicotin-amide Riboside Supplementation Is Well-tolerated and Elevates NAD+ in Healthy Mid-dle-aged and Older Adults." *Nature Communications* 9, no. 1286.

Mascarelli, P. E., R. G. Maggi, S. Hopkins, et al. 2013. "*Bartonella henselae* Infection in a Family Experiencing Neurological and Neurocognitive Abnormalities after Woodlouse Hunter Spider Bites." *Parasites and Vectors* 6: 98.

Mathias, C. J., D. A. Low, V. Iodice, et al. 2011. "Postural Tachycardia Syndrome — Current Experience and Concepts." *Nature Reviews Neurology* 8: 22–34.

Matschke, Jacob, et al. 2020. "Neuropathology of Patients with COVID-19 in Germany: A Post-Mortem Case Series." *The Lancet* 19, no. 11: 919–929. doi: https://doi.org/10.1016/S1474-4422(20)30308-2.

Mattman, L. H. 2000. *Cell Wall Deficient Forms: Stealth Pathogens.* Boca Raton: CRC Press.

Mayo Clinic. 2020. "*Helicobacter pylori* (*H. pylori*) Infection." Mayo Clinic, April 8. https://www.mayoclinic.org/diseases-conditions/h-pylori/symptoms-causes/syc-20356171.

McCall, Becky. 2020. "Vitamin D Deficiency in COVID-19 Quadrupled Death Rate." Medscape, December 11. https://www.medscape.com/viewarticle/942497.

McClure, R., D. Yanagisawa, D. Stec, et al. 2015. "Inhalable Curcumin: Offering the Potential for Translation to Imaging and Treatment of Alzheimer's Disease." *Journal of Alzheimer's Disease* 44, no. 1: 283–295.

Mech, A. W., and A. Farah. 2016. "Correlation of Clinical Response with Homocysteine Reduc-tion during Therapy with Reduced B Vitamins in Patients with MDD Who Are Positive for MTHFR C677T or A1298C Polymorphism: A Randomized, Double-blind, Placebo-con-trolled Study." *Journal of Clinical Psychiatry* 77, no. 5: 668–671.

Meng, Y., J. Li, X. Chen, et al. 2018. "Association between Folic Acid Supplementation and Retinal Atherosclerosis in Chinese Adults with Hypertension Complicated by Diabetes Mellitus." *Frontiers in Pharmacology* 9: 1159.

Middelveen, M. J., K. R. Filush, C. Bandoski, et al. 2019. "Mixed *Borrelia burgdorferi* and *Helico-bacter pylori* Biofilms in Morgellons Disease Dermatological Specimens." *Healthcare* (Basel) 7, no. 2: 70.

Million, M., et al. 2020. "Clinical Efficacy of Chloroquine Derivatives in COVID-19 Infection: Comparative Meta-Analysis between the Big Data and the Real World." *New Microbes New Infect* 38: 100709. doi: 10.1016/j.nmni.2020.100709.

Mirkin, Gabe. 2019. "Barry Marshall, from Quack to Nobel Prize." April 7. https://www.drmir-kin.com

Miziara, C. S. M. G., V. A. Gelmeti Serrano, and N. Yoshinari. 2018. "Passage of *Borrelia burg-dorferi* through Diverse Ixodid Hard Ticks Causes Distinct Diseases: Lyme Borreliosis and Baggio-Yoshinari Syndrome." *Clinics* (São Paolo) 73.

Mohney, Gillian. 2016. "Zika Virus: President Obama Urges Congress to Pass Funding to Fight Virus." ABC News, May 20.

Montoya, J. G., A. M. Kogelnik, M. Bhangoo, et al. 2013. "Randomized Clinical Trial to Evaluate the Efficacy and Safety of Valganciclovir in a Subset of Patients with Chronic Fatigue Syn-drome." *Journal of Medical Virology* (Aug. 19).

Moolgavkar, S. R. 1912. "On Certain Bodies Found in Syphilitic Lesions Demonstrated by the Jelly Method." *British Medical Journal* 2, no. 2711 (December): 1655–1656.

Moritz, E. D., C. S. Winton, L. Tonnetti, et al. 2016. "Screening for *Babesia microti* in the U.S. Blood Supply." *New England Journal of Medicine* 375, no. 23 (December): 2236–2245.

Motamedi, H., E. Darabpour, M. Gholipour, et al. 2010. "In Vitro Assay for the Anti-*Brucella*

Activity of Medicinal Plants Against Tetracycline-resistant *Brucella melitensis.*" *Journal of Zhejiang University Science B: Biomedicine and Biotechnology* 11, no. 7 (July): 506–511.

Mullooly, C., and S. P. Higgins. 2010. "Secondary Syphilis: The Classical Triad of Skin Rash, Mucosal Ulceration and Lymphadenopathy." *International Journal of STD and AIDS* 21, no. 8 (August): 537–545.

Naktin, Jaan Peter. 2017. "Late You Come: Legislation on Lyme Treatment in an Era of Conflicting Guidelines." *Open Forum Infectious Diseases* 4, no. 4 (Fall).

Nasralla, M., J. Haier, and G. L. Nicolson. 1999. "Multiple Mycoplasmal Infections Detected in Blood of Patients with Chronic Fatigue Syndrome and/or Fibromyalgia Syndrome." *European Journal of Clinical Microbiology and Infectious Diseases* 18, no. 12 (December): 859–865.

National Institute of Allergy and Infectious Diseases. 2020."NIH Clinical Trial Shows Remdesivir Accelerates Recovery from Advanced COVID-19." April 29. https://www.niaid.nih.gov/news-events/nih-clinical-trial-shows-remdesivir-accelerates-recovery-advanced-covid-19.

National Institutes of Health. 2019. "Estimates of Funding for Various Research, Condition, and Disease Categories." Table published April 19. https://report.nih.gov

Nijs, Jo, Garth L. Nicolson, Pascale De Becker, et al. 2002. "High Prevalence of Mycoplasma Infections among European Chronic Fatigue Syndrome Patients: Examination of Four Mycoplasma Species in Blood of Chronic Fatigue Syndrome Patients." *FEMS Immunology & Medical Microbiology* 34, no. 3 (November): 209–214.

Noble, Holocomb B. 2000. "3 Suits Say Lyme Vaccine Caused Severe Arthritis." *New York Times,* June 13.

Nouri, Ali. Federation of American Scientists. https://fas.org/expert/ali-nouri/.

Novak, P., D. Felsenstein, C. Mao, et al. 2018. "Association of Small Fiber Neuropathy and Post Treatment Lyme Disease Syndrome." *PLoS One* 14, no 2: e0212222.

Nowakowski, J., R. B. Nadelman, R. Sell, et al. 2003. "Long-term Follow-up of Patients with Culture-confirmed Lyme Disease." *American Journal of Medical Sciences* 115: 91–96.

Nowakowski, J., I. Schwartz, R. B. Nadelman, et al. 1997. "Culture-confirmed Infection and Reinfection with *Borrelia burgdorferi.*" *Annals of Internal Medicine* 127: 130–132.

Nunes, M.A., N.M. Schöwe, K.C. Monteiro-Silva, et al. 2015. "Chronic Microdose Lithium Treatment Prevented Memory Loss and Neurohistopathological Changes in a Transgenic Mouse Model of Alzheimer's Disease." *PLoS One* 10, no. 11: e0142267.

Ocon, A. J., A. V. Kwiatkowski, and R. Peredo-Wende. 2018. "Adult-onset Still's Disease with Haemorrhagic Pericarditis and Tamponade Preceded by Acute Lyme Disease." *BMJ Case Rep.* (Aug) pii: bcr-2018-225517.

O'Dell, J. R., J. R. Elliott, J. A. Mallek, et al. 2006. "Treatment of Early Seropositive Rheumatoid Arthritis: Doxycycline plus Methotrexate versus Methotrexate Alone." *Arthritis and Rheumatology* 54, no. 2 (February): 621–627.

Ogrendik, M. 2007. "Effects of Clarithromycin in Patients with Active Rheumatoid Arthritis." *Current Medical Research and Opinion* 23, no. 3 (March): 515–522.

Ogrendik, M. 2009. "Rheumatoid Arthritis Is Linked to Oral Bacteria: Etiological Association." *Mod Rheumatol.* 19 no. 5: 453–6.

Ogrendik, Mesut. 2014. "Antibiotics for the Treatment of Rheumatoid Arthritis." *International Journal of General Medicine* 7: 43–47.

Ogrendik, M. and N. Karagoz. 2011. "Treatment of Rheumatoid Arthritis with Roxithromycin: A Randomized Trial." *Postgrad Med.* 123 no. 5 (Sep): 220–7.

Ohn, J., S. Y. Park, and J. Moon. 2017. Morgellons disease. *Ann Dermatol.* 29: 223–225.

Oksi, J., H. Kalimo, R. J. Marttila, et al. 1996. "Inflammatory Brain Changes in Lyme Borreliosis." *Brain* 119, Pt. 6 (December): 2143–2154.

Oksi, J., M. Marjamaki, J. Nikoskelainen, and M. K. Vijanen. 1999. "*Borrelia burgdorferi* Detected by Culture and PCR in Clinical Relapse of Disseminated Lyme Borreliosis." *Annals of Medicine* 31, no. 3 (June): 225–232.

Oksi, J., J. Mertsola, M. Reunanen, et al. 1994. "Subacute Multiple-site Osteomyelitis Caused by *Borrelia burgdorferi*." *Clinical Infectious Diseases* 19, no. 5 (November): 891–896.

Oregon Occupational Safety and Health. 2020. "N95 Respirator — How to Put On and Use." June 23. https://www.youtube.com/watch?v=ucmx_hj1SW8.

Parent, Michael D. No date. "The Case for Chronic Infection: Evidential Persistence of *Borrelia* Species Post Antibiotic Exposure in Vivo and in Vitro." https://pdfs.semanticscholar.org/

Parish, Dana. 2016. "'A Slow Slipping Away' — Kris Kristofferson's Long-undiagnosed Battle with Lyme Disease." The Huffington Post, July 6.

Park, Matthew D. 2020. "Macrophages: A Trojan Horse in COVID-19?" *Nature Reviews Immunology* 20: 351. doi: https://doi.org/10.1038/s41577-020-0317-2.

Park, S.C. J.C. Moon, S.Y. Shin, et al. 2016. "Functional Characterization of Alpha-synuclein Protein with Antimicrobial Activity." *Biochem Biophys Res Commun.* 478 no. 2 (Sep): 924–8.

Paul, A. 2001. "Arthritis, Headache, Facial Paralysis: Despite Negative Laboratory Tests *Borrelia* Can Still Be the Cause." *MMW Fortschritte der Medizin* 143, no. 6 (February): 17.

Pearce, A., C. Lockwood, C. van den Heuvel, and J. Pearce. 2017. "The Use of Therapeutic Magnesium for Neuroprotection During Global Cerebral Ischemia Associated with Cardiac Arrest and Cardiac Surgery in Adults: A Systematic Review." *JBI Database of Systematic Reviews and Implement Reports* 15, no. 1 (January): 86–118.

Pfister, H.W., V. Preac-Mursic, B. Wilske, et al. 1991. "Randomized Comparison of Ceftriaxone and Cefotaxime in Lyme Neuroborreliosis." *J Infect Dis.* 163 no. 2 (Feb): 311–8.

Piesman, J. 1995. "Dispersal of the Lyme Disease Spirochete *Borrelia burgdorferi* to Salivary Glands of Feeding Nymphal *Ixodes scapularis* (Acari: Ixodidae)." *Journal of Medical Entomology* 32, no. 4 (July): 519–521.

Pikelj, F., F. Strle, and M. Mozina. 1989. "Seronegative Lyme Disease and Transitory Atrioventricular Block." *Annals of Internal Medicine* 111, no. 1 (July): 90.

Pohl-Koppe, A., E. L. Logigian, A. C. Steere, and D. A. Hafler. 1999. "Cross-reactivity of *Borrelia burgdorferi* and Myelin Basic Protein-specific T Cells Is Not Observed in Borrelial Encephalomyelitis." *Cellular Immunology* 194, no. 1 (May): 118–123.

Poinar, George Jr. 2015. "Spirochete-like Cells in a Dominican Amber *Ambylomma* Tick (Arachnida: Ixodidae)." *Historical Biology* 27, no. 5: 565–570.

Politi, Daniel. 2021. "Concern Increases over Slow Rollout of COVID-19 Vaccines in U.S." *Slate,* January 1. https://slate.com/news-and-politics/2021/01/concern-increases-slow-roll out-covid-vaccines.html

Pothineni, Venkata Raveendra, Dhananjay Wagh, Mustafeez Mujtaba Babar, et al. 2016. "Identification of New Drug Candidates against *Borrelia burgdorferi* Using High-throughput Screening." *Drug Design, Development and Therapy* 10: 1307–1322.

Pozo, Del J. L., M. S. Rouse, and R. Patel. 2008. "Bioelectric Effect and Bacterial Biofilms: A Systematic Review." *International Journal of Artificial Organs* 31, no. 9 (September): 786–795.

Proal, Amy. 2017. "Interview with Evolutionary Biologist Paul Ewald: Infection and Chronic Disease." *MicrobeMinded,* November 11. http://microbeminded.com

———. 2021. (@microbeminded2) "Hey! There are many papers on persistent #coronaviruses. I love this 1979 paper which states, 'The persistent #infections established by some coronaviruses should provide very good experimental models for elucidating the pathogenic mechanisms of some important human #diseases.'" Twitter, January 2. https://twitter.com/microbeminded2/status/1345451224829722626?s=20.

Qureshi, M. Z., D. New, N. J. Zulqarni, et al. 2002. "Overdiagnosis and Overtreatment of Lyme Disease in Children." *Pediatric Infectious Diseases Journal* 21, no. 1 (Jan): 12–14.

Raffalli, J., and G. P. Wormser. 2016. "Persistence of Babesiosis for >2 Years in a Patient on Rituximab for Rheumatoid Arthritis." *Diagnostic Microbiology and Infectious Diseases* 85, no. 2 (June): 231–232.

Randal, Judith, and William Hines. 1987. "Lyme Disease: Focus on a Mysterious 'Imitator.'" *Los Angeles Times*, November 9.

Rebman, Alison W., Kathleen T. Bechtold, Ting Yang, et al. 2017. "The Clinical, Symptom, and Quality-of-life Characterization of a Well-defined Group of Patients with Posttreatment Lyme Disease Syndrome." *Frontiers in Medicine* 4 (December): 224.

Reddy, Sumathi. 2020. "Long-Haul Covid Patients Put Hope in Experimental Drugs." *Wall Street Journal*, last modified December 21. https://www.wsj.com/articles/experimental-drugs-aim-to-treat-long-haul-covid-11608569400?tesla=y.

Relaño-Ginés, A., S. Lehmann, E. Brillaud, et al. 2018. "Lithium as a Disease-modifying Agent for Prion Diseases." *Translational Psychiatry* 8: 163.

Renner, Kerstin, et al. 2020. "T Cell Anergy in COVID-19 Reflects Virus Persistence and Poor Outcomes." *MedRxiv,* September 23. doi: https://doi.org/10.1101/2020.09.21.20198671.

Roberts, A.L., N.J. Johnson, M.E. Cudkowicz, et al. 2016. "Job-related Formaldehyde Exposure and ALS Mortality in the USA." *J Neurol Neurosurg Psychiatry* 87, no 7 (July): 786–8.

Rolain, Jean-Marc, Max Maurin, and Didier Raoult. 2000. "Bactericidal Effect of Antibiotics on *Bartonella* and *Brucella* spp.: Clinical Implications." *Journal of Antimicrobial Chemotherapy* 46, no. 5 (November): 811–814.

Roos, Robert. 2003. "Estimates of SARS Death Rates Revised Upward." Center for Infectious Disease and Policy, May 7. https://www.cidrap.umn.edu/news-perspective/2003/05/estimates-sars-death-rates-revised-upward.

Rosado, M. M., M. Simkó, M. O. Mattsson, and C. Pioli. 2018. "Immune-modulating Perspectives for Low Frequency Electromagnetic Fields in Innate Immunity." *Frontiers in Public Health* 6 (March): 85.

Rosenberg, Ronald, Nicole P. Lindsey, Marc Fischer, et al. 2018. "Vital Signs: Trends in Reported Vector-borne Disease Cases — United States and Territories, 2004–2016." *The Centers for Disease Control and Prevention Morbidity and Mortality Weekly Report* (*MMWR*) 67, no. 17 (May 4): 496–501.

Rossi, S., and A. Pitidis. 2018. "Multiple Chemical Sensitivity: Review of the State of the Art in Epidemiology, Diagnosis, and Future Perspectives." *Journal of Occupational and Environmental Medicine* 60, no. 2: 138–146.

Rudenko, N., M. Golovchenko, M. Vancova, et al. 2016. "Isolation of Live *Borrelia burgdorferi sensu lato* Spirochaetes from Patients with Undefined Disorders and Symptoms Not Typical for Lyme Borreliosis." *Clinical Microbiology and Infection* 22, no. 3 (March): 267.

Saeki, Y., T. Mima, S. Sakoda, et al. 1992. "Transfer of Multiple Sclerosis into Severe Combined Immunodeficiency Mice by Mononuclear Cells from Cerebrospinal Fluid of the Patients." *PNAS* 89 no. 13: 6157–6161.

Salazar, J. C., M. A. Gerber, and C. W. Goff. 1993. "Long-term Outcome of Lyme Disease in Children Given Early Treatment." *Journal of Pediatrics* 122: 591–593.

Sapi, E., R. S. Kadliwala, H. Ismail, et al. 2019. "The Long-term Persistence of *Borrelia burgdorferi* Antigens and DNA in the Tissues of a Patient with Lyme Disease." *Antibiotics* (Basel) 8, no. 4.

Sapi, Eva, et al. 2019. "The Long-Term Persistence of *Borrelia burgdorferi* Antigens and DNA in the Tissues of a Patient with Lyme Disease." *PubMed* 11;8, no. 4: 183, doi: 10.3390/antibiot ics8040183.

Saraiva, Danilo G., Herbert S. Soares, João Fábio Soares, et al. 2014. "Feeding Period Required by *Amblyomma aureolatum* Ticks for Transmission of *Rickettsia rickettsii* to Vertebrate Hosts." *Emerging Infectious Diseases* 20, no. 9 (September): 1504–1510.

Satchell, Graham. 2016. "Autism in Women 'Significantly Underdiagnosed.'" BBC News, August 31.

Saviola, G., L. Abdi-Ali, L. Campostrini, et al. 2013. "Clarithromycin in Rheumatoid Arthritis: The Addition to Methotrexate and Low-dose Methylprednisolone Induces a Significant Additive Value." *Rheumatology International* 33, no. 11 (Nov): 2833–2838.

Schardt, F.W. 2004. "Clinical Effects of Fluconazole in Patients with Neuroborreliosis," *Eur J Med Res* 9, no. 7: 334–6.

Schmidli, J., T. Hunziker, P. Moesli, and U. B. Schaad. 1988. "Cultivation of *Borrelia burgdorferi* from Joint Fluid Three Months after Treatment of Facial Palsy due to Lyme Borreliosis." *Journal of Infectious Diseases* 158, no. 4: 905–906.

Schnyder, G., M. Roffi, R. Pin, et al. 2001. "Decreased Rate of Coronary Restenosis after Lowering of Plasma Homocysteine Levels." *New England Journal of Medicine* 345, no. 22: 1593–1600.

Schwarzwalder, A., M. F. Schneider, A. Lydecker, and J. N. Aucott. 2010. "Sex Differences in the Clinical and Serologic Presentation of Early Lyme Disease: Results from a Retrospective Review." *Gender Medicine* 7, no. 4 (August): 320–329.

Scrimenti, R. 1970. "Erythema Chronicum Migrans." *Archives of Dermatology* 102: 104–105.

Seki, N., S. Kasai, N. Saito, et al. 2007. "Quantitative Analysis of Proliferation and Excretion of *Bartonella quintana* in Body Lice, *Pediculus humanus L.*" *American Journal of Tropical Medicine and Hygiene* 77: 562–566.

Sessa, Ben. 2012. *The Psychedelic Renaissance: Reassessing the Role of Psychedelic Drugs in 21st Century Psychiatry and Society*. London: Muswell Hill Press.

Shadick, N. A., C. B. Phillips, E. L. Logigian, et al. 1994. "The Long-term Clinical Outcomes of Lyme Disease: A Population-based Retrospective Cohort Study." *Annals of Internal Medicine* 121: 560–567.

Shah, Binita, Jonathan D. Newman, Kathleen Woolf, et al. 2018. "Anti-inflammatory Effects of a Vegan Diet versus the American Heart Association–recommended Diet in Coronary Artery Disease Trial." *Journal of the American Heart Association* 7, no. 23: e011367.

Shapiro, Francine. 2014. "The Role of Eye Movement Desensitization and Reprocessing (EMDR) Therapy in Medicine: Addressing the Psychological and Physical Symptoms Stemming from Adverse Life Experiences." *Permanente Journal* 18, no. 1 (Winter): 71–77.

Sharma, B., A. V. Brown, N. E. Matluck, et al. 2015. "*Borrelia burgdorferi*, the Causative Agent of Lyme Disease, Forms Drug-Tolerant Persister Cells." *Antimicrobial Agents and Chemotherapy* 59, no. 8: 4616–4624.

Shor, S., C. Green, B. Szantyr, et al. 2019. "Chronic Lyme Disease: An Evidence-Based Definition by the ILADS Working Group." *Antibiotics* 8, no. 4 (Dec): 269.

Šmajs, D., L. Paštěková, and L. Grillová. 2015. "Macrolide Resistance in the Syphilis Spirochete,

Treponema pallidum ssp. *pallidum*: Can We Also Expect Macrolide-resistant Yaws Strains?" *American Journal of Tropical Medicine and Hygiene* 93, no. 4 (Oct): 678–683.

Small, Gary, Prabha Siddarth, Zhaoping Li, et al. 2018. "Memory and Brain Amyloid and Tau Effects of a Bioavailable Form of Curcumin in Non-demented Adults." *American Journal of Geriatric Psychiatry* 26, no. 3 (March): 266–277.

Smith, A. D., S. M. Smith, C. A. de Jager, et al. 2010. "Homocysteine-lowering by B Vitamins Slows the Rate of Accelerated Brain Atrophy in Mild Cognitive Impairment: A Randomized Controlled Trial." *PLoS One* 5, no. 9: e12244.

Smith, R. P., R. T. Schoen, D. W. Rahn, et al. 2002. "Clinical Characteristics and Treatment Outcome of Early Lyme Disease in Patients with Microbiologically Confirmed Erythema Migrans." *Annals of Internal Medicine* 136: 421–428.

Smiyan, S., I. Galaychuk, I. Zhulkevych, et al. 2019. "Sjögren's Syndrome and Lymphadenopathy Unraveling the Diagnosis of Lyme Disease." *Reumatologia* 57 no. 1: 59–62.

Snowden, J., and S. Stovall. 2011. "Tularemia: Retrospective Review of 10 Years' Experience in Arkansas." *Clinical Pediatrics* (Phila) 50, no. 1 (January): 64–68.

Song, Li, Yu Yangsheng, Yinshi Yue, et al. 2013. "Microbial Infection and Rheumatoid Arthritis." *Journal of Clinical and Cellular Immunology* 4, no. 6 (December): 174.

Soscia, S. J., J. E. Kirby, K. J. Washicosky, et al. 2010. "The Alzheimer's Disease–Associated Amyloid Beta-protein Is an Antimicrobial Peptide." *PLoS One* 5, no. 3 (March): e9505.

Specter, Michael. 2013. "The Lyme Wars." *New Yorker*, July 1.

Spellberg, B., and J. E. Edwards Jr. 2001. "Type 1/Type 2 Immunity in Infectious Diseases." *Clin Infect Dis.* 32, no 1 (Jan): 76–102.

Spiewak, Jim. 2020. "COVID Long-Hauler Study Found 205 Symptoms in 10 Body Organs." KUTV, December 29. https://kutv.com/news/coronavirus/covid-long-hauler-study-found-200-symptoms-in-10-body-organs.

Stanek, G., and F. Strle. 2003. "Lyme Borreliosis." *Lancet* 362: 1639–1647.

Steere, A. C., J. A. Hardin, and S. E. Malawista. 1978. "Lyme Arthritis: A New Clinical Entity." *Hospital Practice* 13, no. 4: 143–158.

Steere, A. C., S. E. Malawista, D. R. Snydman, et al. 1977. "Lyme Arthritis: An Epidemic of Oligoarticular Arthritis in Children and Adults in Three Connecticut Communities." *Arthritis and Rheumatology* 20: 7–17.

Steiner, G. "Guinea Pig Inoculation with MS Tissues." 1918. *Arch. Psychiat. Nervenkrankh Berlin*, 60.

Steiner, G., "MS Agent Inoculation in Monkeys." 1919. *Z. Neurol. Psychiat. Reger Berlin*, XVLL: 491.

Steiner, Gabriel. 1954. "Morphology of *Spirochaeta myelophthora* in Multiple Sclerosis." *Journal of Neuropathology and Experimental Neurology* 13, no. 1 (January): 221–229.

Stoodley, P., D. deBeer, H. M. Lappin-Scott, et al. 1997. "Influence of Electric Fields and pH on Biofilm Structure as Related to the Bioelectric Effect." *Antimicrobial Agents and Chemotherapy* 41, no. 9 (September): 1876–1879.

Stratton, Charles W. 2016. "A Review of Multiple Sclerosis as an Infectious Syndrome." *Journal of Neurology and Neurophysiology*, October 31.

Stricker, R., and L. Johnson. 2007. "Let's Tackle the Testing." *British Medical Journal* 335, no. 7628 (November): 1008.

Strle, F., V. Maraspin, S. Lotric-Furlan, et al. 1996. "Azithromycin and Doxycycline for Treatment of Borrelia Culture-positive Erythema Migrans." *Infection* 24 no 1 (Jan): 64–8.

Sukenik, S., L. Neumann, D. Buskila, et al. 1990. "Dead Sea Bath Salts for the Treatment of

Rheumatoid Arthritis." *Clinical and Experimental Rheumatology* 8, no. 4 (July–August): 353–357.

Tarleton, E. K., B. Littenberg, C. D. MacLean, et al. 2017. "Role of Magnesium Supplementation in the Treatment of Depression: A Randomized Clinical Trial." *PLoS One* 12, no. 6 (June): e0180067.

Temple-Raston, Dina. 2020. "CDC Report: Officials Knew Coronavirus Test Was Flawed but Released It Anyway." NPR, last modified November 6. https://www.npr.org/2020 /11/06/929078678/cdc-report-officials-knew-coronavirus-test-was-flawed-but-released -it-anyway.

Ternyila, Danielle. 2020. "Leronlimab Appears to Prevent Progression to Severe or Critical COVID-19." Targeted Oncology, November 3. https://www.targetedonc.com/view/leron limab-appears-to-prevent-progression-to-severe-or-critical-covid-19.

Tesini, Brenda L. No date. "Congenital Syphilis" entry in *Merck Manual for Professionals*. https:// www.merckmanuals.com/professional/pediatrics/infections-in-neonates/congenital-syphilis

Theel, Elitza S. 2016. "The Past, Present, and (Possible) Future of Serologic Testing for Lyme Disease." *Journal of Clinical Microbiology* 54, no. 5 (April): 1191–1196.

Thelander, H. E. 1941. "Medical History Repeats Itself." *California and Western Medicine* 55, no. 2 (August): 91–94.

Tilley, B.C., G.S. Alarcón, S.P. Heyse, et al. 1995. "Minocycline in Rheumatoid Arthritis. A 48-week, Double-blind, Placebo-controlled Trial." *Ann Intern Med.* 122 no. 2 (Jan): 81–9.

Trevejo, R. T., P. J. Krause, V. K. Sikand, et al. 1999. "Evaluation of Two-test Serodiagnostic Method for Early Lyme Disease in Clinical Practice." *Journal of Infectious Diseases* 179, no. 4 (April): 931–938.

Triulzi, F., and G. Scotti. 1998. "Differential Diagnosis of Multiple Sclerosis: Contribution of Magnetic Resonance Techniques." *Journal of Neurology, Neurosurgery, and Psychiatry* 64 (May): Suppl. 1:S6–14.

Tsiodras, S., T. Kelesidis, I. Kelesidis, et al. 2006. "*Mycoplasma pneumoniae*–associated Myelitis: A Comprehensive Review." *European Journal of Neurology* 13, no. 2 (February): 112–124.

Tufts, D.M. and M.A. Diuk-Wasser. 2018. "Transplacental Transmission of Tick-borne *Babesia microti* in Its Natural Host *Peromyscus leucopus*." *Parasites and Vectors* 11, no. 1 (May): 286.

Tuller, David. 2020. "At 12, She's a Covid 'Long Hauler.'" *New York Times,* last modified December 4. https://www.nytimes.com/2020/10/22/well/family/coronavirus-symptoms-kids -children-long-hauler.html.

Tzeng, N.S., C.H. Chung, F.H. Lin, et al. 2018. "Anti-herpetic Medications and Reduced Risk of Dementia in Patients with Herpes Simplex Virus Infections: A Nationwide, Population-based Cohort Study in Taiwan." *Neurotherapeutics* 15, no. 2 (April): 417–429.

Ullrich, K., N. Saha, and S. Lake. 2012. "Neuroretinitis Following Bull Ant Sting." *BMJ Case Reports.*

Unal, D., R. Coskun, S. Demir, et al. 2017. "Usefulness of In Vivo and In Vitro Diagnostic Tests in the Diagnosis of Hypersensitivity Reactions to Quinolones and in the Evaluation of Cross-Reactivity." *Allergy Asthma Immunol Res.* 9, no 4 (Jul): 347–359.

U.S. Department of Health and Human Services. 2018. "Tick-borne Disease Working Group 2018 Report to Congress." https://www.hhs.gov/

van Dee, L. M. Stehouwer, and T. van Bemmel. 2018. "Systemic Sarcoidosis Associated with Exposure to *Borrelia burgdorferi* in a 21-Year-Old Man." *Eur J Case Rep Intern Med.*5, no.10: 942.

Villanova, N., F. Azpiroz, and J. R. Malagelada. 1997. "Perception and Gut Reflexes Induced by

Stimulation of Gastrointestinal Thermoreceptors in Humans." *Journal of Physiology* 502, Pt. 1 (July): 215–222.

Virtanen, Jussi Oskari, and Steve Jacobson. 2012. "Viruses and Multiple Sclerosis." *CNS and Neurological Disorders—Drug Targets* 11, no. 5 (August): 528–544.

Vitry, M. A., D. Hanot Mambres, M. Deghelt, et al. 2014. "*Brucella melitensis* Invades Murine Erythrocytes During Infection." *Infection and Immunity* 82, no. 9 (September): 3927–3938.

von Hertzen, L. C. 2002. "Role of Persistent Infection in the Control and Severity of Asthma: Focus on *Chlamydia pneumoniae.*" *European Respiratory Journal* 19: 546–555.

Waddell, L.A., J. Greig, L. R. Lindsay, et al. 2018. "A Systematic Review on the Impact of Gestational Lyme Disease in Humans on the Fetus and Newborn." *PLoS One* 13, no. 11: e0207067.

Waddell, Lisa. A., Judy Greig, Mariola Mascarenhas, et al. 2016. "The Accuracy of Diagnostic Tests for Lyme Disease in Humans: A Systematic Review and Meta-analysis of North American Research." *PLoS One* 11, no. 12: e0168613.

Wang, N., L. Parimi, H. Liu, et al. 2017. "A Review on Dapsone Hypersensitivity Syndrome among Chinese Patients with an Emphasis on Preventing Adverse Drug Reactions with Genetic Testing." *American Journal of Tropical Medicine and Hygiene* 96, no. 5 (May): 1014–1018.

Wang, X., X. Qin, H. Demirtas, et al. 2007. "Efficacy of Folic Acid Supplementation in Stroke Prevention: A Meta-analysis." *Lancet* 369, no. 9576: 1876–1882.

Wang, Yeming, et al. 2020. "Remdesivir in Adults with Severe COVID-19: A Randomised, Double-Blind, Placebo-Controlled, Multicentre Trial." *The Lancet* 395, no. 10236: 1569–1578. doi: 10.1016/S0140-6736(20)31022-9.

Warren, J. R., and B. Marshall. 1983. "Unidentified Curved Bacilli on Gastric Epithelium in Active Chronic Gastritis." *Lancet* 1(8336): 1273–1275.

Warthin, A. S., and R. E. Olson. 1930. "The Granular Transformation of *Spirochaeta pallida* in Aortic Focal Lesions." *American Journal of Syphilis* 14: 433–437.

Warthin, A. S., and R. E. Olsen. 1931. "The Apparent Sequence of Spirochetes and Granular Forms in Syphilitic Buboes." *American Journal of Syphilis* 15: 145.

Watts, M.R., Kim, R., Ahuja, V., et al. 2019. "Comparison of Loop-Mediated Isothermal Amplification and Real-Time PCR Assays for Detection of Strongyloides Larvae in Different Specimen Matrices." *J Clin Microbiol* 57, no. 4 (March): pii: e01173–18.

Weber, K., G. Schierz, B. Wilske, et al. 1986. "Reinfection in Erythema Migrans Disease." *Infection* 14: 32–35.

Weinberg, Uri. 2019. "Novocure's Tumor Treating Fields: Innovative Brain Cancer Therapy with Survival and Safety Benefits." Sponsor Feature in *Nature Research.*

Weintraub, Pamela. 2001. "The Bitter Feud over LYMErix." Posted July 6. http://www.whale.to/

Wells, R., A. J. Spurrier, D. Linz, et al. 2018. "Postural Tachycardia Syndrome: Current Perspectives." *Vascular Health and Risk Management* 14: 1–11.

Wertheim, Joel O., et al. 2013. "A Case for the Ancient Origin of Coronaviruses." *J Virol* 87, no. 12: 7039–7045. doi: 10.1128/JVI.03273-12.

Wilson, E. N., S. Do Carmo, and M. F. Iulita. 2017. "BACE1 Inhibition by Microdose Lithium Formulation NP03 Rescues Memory Loss and Early Stage Amyloid Neuropathology." *Translational Psychiatry* 8, no. 8 (August): e1190.

Winblad, N. E., M. Changaris, and P. K. Stein. 2018. "Effect of Somatic Experiencing Resiliency-based Trauma Treatment Training on Quality of Life and Psychological Health as Potential Markers of Resilience in Treating Professionals." *Frontiers in Neuroscience* 12 (February): 70.

Winkelman, M. 2014. "Psychedelics as Medicines for Substance Abuse Rehabilitation: Evaluating Treatments with LSD, Peyote, Ibogaine and Ayahuasca." *Current Drug Abuse Reviews* 7, no. 2: 101–116.

Witkin, S. S., E. Minis, A. Athanasiou, et al. 2017. "*Chlamydia trachomatis*: The Persistent Pathogen." *Clinical and Vaccine Immunology* 24, no. 10 (October): e00203-17.

World Health Organization. 2003. "Consensus Document on the Epidemiology of Severe Acute Respiratory Syndrome (SARS)." November. https://www.who.int/csr/sars/WHOconsensus.pdf?ua=1.

World Health Organization. 2007. Guidelines on Tularemia. https://www.cdc.gov/

World Health Organization. 2020. "WHO Recommends against the Use of Remdesivir in COVID-19 Patients." November 20. https://www.who.int/news-room/feature-stories/detail/who-recommends-against-the-use-of-remdesivir-in-COVID-19-patients.

Wormser, G. P., R. Ramanathan, J. Nowakowski, et al. 2003. "Duration of Antibiotic Therapy for Early Lyme Disease: A Randomized, Double-blind, Placebo-controlled Trial." *Annals of Internal Medicine* 138: 697–704.

Wright, Jessica. 2013. "Epigenetic: Reversible Tags." *Nature* 498 (June): S10–S11.

Wu, Katherine J., and Gina Kolata. 2020. "Remdesivir Fails to Prevent Covid-19 Deaths in Huge Trial." *New York Times,* last updated November 19. https://www.nytimes.com/2020/10/15/health/coronavirus-remdesivir-who.html.

Wu, Katherine J., Carl Zimmer, and Jonathan Corum. 2021. "Coronavirus Drug and Treatment Tracker." *New York Times,* last updated January 21. https://www.nytimes.com/interactive/2020/science/coronavirus-drugs-treatments.html.

Xue, Y. C., R. Feuer, N. Cashman, and H. Luo. 2018. "Enteroviral Infection: The Forgotten Link to Amyotrophic Lateral Sclerosis?" *Frontiers in Molecular Neuroscience* 11 (March): 63.

Yan, Holly. 2020. "Covid-19 Now Kills More Than 1 American Every Minute. And the Rate Keeps Accelerating as the Death Toll Tops 300,000." CNN, last modified December 14. https://www.cnn.com/2020/12/14/health/us-COVID-deaths-300k/index.html.

Yang, M., W. Guo, C. Yang, et al. 2017. "Mobile Phone Use and Glioma Risk: A Systematic Review and Meta-analysis." *PLoS One* 12, no. 5 (May): e0175136.

Yardley, William. 2014. "Willy Burgdorfer, Who Found Bacteria That Cause Lyme Disease, Is Dead at 89." *New York Times,* November 19.

Yong, Ed. 2020. "Long-Haulers Are Redefining COVID-19." *The Atlantic,* August 19. https://www.theatlantic.com/health/archive/2020/08/long-haulers-covid-19-recognition-support-groups-symptoms/615382/.

Yoon, E. C., E. Vail, G. Kleinman, et al. 2015. "Lyme Disease: A Case Report of a 17-Year-Old Male with Fatal Lyme Carditis." *Cardiovascular Pathology* 24, no. 5: 317–321.

Yu, Ignatius T. S., et al. 2004. "Evidence of Airborne Transmission of the Severe Acute Respiratory Syndrome Virus." *New England Journal of Medicine* 350: 1731–1739. doi: 10.1056/NEJMoa032867.

Zeratsky, Katherine. 2020. "What Is Vitamin D Toxicity? Should I Be Worried about Taking Supplements?" Mayo Clinic, April 17. https://www.mayoclinic.org/healthy-lifestyle/nutrition-and-healthy-eating/expert-answers/vitamin-d-toxicity/faq-20058108.

Zerbo, O., A. M. Iosif, C. Walker, et al. 2013. "Is Maternal Influenza or Fever During Pregnancy Associated with Autism or Developmental Delays? Results from the CHARGE Study." *Journal of Autism and Developmental Disorders* 43, no. 1 (January): 25–33.

Zhan, L., Q. Xie, and R. Tibbetts. 2015. "Opposing Roles of p38 and JNK in a Drosophila Model of TDP-43 Proteinopathy Reveal Oxidative Stress and Innate Immunity as Pathogenic Components of Neurodegeneration." *Human Molecular Genetics* 24, no. 3 (February): 757–772.

Zhao, M., X. Wang, M. He, et al. 2017. "Homocysteine and Stroke Risk: Modifying Effect of Methylenetetrahydrofolate Reductase C677T Polymorphism and Folic Acid Intervention." *Stroke* 48, no. 5: 1183–1190.

Zhou Wenting. 2020. "Shanghai Officials Reveal Novel Coronavirus Transmission Modes." *China Daily*, February 8. https://www.chinadaily.com.cn/a/202002/08/WS5e3e7d 97a310128217275fc3.html.

Zimmerman, J. W., M. J. Pennison, I. Brezovich, et al. 2012. "Cancer Cell Proliferation Is Inhibited by Specific Modulation Frequencies." *British Journal of Cancer* 106, no. 2 (January): 307–313.

Notes

The notes below refer to the book's bibliography, which is a partial list of scientific papers and other references that you might find helpful for learning more about some of the facts and concepts mentioned in this book. If we had our wish, we'd cite every paper we've read on Lyme disease and other vector-borne illnesses, but that would be impossible because the list would come to thousands of entries. At the least, these notes can open doors to further research and inquiry. In addition to published studies, many of which are listed here, this book is also based on numerous interviews we conducted with authors of high-profile research and formally published papers, as well as experts in the subject area of Lyme+ with first-hand knowledge of facts. These people were all gracious enough to grant us permission to quote them directly, either using their names, or anonymously for a variety of reasons.

INTRODUCTION

1. Rosenberg, Lindsey, Fischer, et al. 2018.
2. Global Lyme Alliance, no date, "What Is Lyme?"
3. www.cdc.gov.
4. DeLong, Hsu, and Kotsoris 2019.
5. LymeDisease.org 2015.
6. Randal and Hines 1987.
7. Davidsson 2018.
8. U.S. Department of Health and Human Services 2018.
9. van Dee, Stehouwer, and van Bemmel 2018.

10. Smiyan, Galaychuk, Zhulkevych, et al. 2019.
11. Novak, Felsenstein, Mao, et al., 2018.
12. Ocon, Kwiatkowski, and Peredo-Wende 2018.

1. A WILD FAMILY OF INFECTIONS

1. Global Lyme Alliance, no date, "What Is Lyme?"
2. Spider bites: Mascarelli, Maggi, Hopkins, et al. 2013. Ant bites: Guru, Agarwal, and Fritz 2018; Ullrich, Saha, and Lake 2012.
3. Waddell, Greig, Lindsay, et al. 2018; Lavelle 2014; Tufts and Diuk-Wasser 2018; Breitschwerdt, Maggi, Farmer, and Mascarelli 2010.
4. Stratton 2016.
5. Johnson 2016.
6. Keller, Graefen, Ball, et al. 2012.
7. Poinar 2015.
8. Garfield 1989.
9. Specter 2013.
10. Dennis and Hayes 2002.
11. Scrimenti 1970.
12. Steere, Malawista, Snydman, et al. 1977.
13. Bauer 2015.
14. Yardley 2014.
15. Burgdorfer, Barbour, Hayes, et al. 1982.
16. Garin and Bujadoux 1922.
17. Scrimenti 1970.
18. Steere, Hardin, and Malawista 1978.
19. Shor, Green, Szantyr, et al. 2019.
20. Centers for Disease Control and Prevention 2011.
21. Stanek and Strle 2003.
22. Hollström 1958; Weber, Schierz, Wilske, et al. 1986; Cartter and Hadler 1989; Gustafson, Svenungsson, Forsgren, et al. 1992; Salazar, Gerber, and Goff 1993; Shadick, Phillips, Logigian, et al. 1994; Aberer, Kehldorfer, Binder, and Schauperi 1999; Nowakowski, Nadelman, Sell, et al. 2003; Bennet and Berglund 2002; Gerber, Shapiro, Burke, et al. 1996; Nowakowski, Schwartz, Nadelman, et al. 1997; Golde, Robinson-Dunn, Stobierski, et al. 1998; Smith, Schoen, Rahn, et al. 2002; Luger, Paparone, Wormser, et al. 1995; Wormser, Ramanathan, Nowakowski, et al. 2003; Krause, Foley, Burke, et al. 2006.
23. Steere, Malawista, Snydman, et al. 1977.
24. Lobraico, Butler, Petrini, and Ahmadi 2014.
25. To access a list of over 700 peer-reviewed articles that support the evidence of persistence of Lyme and other tick-borne diseases, go to the ILADS's website at www.ilads.org and download the file: https://www.ilads.org/wp-content/uploads/2018/07/CLDList-ILADS.pdf; also see Parent (no date).

26. Embers, Hasenkampf, Jacobs, et al. 2017; Crossland, Alvarez, and Embers 2017.
27. Rudenko, Golovchenko, Vancova, et al. 2016; Oksi, Marjamaki, Nikoskelainen, and Vijanen 1999.
28. Battafarano, Combs, Enzenauer, and Fitzpatrick 1993.
29. Cabello, Godfrey, Bugrysheva, and Newman 2017; Caskey, Hasenkampf, Martin, et al. 2019; Feng, Li, Yee, et al. 2019; Sharma, Brown, Matluck, et al. 2015.
30. Rebman, Bechtold, Yang, et al. 2017.
31. Johns Hopkins Newsroom 2018.
32. Sapi, Kadliwali, Ismail, et al. 2019.
33. Stricker and Johnson 2007.
34. Chou, Huffman, Fu, et al. 2005.
35. Gutierrez, Krasnov, Morick, et al. 2015; Guru, Agarwal, and Fritz 2018; Ullrich, Saha, and Lake 2012; Mascarelli, Maggi, Hopkins, et al. 2013.
36. Cheslock and Embers 2019.
37. National Institutes of Health 2019.

2. THE MYTHS THAT GET IN THE WAY

1. Chomel, Boulouis, Breitschwerdt, et al. 2009; Billeter, Levy, Chomel, and Breitschwerdt 2008; Chomel, Kasten, Floyd-Hawkins, et al. 1996; Finkelstein, Brown, O'Reilly, et al. 2002; Seki, Kasai, Saito, et al. 2007; Lulu, Araj, and Khateeb 1988.
2. Boggs 2001.
3. "Parasite Immune Evasion," Nature.com, https://www.nature.com/subjects/parasite-immune-evasion
4. Fatmi, Zehra, and Carpenter 2017.
5. Centers for Disease Control and Prevention, no date, "Heartland and Bourbon Virus Diseases."
6. Chu, Chen, Hsu, et al. 2019.
7. Tsiodras, Kelesidis, Kelesidis, et al. 2006.
8. Banerjee and Petersen 2009; Tsiodras, Kelesidis, Kelesidis, et al. 2006.
9. Constantino, Rivera, Banuelos, et al. 2009.
10. Nijs, Nicolson, De Becker, et al. 2002.
11. Endresen 2003; Nasralla, Haier, and Nicolson 1999.
12. Ahmadi, Mirsalehian, Sadighi Gilani, et al. 2017.
13. Eddie, Radovsky, Stiller, and Kumada 1969.
14. Croxatto, Rielle, Kernif, et al. 2014.
15. Hokynar, Sormunen, Vesterinen, et al. 2016.
16. Facco, Grazi, Bonassi, et al. 1992.
17. Filardo, Di Pietro, Farcomeni, et al. 2015.
18. Fainardi, Castellazzi, Seraceni, et al. 2008.
19. Endo, Shirai, Saigusa, and Mochizuki 2017.

20. Hahn and McDonald 1998.
21. Johnston 2001.
22. von Hertzen 2002.
23. Bachmaier and Penninger 2005.
24. Witkin, Minis, Athanasiou, et al. 2017.
25. World Health Organization 2007.
26. Feldman, Stiles-Enos, Julian, et al. 2003.
27. Mascarelli, Maggi, Hopkins, et al. 2013; Guru, Agarwal, and Fritz 2018; Ullrich, Saha, and Lake 2012.
28. Breitschwerdt, Greenberg, Maggi, et al. 2019.
29. The Centers for Disease Control and Prevention, https://www.cdc.gov/dpdx/babesiosis/index.html
30. Hasanjani Roushan, Mohrez, Smailnejad Gangi, et al. 2004.
31. Vitry, Hanot Mambres, Deghelt, et al. 2014.
32. Derrick 1983.
33. Gürtler, Bauerfeind, Blümel, et al. 2014.
34. Centers for Disease Control 2019c.
35. Brant and Loker 2009.
36. Ebel and Kramer 2004.
37. Saraiva, Soares, Soares, et al. 2014.
38. Cook 2015.
39. Piesman 1995.
40. Qureshi, New, Zulqarni, and Nachman 2002.
41. Paul 2001; Pikelj, Strle, and Mozina 1989; Fraser, Kong, and Miller 1992; Oksi, Mertsola, Reunanen, et al. 1994; Honegr, Hulinska, Dostal, et al. 2001; Pfister, Preac-Mursic, Wilske, et al. 1991; Lawrence, Lipton, Lowy, et al. 1995; Oksi, Kalimo, Marttila, et al. 1996.
42. Pfister, Preac-Mursic, Wilske, et al., 1991; Lawrence, Lipton, Lowy, et al., 1995; Oksi, Klaimo, Marttila, et al., 1996.
43. Trevejo, Krause, Sikand, et al. 1999.
44. Luft, Steinman, Neimark, et al. 1992.
45. Steiner 1954; Stratton 2016.
46. Embers, Hasenkampf, Jacobs, et al. 2017.
47. Crossland, Alvarez, and Embers 2018.
48. Schmidli, Hunziker, Moesli, and Schaad 1988.
49. Battafarano, Combs, Enzenauer, and Fitzpatrick 1993.
50. Warren and Marshall 1983.
51. Abbott 2005.
52. Freedberg and Baron 1940; Mirkin 2019.
53. Kim 2018.
54. See LymeHope's downloadable compilation of evidence/literature on transplacental transmission of Lyme+ at https://www.lymehope.ca/resources.html

55. LymeHope.com, News and Updates: https://www.lymehope.ca/news-and
    -updates/world-health-organization-recognizes-congenital-lyme-borreliosis;
    also https://www.lymehope.ca/news-and-updates/world-health-organization
    -who-removes-congenital-lyme-borreliosis-from-icd-11-codes
56. See LymeHope's downloadable compilation of evidence/literature at https://
    www.lymehope.ca/resources.html
57. Waddell, Greig, Robbin, Lindsay, et al. 2018; Lapenta 2018.
58. Azoulay, Fons-Rosen, and Graff Zivin 2019.

3. BITTEN AND BROKEN

1. Unal, Coskun, Demir, et al. 2017.
2. Ohn, Park, and Moon 2017.
3. Aung-Din, Sahni, Jorizzo, and Feldman 2018.
4. Middelveen, Flush, Bandoski, et al. 2019.
5. Tesini, no date; see also the entry for "Syphilis" at The Mayo Clinic's website:
   https://www.mayoclinic.org/diseases-conditions/syphilis/symptoms-causes/syc
   -20351756
6. See the World Health Organization's Fact Sheet for Leptospirosis: http://www
   .searo.who.int/about/administration_structure/cds/CDS_leptospirosis-Fact
   _Sheet.pdf
7. Centers for Disease Control 2019a.
8. Centers for Disease Control 2019b.
9. Farmer, Beltran, and Choi 2017; Centers for Disease Control 2019b.
10. Cong, Zhang, Zhou, et al. 2014.
11. Khademvatan, Khajeddin, Izadi, and Yousefi 2014.
12. Lawton and Sharma 2017.
13. Cox 2001.
14. Spellberg and Edwards 2001.
15. Loria-Kohen, Marcos-Pasero, de la Iglesia, et al. 2017.
16. Briones-Vozmediano and Espinar-Ruiz 2019.
17. Rossi and Pitidis 2018; Katoh 2018; Azuma, Uchiyama, Tanigawa, et al. 2019.
18. Tzeng, Chung, Lin, et al. 2018.
19. Montoya, Kogelnik, Bhangoo, et al. 2013.
20. Kloppenburg, Breedveld, and Terwiel 1994; Tilley, Alarcón, Heyse, et al. 1995;
    Ogrendik 2009; Ogrendik and Karagoz 2011; Gompels, Smith, and Charles 2006.
21. Ogrendik 2007; O'Dell, Elliott, Mallek, et al. 2006; Saviola, Abdi Ali, Cam-
    postrini, et al. 2013.

4. HOW THE MEDICAL WORLD GOT IT SO WRONG

1. Thelander 1941.
2. Centers for Disease Control 2015.

3. Diethelm and McKee 2009.
4. Infectious Diseases Society of America, no date.
5. Jacquet and Sézary 1907; Warthin and Olson 1930; Manouélian 1930; Manouélian 1935; Warthin and Olson 1931; Mattman 2000; Moolgavkar 1912.
6. Feng, Yi, Lee, et al. 2019.
7. Moolgavkar 1912.
8. Shadick, Phillips, Logigian, et al. 1994.
9. Klempner, Hu, Evans, et al. 2001; Delong, Blossom, Maloney, and Phillips 2012.
10. Hakim and Richtel 2019.
11. Mohney 2016.
12. National Institutes of Health 2019.
13. Callahan and Tsouderos 2010.
14. https://www.lymedisease.org/15/
15. Schwarzwalder, Schneider, Lydecker, and Aucott 2010.
16. Parish 2016.
17. Oksi, Kalimo, Marttila, et al. 1996; Oksi, Marjamaki, Nikoskelainen, et al. 1999; Donta 1997.
18. Feng, Li, Yee, et al. 2019.
19. Klempner, Noring, and Rogers 1993; Strle, Maraspin, Lotric-Furlan, et al. 1996; Shadick, Phillips, Logigian, et al. 1994.
20. Naktin 2017.
21. Hook, Nelson, and Mead 2015.
22. See https://underourskin.com/resources
23. See https://static1.squarespace.com/static/53498f16e4b01ce82d4b2228/t/579a8 6e46a49638f9c8366b6/1469744869866/UOS2_claim_references_3.pdf
24. Herman 2019.
25. Blankenship 2019.
26. American Autoimmune Related Diseases Association, Inc., "Autoimmune Disease Statistics," www.aarda.org.
27. Kuchynka, Palecek, Havranek, et al. 2015.
28. Yoon, Vail, Kleinman, et al. 2015; Jensen, Dalsgaard, and Johansen 2014.
29. Centers for Disease Control 2019d.
30. Dysautonomia International, no date, "Postural Orthostatic Tachycardia Syndrome (POTS)."
31. Mathias, Low, and Iodice 2011.
32. Kanjwal, Karabin, Kanjwal, and Grubb 2011.
33. Kanjwal, Karabin, Kanjwal, and Grubb 2011.
34. Dysautonomia International, no date, "Instructions for POTS Exercise Program."
35. Dysautonomia International, no date, "Lifestyle Adaptations for POTS."
36. Kuhn and Steiner 1917; Kuhn and Steiner 1920.

5. MODERN PLAGUES CAUSED BY UNDERLYING INFECTION

1. Garson, Usher, Al-Chalabi, et al. 2019.
2. Xue, Feuer, Cashman, and Luo 2018.
3. Gunnarsson and Bodin 2019.
4. Roberts, Johnson, Cudkowicz, et al. 2016.
5. Cox, Kostrzewa, and Guillemin 2018.
6. Bradley, Miller, and Levine 2018.
7. Hänsel, Ackerl, and Stanek 1995.
8. Halperin, Kaplan, Brazinsky, et al. 1990.
9. Argyriou, Karanasios, Papapostolou, et al. 2018.
10. Garcia-Monco, Miro Jornet, Fernandez Villar, et al. 1990; Kohler, Kern, Kasper, et al. 1988; Pohl-Koppe, Logigian, Steere, and Hafler 1999; Halperin, Luft, Anand, et al. 1989; Triulzi and Scotti 1998.
11. Kuhn and Steiner 1917; Steiner 1918; Steiner 1919; Adams 1948; Saeki, Mima, Sakoda, et al. 1992.
12. Brorson, Brorson, Henriksen, et al. 2001.
13. Virtanen and Jacobson 2012.
14. Wright 2013.
15. Song, Yangsheng, Yue, et al. 2013.
16. Fox 2005; Condemi 1992; Balandraud, Roudier, and Roudier 2004.
17. MacDonald and Miranda 1987.
18. Kumar, Choi, Washicosky, et al. 2016.
19. Soscia, Kirby, Washicosky, et al. 2010.
20. Kolata 2016.
21. Itzhaki, Lathe, Balin, et al. 2016.
22. Park, Moon, and Shin 2016; Beatman, Massey, and Shives 2015.
23. Zhan, Xie, and Tibbetts 2015.
24. Proal 2017.
25. Lorber 1996.
26. Ogrendik 2014.
27. Chen, Du, Zheng, et al. 2018.
28. Tzeng, Chung, Lin, et al. 2018.
29. McClure, Yanagisawa, Stec, et al. 2015.
30. Fallon and Nields 1994.
31. Fallon and Nields 1994.
32. Bullmore 2018.
33. Chamberlain, Cavanagh, de Boer, et al. 2019.
34. Berk, Williams, Jacka, et al. 2013.
35. Marcin 2019.
36. Zhao, Wang, He, et al. 2017.
37. Wang, Qin, Demirtas, et al. 2007.
38. Meng, Li, Chen, et al. 2018.
39. Smith, Smith, de Jager, et al. 2010; Douaud, Refsum, de Jager, et al. 2013.

40. de Jager, Oulhaj, Jacoby, et al. 2012.
41. Mech and Farah 2016.
42. Loria-Kohen, Gómez-Candela, Palma-Milla, et al. 2013.
43. Schnyder, Roffi, Pin, et al. 2001.
44. Lonn, Yusuf, Arnold, et al. 2006.
45. Satchell 2016.
46. Hornig, Bresnahan, Che, et al. 2017.
47. Zerbo, Iosif, Walker, et al. 2013.
48. Kuhn and Bransfield 2014.

6. THE DIFFICULTY IN DIAGNOSIS

1. Weintraub 2001.
2. Marks 2011; Latov, Wu, Chin, et al. 2004; Noble 2000.
3. Centers for Disease Control 2013a.
4. Lyme Disease Association 2002.
5. Noble 2000.
6. Theel 2016.
7. Bozbaş, Ünübol, and Gürer 2016; El-Diasty, Wareth, Melzer, et al. 2018; Bharathan, Backhouse, Rawat, et al. 2016.
8. Chaignat, Djordjevic-Spasic, Ruettger, et al. 2014; Snowden and Stovall 2011.
9. Raffalli and Wormser 2016; Herwaldt, Persing, Précigout, et al. 1996; Moritz, Winton, Tonnetti, et al. 2016.
10. Centers for Disease Control 2013b.
11. Fillaux and Magnaval 2013; Alabiad, Albini, Santos, and Davis 2010.
12. Watts, Kim, Ahuja, et al. 2019.
13. Embers, Hasenkampf, Jacobs, et al. 2017; Kalish, McHugh, Granquist, et al. 2001; Craft, Fischer, Shimamoto, and Steere 1986.
14. Embers, Hasenkampf, Jacobs, et al. 2017.
15. Oksi, Marjamaki, Nikoskelainen, and Vijainen 1999; Oksi, Kalimo, Marttila, et al. 1996; Haupl, Hahn, Rittig, et al. 1993.
16. Dattwyler, Volkman, Luft, et al. 1988.
17. Drummond, dos Santos, da Silva, et al. 2019.
18. Global Lyme Alliance, no date, "Lyme Disease Testing"; Waddell, Greig, Mascarenhas, et al. 2016.
19. Center for Food Security and Public Health, no date.
20. Lee, Healy, and Lambert 2019.
21. Landford 2017.

7. THE ROAD TO RECOVERY

1. Baker, Ferrari, and Shea 2018.
2. Hassler, Riedel, Zorn, and Preac-Mursic 1991.

3. Feng, Zhang, Shi, and Zhang 2016.
4. Šmajs, Paštěková, and Grillová 2015.
5. Feng, Auwaerter, and Zhang 2015; Rolain, Maurin, and Raoult 2000.
6. Feng, Zhang, Shi, et al. 2017.
7. Ma, Shi, and Zhang 2019.
8. Motamedi, Darabpour, Gholipour, and Seyyed Nejad 2010.
9. Goc, Niedzwiecki, and Rath 2017; Goc, Niedzwiecki, and Rath 2015.
10. Goc, Niedzwiecki, and Rath 2015; Goc, Niedzwiecki, and Rath 2017.
11. Schardt 2004.
12. Feng, Weitner, Shi, et al. 2015; Li, Feng, Xiao, et al. 2019.
13. Private communication by email with Dr. Ying Zhang of Johns Hopkins, cited with permission of Dr. Zhang.
14. Breitschwerdt, Greenberg, Maggi, et al. 2019.

8. MENDING YOUR MIND

1. EMDR Institute, no date.
2. Marcus, Marquis, and Sakai 1997.
3. Shapiro 2014.
4. Brom, Stokar, Lawi, et al. 2017.
5. Winblad, Changaris, and Stein 2018.
6. Feng, Leone, Schweig, and Zhang 2019.
7. Feng, Zhang, Shi, et al., 2017.
8. Al-Mariri and Safi 2013.
9. Ma, Shi, and Zhang 2019.
10. Shah, Newman, Woolf, et al. 2018.
11. Villanova, Azpiroz, and Malagelada 1997.
12. Chandrasekaran, Sanchez, Mohammed, et al. 2016.
13. Sukenik, Neumann, Buskila, et al. 1990.
14. Tarleton, Littenberg, MacLean, et al. 2017.
15. Boyle, Lawton, and Dye 2017.
16. Han, Fang, Wei, et al. 2017.
17. Pearce, Lockwood, van den Heuvel, and Pearce 2017.
18. See the entry on Royal Raymond Rife at Spencorp Media: https://www.spencorp.info/royal-raymond-rife
19. American Cancer Society 1994.
20. Weinberg 2019.
21. ASCO Post 2019.
22. Crocetti, Beyer, Schade, et al. 2013; Zimmerman, Pennison, Brezovich, et al 2012.
23. Rosado, Simkó, Mattsson, and Pioli 2018.
24. Stoodley, deBeer, Lappin-Scott, et al. 1997; Pozo, Rouse, and Patel 2008; Harrill 2000.

25. Yang, Guo, Yang, et al. 2017.
26. Pothineni, Wagh, Babar, et al. 2016.
27. Liegner 2019.
28. Horowitz and Freeman 2019.
29. Wang, Parimi, Liu, and Zhang 2017.
30. Liu, Wang, Bao, et al. 2019.
31. Feng, Weitner, Shi, et al. 2015; Li, Feng, Xiao, et al. 2019.
32. Bozkurt, Dumlu, Tokac, et al. 2015.
33. https://www.accessdata.fda.gov/drugsatfda_docs/nda/2016/204630Origi
s000PharmR.pdf
34. Sessa 2012; Winkelman 2014; American Psychological Association 2018.
35. Small, Siddarth, Li, et al. 2018.
36. Martens, Denman, Mazzo, et al. 2018. Also see the work of David Sinclair's lab:
https://genetics.med.harvard.edu/sinclair/research.php
37. Relaño-Ginés, Lehmann, Brillaud, et al. 2018; Diniz, Machado-Vieira, and Forlenza 2013; Wilson, Do Carmo, and Iulita 2017; Nunes, Schöwe, Monteiro-Silva,
et al. 2015.
38. For more about Rick Osfeld's Tick Project, go to the Carey Institute at http://
www.careyinstitute.org.

9. COVID

1. Holly Yan 2020.
2. Kaplan 2020.
3. Temple-Raston 2020.
4. Feuer 2020.
5. Zhou 2020.
6. CNBC Television 2020.
7. Nouri, https://fas.org/expert/ali-nouri/.
8. Politi 2021.
9. Oregon Occupational Safety and Health 2020.
10. Wertheim et al. 2013.
11. Centers for Disease Control 2013.
12. Roos 2003.
13. World Health Organization 2003.
14. Yu et al. 2004.
15. Alsolamy et al. 2015.
16. Liu et al. 2020.
17. Gonzalez Gompf, Jones, and Davis, no date.
18. The Angiogenesis Foundation, https://angio.org/who-we-are/.
19. Yong 2020.
20. Spiewak 2020.

21. Iacobucci 2020.
22. Wudan Yan 2020.
23. Tuller 2020.
24. Mayo Clinic 2020.
25. Anderson 2013.
26. Arbour et al. 2000.
27. Arbour et al. 1999.
28. Healio 2019.
29. Proal 2021.
30. Matschke et al. 2020.
31. Park 2020.
32. Gupta et al. 2020.
33. Cheung et al. 2020.
34. Dias De Melo et al. 2020.
35. Choi et al. 2020.
36. Renner et al. 2020.
37. Belluck 2020.
38. Chopra et al. 2020.
39. Reddy 2020.
40. Ternyila 2020.
41. Drago et al. 2020.
42. Krause et al. 2020.
43. Mansueto et al. 2012.
44. Sapi et al. 2019.
45. McCall 2020.
46. Hancocks 2020.
47. Zeratsky 2020.
48. Wang et al. 2020.
49. National Institute of Allergy and Infectious Diseases 2020.
50. Wu and Kolata 2020.
51. World Health Organization 2020.
52. Lupkin 2020.
53. Wu, Zimmer, and Corum 2021.
54. Joyner et al. 2021.
55. Hill 2020.
56. Million et al. 2020.

CONCLUSION

1. For all of Dana Parish's entries on the Huffington Post, see https://www.huffpost.com/author/thedanaparish-150
2. Miziara, Gelmeti Serrano, and Yoshinari 2018.

3. https://leitesculinaria.com
4. https://norvect.no
5. These statements are reprinted with permission from an interview Dr. Perronne gave to Huib Kraaijeveld, who runs the site On-Lyme.org. See Kraaijeveld 2017.
6. Ashiru 2019.
7. This statement is attributed to the artist Ed Ruscha.

Acknowledgments

We have been immensely lucky to know you and will always be in your debt.

FROM STEVE

To my mother: Thank you for gracing me with your boundless heart, resilience, and voice. Without you, I could never have found the strength to speak the truth.

To my father, in whose eyes I could do no wrong: Thank you for gifting me with your love of science and sense of wonder for the universe.

To my stepfather: You're a knight in shining armor. Thank you for coming into our lives.

To my brothers: Thank you for being my tireless advocates and voices of reason.

Tom Salemo: Thank you for stepping up like nobody else could.

Barbara and Jack Blossom: Thank you for your wisdom, light, and 8th-grade humor.

Greg Carlon: Thank you for being good. For being true. You're an inspiration to everyone who's been lucky enough to cross your path, myself included.

FROM DANA

Mom: Thanks for making me laugh every day of my life, for instilling my steely reserve, and for always reminding me to chart my own path. I love you with a passion.

Daddio: You are the first love of my life, my wisest sage, and the guy who keeps me outta trouble. Love you so much.

G: My darling brother. I hope I've made you proud.

Andy: For never letting me see you sweat; making me a billion sandwiches; for listening, learning, caring, and dropping everything when I needed you. All my love and appreciation.

Katy McBride and Joy Devins: My angels. I would never have made it without you.

FROM BOTH OF US

Kristina Grish: Eternal thanks for following through on your wild 3:00 a.m. vision and for making the introduction of a lifetime. You're an exceptional friend and human.

Bonnie Solow: our agent extraordinaire, lioness, and North Star. Thank you for holding the rope every step of the way.

Kristin Loberg: You're the ultimate alchemist and we're humbled by your gifts. We couldn't have done it without you and wouldn't have wanted to.

Deb Brody and our amazing team at HMH: We couldn't have asked for a better home. Thank you for walking with us on this path to change the world.

Linda Giampa of Bay Area Lyme Foundation: Our fierce, savvy, un-flappable champion and friend. Thank you for all that you do, and all that you are.

Huge thanks to Laure Woods, Wendy Adams, Lia Gaertner, Bon-nie Crater, and all at Bay Area Lyme Foundation for your unwavering support.

Neil Spector: For your friendship, goodness, brilliance, bravery, in-tegrity, and the endless gifts you give to the world, thank you.

Emily and Malcolm Fairbairn and family: You push us in all the right directions and we will never cease to be amazed by your fearless-ness, brilliance, and generosity.

Brandi Dean: For always coming through. Thank you for your never-ending faith in us.

Thanks, also, to all of the following people, who have contributed to our lives and our mission. This list could never be complete: Alex Cohen, Jeanne Melino, Ben Nemser and and all at the Steven & Alexandra Cohen Foundation, Sandi Mendelson, Spector family, Dr. Charlotte Mao, all at The Dean Center, Sue Faber, LymeHope, Karen Guadian and Jennifer Reid of Lyme Connection, Lew and Wendy Leone, all at FOX5 NY, the Needleman and Armintor families, Fogelman-Selby family, Jill and Alain Rothstein, Laurie Soriano, Jeff Silberman, Pete and Lisa Najarian, Twin Cities Lyme Foundation, Millon family, Mark Donofrio and Alex Lach, Fay Ann Lee and Matt "Biff" Jozoff, Camille Zamora and Tom Whayne, Walsey family, Karin Weinberg, Buchwald family, Peter and Heather Lloyd, Chely Wright, Karen Cage, Jeff and Carla Nugent, the Stachers, Pam Weintraub, Lisa and Kris Kristofferson, Mary Beth Pfeiffer, Kris Newby, Dr. Ed Breitschwerdt, Dr. Amanda Elam, Dr. Jen Miller and all at Galaxy Labs, Dr. Monica Embers, Lyme Disease.org, Project Lyme, the LivLyme Foundation, Focus on Lyme, Huib Kraaijeveld, SonyATV, Clio Massey, Marla Maples, the Hollander, Newman and Clark families, Melanie Ciccone, Heather Hearst, Ashley Greenfield and family, Chrissy and Pat Irving, Lindsay Keys, Ivan Shaw and Lisa Von Weise, Winslow Murdoch, Rob and Pru Sternin, Dr. Melissa Duperval, Dr. Katherine Keil, Melissa Ferwerda Bell, Dr. Kristen Honey, Dr. Richard Horowitz, Dr. Ken Liegner, Dr. Robert Bransfield, ILADS, LymeLight Foundation, Isabel Rose, Laura Lynne Jackson, Enid Haller, David Conner, David Leite, Elizabeth Lunny, Ross Douthat, Kelly Melchionno, Caitlin Doody, Deb Defeo, Dr. Lisa Valow-Picarello, Dr. Thomas Moorcroft, the Barboshis, NorVect, FSI Sweden, Swedish Lyme Association, Joe Adjei, Ally Hilfiger, Yolanda Hadid, Bonnie Bennett, NatCapLyme, Franzel family, Jeff and Jamie Rosen, Carrie Perry, Nicole Greene, Bruce Fries, and Nicole Malachowski.

Infinite thanks to all who agreed to be interviewed for our book, cheered us on, and shared their stories for the first time. To the doctors, researchers, universities, foundations, and advocates who light the way, bless you. And to Dr. Phillips' amazing patients and the entire Lyme+ community—your journey, wisdom, and support are our inspiration. This is for you.

Index

doxycycline (*continued*)
  research on, 11, 13
  for specific diseases, 27, 45
droplets (COVID), 215–216
Dynamic Neural Retraining System
  (DNRS), 192–193

E
Ebel, Gregory, 32
echinococcus, 31
electromagnetic field machines, 203–204
ELISA (test), 149–153, 181
emergency medical treatment, 174, 175
epigenetics, 117–118
epsom salt baths, 201
Epstein-Barr virus (EBV), 83–84, 116,
  118, 122
Erikson, Marna, xi–xii
Ewald, Paul W., 124–126
exercise, 198–200
expectations, unrealistic, 91–93
eye movement desensitization and
  reprocessing (EMDR), 187–189
eye problems. *see* symptoms
eye protection for COVID, 217

F
Faber, Sue, 49–50
fallacies, 93
Fallon, Brian, 131
false-negative tests, 35, 64, 67, 78, 110,
  149–154
FDA (Food and Drug Administration),
  43, 119, 145–147, 149, 178, 203–204,
  206, 226, 236
Federation of American Scientists, 216
fibromyalgia, 109–110
filaria, 21, 30
Flannery, Maggie, 220
flu, 124, 136
fluconazole, 177
Freedberg, A. Stone, 42
friends, support from, 209–210

G
GABA (gamm-aminobutyric acid),
  199–200
Galaxy Diagnostics, 154
gastrointestinal problems. *see* symptoms
Gehrig, Lou, 6
genetic issues
  autoimmunity and, 117–118
  MTFHR gene variant, 133–134
  recombinant vaccines, 145
genitourinary problems. *see* symptoms
germ theory, 93–94
Gilead Sciences, 226
Gone in a Heartbeat (Spector), 106
Greenberg, Rosalie, 75–76
Guion, Constance, 42
gut. *see* microbiome

H
Haller, Enid, 160
Hawkins, Ralph, 51
heart issues. *see also* symptoms
  drug precautions for, 177
  examples of symptoms, 55–59,
    106–108
  inflammation and, 132–133
heavy metals, 84–85
Heffernan, Margaret, 51–52
Helicobacter pylori, 41–43, 122
herbals, 179, 195–203
herpes, 83–84, 116, 118, 127, 136
Herxheimer reactions
  blebbing *vs.*, 63
  defined, 17
  expectations for, 171–175
  psychiatric symptoms of, 128
Hilfiger, Ally, 128
homocysteine, 134
Hoofnagle, Chris and Mark, 91
Hopper, Annie, 193
Horowitz, Richard, 205
How to Change Your Mind (Pollan),
  207